Writing Case Reports

A HOW-TO MANUAL
FOR CLINICIANS

Second Edition

**For physical therapists and other health care professionals
who want to contribute descriptions of practice
to their profession's body of knowledge**

Edited by Irene McEwen, PT, PhD

**A Publication of the
American Physical Therapy Association
Alexandria, Virginia**

ISBN # 1-887759-98-0

For more information about this and other APTA publications, contact the American Physical Therapy Association, 1111 North Fairfax Street, Alexandria, VA 22314-1488, or access APTA's Online Resource Catalog via APTA's Web site, www.apta.org. [Publication No. C-12]

Staff Editors: Jan P Reynolds, Steven Glaros
Book Designer: Linda Silk

Contributors

Vincent Basile, PT, OCS, is Co-owner, Basile Physical Therapy Associates, Berwick, Pennsylvania, which provides outpatient and home health physical therapy services. A practitioner in the area of orthopedic physical therapy for more than 25 years, he has published articles in *Physical Therapy* and the *Journal of Orthopaedic and Sports Physical Therapy*.

G Kelley Fitzgerald, PT, PhD, is Assistant Professor, Department of Physical Therapy, School of Health and Rehabilitation Sciences, University of Pittsburgh, Pittsburgh, Pennsylvania, and has published case reports, research reports, clinical perspectives, and book chapters on topics related to orthopedic physical therapy, his primary area of practice. He is a manuscript reviewer for *Physical Therapy*.

Gail M Jensen, PT, PhD, is Professor and Director of the Transitional DPT Program, Department of Physical Therapy, School of Pharmacy and Allied Health, and Faculty Associate, Center for Health Policy and Ethics, Creighton University, Omaha, Nebraska. She previously served on the Editorial Boards of *Physical Therapy* and the *Journal of Physical Therapy Education* (published by the Section for Education of APTA) and is Deputy Editor for *Physiotherapy Research International*. A recipient of APTA's Golden Pen Award, she has published research reports, perspectives, and books in the areas of professional education, reflective practice, clinical expertise, and qualitative research.

Irene McEwen, PT, PhD, is Professor, Department of Physical Therapy, College of Allied Health, University of Oklahoma Health Sciences Center, Oklahoma City, Oklahoma, and is Associate Editor for Case Reports and Deputy Editor, *Physical Therapy*. A recipient of APTA's Dorothy Briggs Memorial Scientific Inquiry Award [Postprofessional Doctoral Level], she has published research articles, clinical perspectives, and book chapters in the area of pediatric physical therapy and has edited books on physical therapy and occupational therapy in education environments.

Daniel Riddle, PT, PhD, is Associate Professor, Department of Physical Therapy, School of Allied Health Professions, Virginia Commonwealth University, Richmond, Virginia. A recipient of APTA's Chattanooga Research Award, he has published case reports and research reports on reliability and validity and on clinical decision making and serves on the Editorial Board of *Physical Therapy*.

Lisa Riolo, PT, PhD, NCS, is Assistant Professor, Emory University School of Medicine, Atlanta, Georgia, and Senior Scientist at the Veterans Affairs Center of Excellence in Geriatric Rehabilitation R&D Center in Atlanta. She is President, Neurology Section of APTA; is a manuscript reviewer for *Physical Therapy* and for *Neurology Report* (published by the Neurology Section); and serves on the Editorial Board of the *Journal of Physical Therapy Education* (published by the Section for Education). She has published research reports on cognitive aspects of mobility and intervention. Her clinical practice has focused on neurological rehabilitation, particularly cerebrovascular accidents and brain injury.

Preface to the Second Edition

When we wrote the first edition of *Writing Case Reports: A How-to Manual for Clinicians*, we wanted it to be a user-friendly resource for clinicians. We envisioned our audience as physical therapy practitioners who had wonderful descriptions of practice to contribute to the professional literature but who needed some help in preparing a case report for publication. The increase in the number of good case reports submitted to *Physical Therapy* and other journals suggests that clinicians are responding to calls for case reports and that they are using the advice in this manual.

Perhaps an even larger audience for the manual—which we didn't anticipate—is students. *Writing Case Reports* is used as a text in many education programs that require professional and postprofessional students, residents, and fellows to write case reports as a culminating and scholarly product of their educational experiences.

Because so many education programs require the writing of case reports, we solicited input from faculty as we were planning this second edition. Many responded, and we are grateful for their input. The most common recommendation was to use terminology that is consistent with the second edition of the *Guide to Physical Therapist Practice*. The second most common recommendation was to provide more information about how to write about the diagnosis and prognosis elements of patient/client management. Several faculty members said they would like the book to include an "imperfect" manuscript of a case report for students to review, and others recommended adding a checklist of the important components of a case report. Many suggested that we update the chapter about searching for literature and the appendix that lists reliability and validity studies. We responded to all of these suggestions in this second edition.

We also tried to make the second edition more useful for occupational therapy practitioners and students. We added content from the *Guide to Occupational Therapy Practice* and included more references to case reports that have been published in the occupational therapy literature. As a faculty member of an education program that requires both physical therapist and occupational therapist students to write case reports, I look forward to using the second edition with all of my students.

Irene R McEwen, PT, PhD

Foreword to the First Edition

You're holding a dream in your hands. Almost 10 years ago, the late Dr Steve Rose—my predecessor as Editor of *Physical Therapy*—and I talked about the need for a book like this. We shared a love of physical therapy practice and wanted to see our colleagues communicating more effectively and efficiently. We longed for a public body of knowledge where ideas could be exchanged and therapists could learn from each other while revealing to the world what we do every day in our clinical settings.

Perhaps the vision that Steve and I shared was a function of our career paths. We both had spent many years in private practice before returning to school to get our doctorates and advanced training in the sciences. As a result, we never lost sight of the fact that physical therapists exist to take care of patients and clients and that there is no more important activity than high-quality patient care. We also knew that few of us were prepared to communicate about practice in a scientifically credible manner.

The vagaries of patient care are too important to be left to random communications, jargon-laden continuing education courses, or accidental dialogues. We should agree and disagree in public and grow through that discourse. We should talk to each other about what we do, and do so using clear language. We should write so that we can refine our descriptions, agree on terms and definitions, and evolve a common language of practice.

That is, we should write case reports!

Since becoming Editor of *Physical Therapy* in 1988, I have been a staunch advocate of case reports, seeking them everywhere I go. (Tony Delitto, Journal Editorial Board member and Chair of the Department of Physical Therapy at the University of Pittsburgh, also shares the vision, and together we have made a number of presentations on writing case reports.) I have even suggested that the ability to communicate scientifically is a professional skill and that everyone graduating from a physical therapy education program should be able to write a case report. (Not everyone has agreed.)

Case reports aren't just a means by which we can all "talk shop" with each other. They are an essential part of our literature. They do not replace research reports; as you will see when you read this manual, case reports and research reports are complementary. Case reports aren't something to be taken lightly or to be published with little scrutiny. Our business is practice, and anything that describes practice must be done well. In addition, case reports provide researchers with the background they need to design outcomes studies. For these reasons, case reports, like research, must undergo peer review.

As Editor, I often am asked by authors, "Shouldn't case reports receive a less stringent review than research articles do?" Clinicians who have achieved what they believe to be exciting patient outcomes understandably want to share what they have observed. Researchers feel the same way, but they have to take part in a process that leads to refinement—the peer-review process. Taking shortcuts in this process is a lot like taking shortcuts in patient care. The results are not pretty.

I won't lie to you: Peer review isn't easy on authors. Most of us find that criticism is a lot like the flu—it is far easier and less painful to give to others than to receive it. But if you follow the guidelines in this manual, you cannot lose. Whether or not your papers are published (and odds are that they will be published if you keep trying to work out the problems), the process of writing and being reviewed is a means to professional growth. Recognize that criticism is just part of the process, and that peer review is a system in which people not only evaluate what you have done but help you make something better. Remember, too, that they are evaluating what you have done—not you, the person.

Our challenge in the coming years is to work together to establish a common body of literature. A body of literature that describes practice. A body of literature that helps new therapists know what to expect, researchers know what questions to ask, and health care managers know what we do. A body of literature that makes each of us identify with each other and understand each other better than ever before.

Thanks to the efforts of Vince Basile, Kelley Fitzgerald, Gail Jensen, Dan Riddle, Lisa Riolo, and Irene McEwen—both in her role as *Physical Therapy's* Associate Editor for Case Reports and as this manual's editor—*Writing Case Reports* is not only a dream come true. It is a means by which even more dreams will be fulfilled for the growth of our profession.

Jules M Rothstein, PT, PhD, FAPTA

Table of Contents

Part 2: Start Writing!

Introduction

Real Clinicians *Do* Write Case Reports!

Maybe you've developed a treatment that gets excellent results, perfected an especially useful management technique, or noted a set of similarities among certain patients that allows you to approach those patients in a unique and effective way. You describe your idea to a few colleagues, and they express interest and enthusiasm. You present it at an informal meeting or an in-service program, and again the feedback is positive. Then, just as you've begun to enjoy that warm glow of satisfaction, someone utters the dreaded words:

"You really ought to write that up for a journal."

Suddenly, there isn't enough air in the room. You think about how much you enjoy direct patient contact. "Real" clinicians, you say to yourself, spend their time treating or managing patients, not writing.

For most of us, "putting it down on paper" ranks among our biggest fears. The feeling of competence we have in the clinic or the classroom fades when we are faced with the great unknown of writing for publication. We remember stories of colleagues who submitted articles to journals and were "savaged" by the editorial review process. We fear that if we write, the same thing will happen to us. We also fear that if our ideas are actually published, we will be exposing ourselves to ridicule. What's the result of this collective phobia? A profession that fails to share basic information—the kind of information required to develop the concepts, methods, and proofs that can improve patient care, help justify our treatments to payers, and distinguish us from faith healers and faddists.

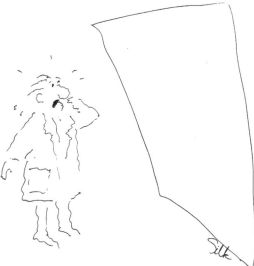

Fear of the Blank Page

The irony is that we clinicians consider ourselves to be the Great Practical Communicators. Talk with any group of us, and you immediately strike a vein of common concern for communication and teaching. And we do communicate effectively—even passionately—on a one-to-one, day-to-day basis. But we still fail to share information effectively. We consider documentation to be a routine aspect of practice, but we don't take the next step to expand that documentation to its logical conclusion: writing a case report for publication in the peer-reviewed literature, where it can become a part of the professional body of knowledge.

You may not realize it, but you already have many of the skills required to write successful case reports. All you need is a practical tool to help you refine and apply those skills. This how-to manual is designed to do just that.

Reading this book isn't like reading a novel; you don't have to begin at the beginning. But you may find it helpful to do so, especially if you have limited experience in writing for publication. Part I shows you how to prepare for writing a case report; Part II takes you through the writing process and explains peer review. We've left plenty of room for you to write in the margins! Running throughout the book are excerpts from a fictional case report to highlight major points. For readers who want more details, **Appendix 1** contains sample author guidelines; **Appendix 2**, references to some studies that have been published on the reliability and validity of measurements; **Appendix 3**, a "case report checklist" that will help you keep track of the essentials as you write your report; **Appendix 4**, a reference list of selected case reports in physical therapy, occupational therapy, and other rehabilitation literature; **Appendix 5**, three published case reports that have been annotated to show how the authors dealt with each component of the case report; and **Appendix 6**, a review of a "submitted" case report that gives you tips on how *not* to write a case report!

Whether you decide to work on your own or with others, the writing process will offer you many opportunities. You'll be able to examine your own clinical observations and reasoning, share your work with a larger audience, give something back to a profession that is so much a part of you—and ultimately do what all "real" clinicians want to do: improve patient care.

Good luck!

Irene McEwen, PT, PhD, Editor

Vincent Basile, PT, OCS

G Kelley Fitzgerald, PT, PhD, OCS

Gail Jensen, PT, PhD

Daniel Riddle, PT, PhD

Lisa Riolo, PT, PhD, NCS

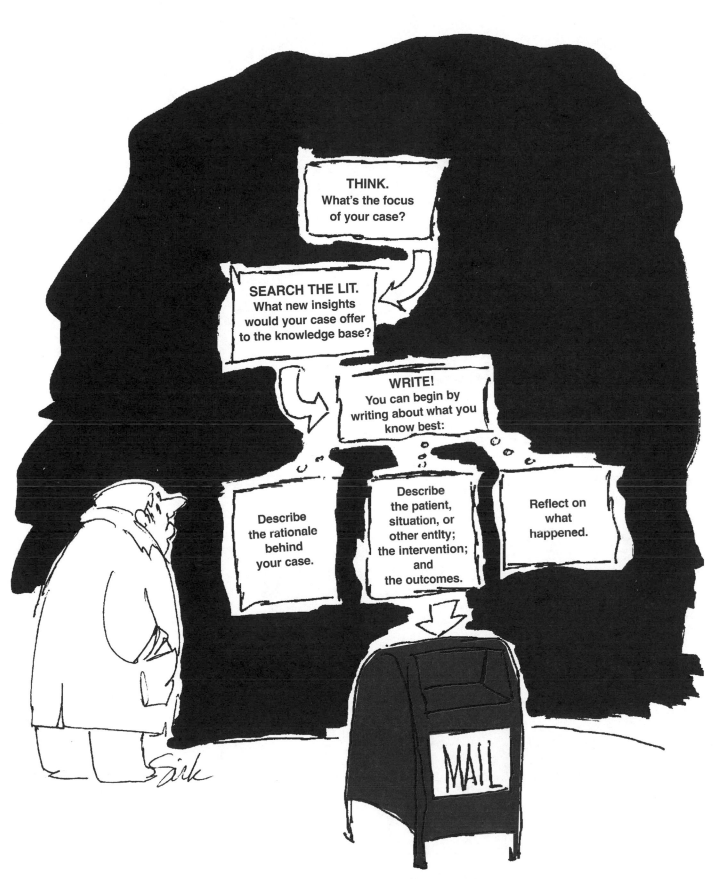

The Case Report Writing Process

Part 1

BEFORE YOU WRITE

"The whole of science is nothing more than a refinement of everyday thinking."

Albert Einstein

Chapter 1

Why Write Case Reports?

ase reports look a lot like research reports. They have a title, an abstract, and an introduction that reviews related literature to provide rationale for the management of the case. They also have a case description that provides information about the patient (or other entity) and the intervention, a section on outcomes, and a discussion. These components are covered in detail later on.

Although case reports *look* a lot like research reports, they aren't. That is, they can't establish cause-and-effect relationships between interventions and outcomes, and their outcomes can't be generalized to other patients or entities. So, why write case reports?

Case reports do play an important role in the professional literature. In fact, they can serve more than one purpose. They might convey experiences to other clinicians while revealing hypotheses for future research, or they might provide material for teaching and learning, assist in the evolution of theory, persuade or motivate other practitioners, or help develop practice guidelines and critical pathways.

Play an Important Role in the Professional Literature

Unlike randomized controlled trials and other experimental studies, case reports are solely descriptions of practice. They don't use the controls demanded by research to determine cause-and-effect relationships. Experimental designs (**Table 1**) have controls that allow identification of cause-and-effect relationships

Case reports can't prove effectiveness—but they can lead researchers to do the kinds of studies that will.

Table 1. Categories of Scientific Inquiry

Experimental Designs

The structure of experimental designs allows researchers to identify cause-and-effect relationships between independent and dependent variables. The strength of the evidence depends on the characteristics of the design, which fall into these classic categories[a]:

True experimental design	Subjects are randomly assigned to experimental and comparison groups. Provides the strongest evidence of cause-and-effect relationships.
Quasi-experimental design	Lacks random assignment of subjects, a comparison group, or both. Often used in clinical research when already existing groups are studied or when random assignment is not possible or both.
Single-subject design	A type of quasi-experimental design that lacks the generalizability of group designs. There are many different types of single-subject designs.

Nonexperimental Designs

Nonexperimental designs do not manipulate the independent variable and cannot determine cause-and-effect relationships. There are three general types[b]:

Descriptive research	Discloses existing conditions or examines relationships among variables, using such means as direct observation, surveys, and interviews. Includes correlational studies, case studies, investigations to identify normative values or developmental patterns, and epidemiological studies, which describe and predict health risks.
Evaluation research	Objectively assesses how well a program or a policy is meeting its goals and objectives. Can provide a means to document quality of care and program effectiveness or efficiency.
Methodological research	Involves the development of measurement tools and the assessment of their reliability, validity, and usefulness in answering clinical questions.

Case Reports

Case reports describe practice. Their credibility is enhanced by attempting to control, rule out, or acknowledge alternative explanations for outcomes, but case reports do not impose the controls required to identify cause-and-effect relationships among variables. Case reports often focus on a patient or a group of patients, but they also may focus on institutions, facilities, education programs, or other definable units. Issues can include patient/client management, ethical dilemmas, use of equipment or devices, or administrative or educational concerns.

[a]Campbell D, Stanley J. *Experimental and Quasi-Experimental Designs for Research.* Chicago, Ill: Rand McNally; 1963.
[b]Portney LG, Watkins MP. *Foundations of Clinical Research: Applications to Practice.* 2nd ed. Upper Saddle River, NJ: Prentice Hall; 2000.

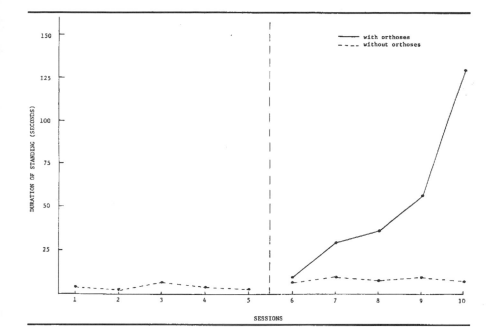

Figure 1. *Unlike case reports, single-subject studies use experimental controls and repeated measures and therefore can show cause-and-effect relationships among variables. This figure, reprinted from a single-subject study by Harris and Riffle,[6] shows the baseline measures of a child's standing time without orthoses and alternately with and without orthoses. By alternately measuring standing time under identical conditions except for the use of orthoses, the researchers controlled for rival explanations and were able to show that the orthoses caused the increased duration of standing.*

between the independent variable (the intervention) and the dependent variable (the observed response or result). Lacking such controls, case reports can be viewed as "pre-experimental," with their value being in the generation of ideas, hypotheses, and techniques that can be studied later through controlled experiments.[1,2]

The terms "case report" and "case study" sometimes are used interchangeably, and their definitions tend to overlap. For the purposes of this manual, the term "case report" refers to descriptions of practice that do not involve research methodology. A "case study," which may be similar in appearance to a case report, refers to a type of research methodology and has procedures and standards of its own; it is included as a type of "descriptive research" in **Table 1**. Schmoll[3] and Merriam[4] included the case study as one of the major types of research designs in qualitative research, whereas other authors have described case studies as yielding both qualitative and quantitative data that can be used to explore, describe, or predict various phenomena.[5] In the past, *Physical Therapy* has published case reports in which authors referred to their work as "case studies" or "studies." *Physical Therapy* now reserves the terms "case study" and "study" for types of research reports.

Case reports also have been confused with single-subject designs. Unlike case reports, single-subject studies use experimental controls and repeated measures and therefore can show cause-and-effect relationships among variables. Harris and Riffle,[6] for example, used an "alternating-treatment" type of single-subject design to demonstrate that ankle-foot orthoses (the independent variable) caused the effect of increasing the length of time a child with cerebral palsy could stand without falling (the dependent variable). **Figure 1** shows the baseline measurements of the child's standing time when he was not wearing the orthoses, followed by measurements of his standing time when he alternately wore and did not wear the orthoses. By alternately measuring standing time under identical

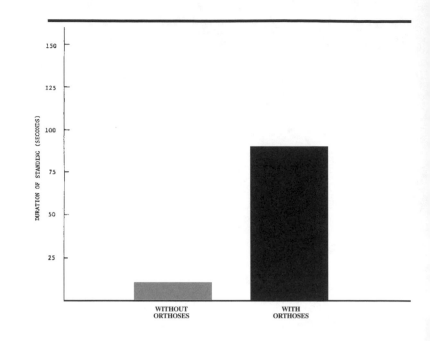

Figure 2. *The data that Harris and Riffle[6] might have collected—if they had written a case report instead of a single-subject study. Adapted with permission of the American Physical Therapy Association from Harris SR, Riffle K. Effects of inhibitive ankle-foot orthoses on standing balance in a child with cerebral palsy: a single-subject design.* Phys Ther. *1986;66:663-667.*

conditions except for the orthoses, the researchers controlled for rival explanations and were able to show that the orthoses caused the increased duration in standing time.

If Harris and Riffle had taken baseline measurements when the child was not wearing orthoses, followed only by a series of measurements when the child was wearing orthoses, their study would have been an "A-B" single-subject design ("A" refers to a baseline phase; "B" refers to an intervention phase). The data for an A-B design would look the same as that in Figure 1, except that the graph would have only the solid "with orthoses" line for sessions 6 through 10. An A-B design is a weak design because something other than the orthoses might have caused the change in the length of time the child could stand. He might, for example, have had an ear infection during the baseline phase, or he might have started a new balance program in physical education class just as the orthoses were introduced. By alternating the measures, however, Harris and Riffle controlled for such extraneous variables that would have affected his balance under both conditions—that is, when he was and was not wearing the orthoses.

Case reports are much like an A-B single-subject design, except that outcome measurements are not taken as repeatedly or as systematically as they are for an A-B design. Case reports often have only one preintervention measurement and one postintervention measurement, which is what usually happens in practice. Some authors, however, may report intermediate measurement data. **Figure 2** shows the data that Harris and Riffle *might* have collected if they had written a case report. As with an A-B design, variables other than the orthoses could have caused or contributed to the outcomes.

Although the purpose of a case report is to describe practice, not to determine cause and effect, some features of the A-B design are useful for case reports. Kazdin[2] suggested several ways to strengthen the credibility of case reports and make them similar to an A-B design:

1) Systematically collect reliable data.

2) Take several measurements over time, before and after the intervention.

3) Use interventions with strong, immediate effects.

4) Report application of the intervention with several patients (or other entities, depending on the focus of your report).

Share Clinical Experiences

Regardless of whether you function primarily as a clinician, an administrator, an academician, or a researcher, you spend most of your professional life asking questions. Clinicians ask such questions as: How often should a 2-year-old child with spastic diplegia receive what type of intervention to accomplish which goals? How does the evaluation lead to determining the diagnosis and prognosis for a 45-year-old man following severe hand trauma? What are the pitfalls to be avoided in the transition of a professional education program from the baccalaureate level to the postbaccalaureate level? What independent and dependent variables are most likely to provide useful information in a study of intervention for conditions related to stroke?

It isn't easy to find answers to these and countless other questions that are asked every day in clinics, classrooms, and laboratories. Research articles, textbooks, continuing education courses, and other sources of information can contribute to our knowledge base; however, these sources are likely to provide only partial answers—and they may not wrestle with how to make those answers work in the real world.

The very nature of the case report requires the kind of details that would be necessary for another clinician to implement the approach or intervention discussed in the report. Riddle and Freeman,[7] for example, related their experience with an aerobic dance instructor who had bilateral plantar fasciitis and Achilles tendinitis. They began with a carefully detailed account of the patient's 8-month history of foot pain and the unsuccessful interventions that she received prior to her referral to the authors' clinic. The authors then clearly described their examination of the patient, including differences in the observations of the two examiners and how they dealt with those differences. Such differences are common in the real world, but they usually are meticulously avoided in research and are rarely confronted in textbooks or continuing education courses.

The outcomes desired by the patient also are rarely considered in research, textbooks, or continuing education courses; however, in daily practice, they must be identified and addressed directly. As a component of their evaluation, Riddle and Freeman determined and reported the goal that their patient wanted to accomplish. They described their decision making as they worked their way through the hypothesis-oriented algorithm for clinicians (HOAC)[8] to design, implement, evaluate, and modify the intervention. Each step of their decision-making process could provide information or inspiration for other clinicians managing patients with similar conditions.

> Case reports are similar to sharing experiences through conversation—with important differences. When published in a peer-reviewed journal, the case report represents the consensus of a small panel of experts.

Sharing experiences through case reports is similar to sharing experiences through conversation with colleagues. Ideas are stimulated; new insights are provided. There are two important differences, however. First, the case report provides sufficient detail to allow colleagues who are not involved in the conversation to replicate the clinical reasoning process. Second, a case report published in a peer-reviewed journal represents the consensus of a small panel of experts. No, case reports cannot give definitive answers about effectiveness of interventions, but they do allow readers to benefit not only from the experiences of the authors but also from the knowledge of the reviewers.

Illustrate Evidence-Based Practice

> Evidence-based practice combines the best available research evidence, clinical experience, and patient choice. Case reports are an excellent method of integrating these three elements.

"Evidence-based practice" is now widely advocated among the health care professions, but what does it mean? Does it mean that all patient/client management decisions have to be based on research? Does it mean that if evidence doesn't exist, clinicians should do nothing until it does? Does it mean that clinicians are free to continue to do what they've always done if research evidence isn't available? The answer to all of these questions is "no"!

The most widely used definition of "evidence-based practice" (really of "evidence-based medicine," which started it all) comes from Sackett and colleagues: "The integration of best research evidence with clinical expertise and patient values.... When these three elements are integrated, clinicians and patients form a diagnostic and therapeutic alliance which optimizes clinical outcomes and quality of life."[9(p1)] Remember, "evidence-based practice means using the best possible data to make a decision—not to justify a decision that's already been made."[10(p7)]

Case reports are an ideal mechanism to illustrate how clinicians integrate the best available research evidence, clinical experience, and patient choice. Parker[11] wrote an excellent example of a case report that illustrates the process of providing care based on research evidence. The patient was an older woman with a fractured femur, and the author needed to decide on medical and surgical management. At the beginning of the report, Parker defined a limit of spending no more than 4 hours on an office computer to identify the evidence. The report first described the computerized databases that the author explored and the types of articles that the author read (reviews of randomized trials, when available). The report then described the evidence found for decision making about initial management; whether to operate and, if so, when and what implant to use; anticoagulation prophylaxis; postoperative care and rehabilitation; and prevention of further fractures.

The rehabilitation portion of Parker's case report[10] is limited and basically concluded that discharge to home and "community services" may be beneficial. Imagine the contributions that case reports about evidence-based rehabilitation for this and other patients would make to the literature! **Chapter 3** provides helpful information about how to search the literature to find evidence to support your patient/client management decisions.

Develop Hypotheses for Research

Case reports can make an important contribution to the process of scientific inquiry by providing a broad base of descriptive information that researchers can test empirically.[1,2] The description that case reports provide usually is not possible in research investigations that examine a limited number of variables under controlled conditions. Each detail of a case report has the potential to become a variable for future research that in turn could help provide definitive answers to questions about practice.[12] If research is to answer the questions that practitioners are asking in the clinic, neither the generating nor the testing of ideas can be left solely to the researcher's imagination.

The case report by Beattie[13] about a pole vaulter with low back pain illustrates how a case report can help identify research variables and hypotheses. Beattie's examination involved many components that may or may not have contributed information essential for diagnosis of the patient's problem. Did pelvic asymmetry in the transverse plane and lower-extremity range of motion relate to the type of back pain reported by the patient? The answer to this potential research question obviously could help improve the effectiveness and efficiency of patient/client management.

Beattie's description of the intervention also suggests variables for future study. The pole vaulter was treated with a combination of joint mobilization, exercise, and use of a lumbar roll during sitting. Beattie commented that the relative effectiveness of each type of intervention could not be determined, but he believed that extension exercises and modification of the patient's typical sitting posture were the most critical factors. Researchers could transform this clinical observation into hypotheses for clinical research. Beattie also reflected on the problems associated with the lack of reliable and valid measurements of spinal movement—yet another potential research focus.

> Through case reports, clinicians can inform researchers about the questions being asked in the clinic—and about the potential answers.

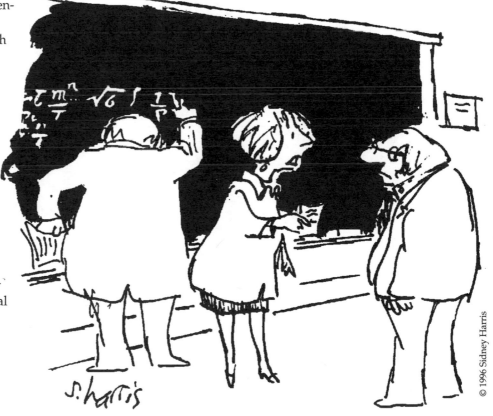

"WE COLLABORATE. I'M AN EXPERT, BUT NOT AN AUTHORITY, AND DR. GELBIS IS AN AUTHORITY, BUT NOT AN EXPERT."

Build Problem-Solving Skills

Case reports are used extensively in the academic programs of such professions as business and law to help students develop critical-thinking and problem-solving skills. Academicians in these fields promote the "case study method," that is, the use of real or fictional case studies that provide opportunities to become familiar with a variety of facts and practices, to identify critical problems and issues, to make decisions, to devise courses of action, and to explore possible outcomes and alternatives.[14,15] Because these are the same skills that professional education programs strive to develop in their students, case reports could be of similar value in professional education courses. A greater number and variety of case reports must be published, however, before this purpose can be served.

Another valuable learning experience for students—and for practitioners—is the *process* of writing a case report.[16,17] During the search for literature to support the case report, not only does the writer gain knowledge directly related to the topic, but the process of locating and synthesizing related information to justify or question a procedure can be even more informative. Students and clinicians who have had little experience in reviewing the literature may be astounded to find scant support for even the most common of clinical procedures—a valuable lesson in itself.

Opportunities for this kind of inspection of your own practice are rare in the midst of day-to-day responsibilities.

Learning continues as the writer describes each step in patient/client management. To be understood by the reader, these descriptions must be clear, complete, jargon-free, and justified—which requires the writer to identify all of the relevant details and reveal the decision-making process. Such opportunities for inspection of our own individual practice are rare in the midst of most practitioners' and students' day-to-day responsibilities. Just as educational is the process of reflection. Reflection is required to write the discussion section, which shows how a case illuminates what is known about the clinical problem and how the case relates to other literature.[18]

Perhaps the most valuable learning experience comes from submitting the case report for publication. Although the peer-review process may seem intimidating at first, writers should remember that it is designed to help them communicate their ideas as effectively and as credibly as possible. If the writer thoughtfully answers the reviewers' questions and carefully considers their suggestions, the writer, the literature, and the profession will be enlightened.

Support, Enhance, or Cast Doubt on Theory Underlying Practice

Theory can be described as a body of related knowledge that serves as a framework for organizing complex and diverse information. Such a framework allows us to fit fragments of information into a larger picture and to predict beyond what we personally have experienced.

Theories are never finished. They are continually expanded and modified to accommodate new information that supports or refutes the theoretical constructs. Some theories encompass a large body of knowledge; others have a much more narrow scope. Dynamic systems theory—discussed by Heriza[19] in the context of movement, for example—is so broad that it has application to such diverse phenomena as weather forecasting and infant development. Other theories, such as the convex-concave theory of arthrokinematic motion,[20] are much more focused.

How can case reports support or enhance theory? By providing real-life examples of a theory's application, or, as Lazarus and Davison[21] described it, by putting "the 'meat' on the theoretical skeleton." This meat is especially important for broad theories that can be difficult to apply in practice. Many clinicians would eagerly read case reports that describe application of motor learning theory to management of a child with cerebral palsy or application of dynamic systems theory to management of a patient with arthritis. Case reports also can enhance theory by describing experiences that go beyond current theory and can suggest hypotheses that could be tested by researchers to advance the theoretical framework.

Case reports may cast doubt on theory. In a case report about a patient with limited shoulder motion, McClure and Flowers[22] challenged the convex-concave theory of arthrokinematic movement by reviewing literature to support their contention that humeral translation may be a function of tension in capsular tissues rather than of joint surface geometry. This challenge could easily lead to a debate about the causes of shoulder motion limitation and raise questions for future investigations.

Persuade and Motivate

Almost every health care profession experienced drastic change during the 1990s. Rehabilitation practices certainly are very different from what they were prior to 1990. These changes have occurred as a result of events both within and outside the rehabilitation professions. II STEP: Contemporary Management of Motor Control Problems—a conference cosponsored by the Foundation for Physical Therapy and the American Physical Therapy Association's Section on Pediatrics and Neurology Section in 1990—is an example of an internal event that had a major impact on practice. The conference and its published proceedings[23] caused many clinicians and researchers to view motor development and motor control very differently from the way they viewed them during the 30 years before the conference. Health care reform efforts initiated during the 1990s are examples of external events; in a relatively short period of time, they had a major impact on the way in which we practice, teach, and conduct research.

Resistance to change is natural, particularly when we are comfortable with the way we have "always done things" and are not certain what to do instead. Case reports give how-to-do-it examples, and, because they are story-like and transparently applicable, they can be an appealing way to begin the change process. The two-part case report by Carmick[24,25] on the use of neuromuscular electrical stimulation (NMES) with children who have cerebral palsy is one example of how a case report can help persuade clinicians to try something new.

Case reports can put "the 'meat' on the theoretical skeleton," describing the application of theory, such as the application of motor learning theory to management of a child with cerebral palsy.

Case reports can help practitioners deal with change, influence administrators, and persuade physicians and insurers of the value of services for particular patients.

Most interventions that were prevalent before the II STEP conference would have rejected use of electrical stimulation with children with cerebral palsy. The II STEP conference taught us that our approaches for people with motor control problems probably need to be modified—and Carmick described one alternative. This case report also generated controversy, and a subsequent letter to the editor cautioned against uninformed use of NMES with children, which the letter writer believed could lead to serious musculoskeletal problems and fatigue.[26] The letter provided yet another opportunity for persuasion, education, and development of research hypotheses.

Another change for many clinicians has been the need to consider context when applying motor learning and dynamic systems principles. Context has long been an important factor in occupational therapy, which Head and Patterson[27] illustrated in their case report of a 79-year-old man with a variety of health-related problems that limited his function. The case report compared evaluation in the clinic setting with evaluation in his home—and highlighted the value of evaluation and intervention within the context of the natural, home environment. This case report could help other clinicians to see the importance of context and could promote an increase in service delivery in patients' natural environments.

Convincing case reports also could help persuade third-party payers to reimburse for certain services for individual patients. One 1995 American Physical Therapy Association–sponsored advertisement for consumer magazines showed a white-haired woman in a wet suit holding a surfboard, declaring, "It's almost impossible to worry about osteoporosis and ride a killer wave at the same time." Did this woman receive physical therapy? If so, imagine the persuasive case report that her story would make! Such a case report could be used to show potential patients, their physicians, and their insurers the value of physical therapy.

Other case reports might help persuade administrators to agree to clinicians' proposals for organizational change. A case report, for example, might clearly illustrate the implementation of a computer-based documentation system to reduce costs, improve patient care, and collect outcomes data. Case reports giving real-life solutions to common professional education problems also could inspire change. Faculty might be persuaded to try innovative ways to select students for admission, provide clinical education, schedule laboratory sessions for large numbers of students, or improve students' professional writing skills.

Case reports can provide critical information about patient/client management and practice variation.

Help Develop Guidelines and Pathways

Because our health care environment has become increasingly complex, practitioners, academicians, researchers, third-party payers, and policymakers must determine with greater accuracy what works for whom and how long it takes.[5] Success (and even professional survival) depends on the accuracy of patient/client management predictions—and currently there is little research on which to base these decisions. Again, case reports cannot provide definitive answers about effectiveness, but the descriptions of clinical practice that they provide can be a rich source of experience (eg, observations of the natural history of conditions and sug-

The Value of Reporting on Nonpatients

Because the preponderance of published case reports involves patients, this manual focuses on patient-related case reports. But case reports that do not involve patients or that involve patients only peripherally also can make a valuable contribution to the professional knowledge base. For instance:

In a case report that could be of value to academicians and clinical educators, Kramer and Stern[1] wrote a multiple-participant case report involving occupational therapy students who did well academically but had trouble meeting clinical performance expectations. Because they reported on several students, they were able to "classify" students by identifying common characteristics among them. The students who had problems in the clinic generally had difficulty accepting responsibility for their behaviors and did not receive feedback well in the classroom or in the clinic. The report goes on to describe the interventions used by the clinical and academic instructors to handle the students' problems. Although the case report does not

"prove" that students who have difficulty accepting feedback or responsibility for their behaviors in the academic setting will have problems in the clinic, the description of the academic-setting behaviors of the students who did have problems in the clinic could alert other academic instructors to the possibility that students with similar behaviors might have similar problems. The described interventions also might be useful to other clinical or academic educators who are trying to help students with similar characteristics.

Case reports also can focus on patient-related equipment or procedures. They should include a detailed description of at least one patient with whom the equipment or procedures were used. McCulloch and Kemper[2] described the use of a vacuum-compression device to treat a patient with a lengthy history of ischemic ulcers. Their intent was to share information with clinicians

about the new vacuum-compression device by illustrating its application with one of their patients. McClure and Flowers[3] described the application of a splint designed to improve a woman's shoulder range of motion, stating the theoretical rationale for maintaining the woman's arm in an elevated position and clearly describing the construction and use of the elevation splint. A case report written by Canélon[4] focused on a description of job-site analysis to determine essential functions required in workplaces. He illustrated the approach by reporting on the successful workplace reintegration of three clients with neurological and orthopedic conditions.

References

1 Kramer P, Stern K. Approaches to improving student performance on fieldwork. *Am J Occup Ther*. 1995;49:156-159.

2 McCulloch JM, Kemper CC. Vacuum-compression therapy for the treatment of an ischemic ulcer. *Phys Ther*. 1993;73:165-169.

3 McClure PW, Flowers KR. Treatment of limited shoulder motion: a case study based on biomechanical considerations. *Phys Ther*. 1992;72:929-936.

4 Canélon MF. Job site analysis facilitates work reintegration. *Am J Occup Ther*. 1995;49:461-467.

gestions about the ways in which patients can be classified) from which practice guidelines, critical pathways, and other patient/client management approaches can be developed.

Two documents on patient/client management that are important for rehabilitation professionals are the American Physical Therapy Association's *Guide to Physical Therapist Practice*[28] and the American Occupational Therapy Association's *Guide to Occupational Therapy Practice.*[29] Primary purposes of both documents include improvement of quality of care and reduction of costs. Case reports that provide information pertinent to the natural history of various conditions and to diagnostic classification, prognosis, and intervention have contributed and will continue to contribute to the development and revision of these association documents.

Case reports also can be used to help identify and reduce variations in practice. Although research is required to establish cause-and-effect relationships, information from an accumulation of case reports can be useful for the purposes of comparison. If the interventions and outcomes described by case reports seem to be superior to other approaches, a closer look at those other approaches may be warranted, with the purpose to implement approaches that others suggest may be more effective. Managed care organizations often collect outcomes data for the purpose of comparing clinics and individual therapists. An accumulation of case reports may provide a way to support or cast doubt on some of the conclusions that those managed care organizations draw from their comparisons.

Next: What Kind of Case Do *You* Have in Mind?

It's worth saying one more time: Case reports cannot identify cause-and-effect relationships between interventions and outcomes. They do, however, give us meticulous descriptions of practice that make important contributions to the professional literature. The first key to success in writing case reports is to choose your case wisely.

References

1   Barlow DH, Hersen M. *Single Case Experimental Designs.* 2nd ed. New York, NY: Pergamon Press; 1984.

2   Kazdin AE. Drawing valid inferences from case studies. *Journal of Counseling and Clinical Psychology.* 1981;19:183-192.

3   Schmoll BJ. Qualitative research. In: Bork CE, ed. *Research in Physical Therapy.* Philadelphia, Pa: JB Lippincott Co; 1993:83-124.

4   Merriam S. *Case Study Research in Education: A Qualitative Approach.* San Francisco, Calif: Jossey-Bass Inc Publishers; 1988.

5   DePoy D, Gitlin LN. *Introduction to Research: Multiple Strategies for Health and Human Services.* St Louis, Mo: CV Mosby Co; 1994.

6   Harris SR, Riffle K. Effects of inhibitive ankle-foot orthoses on standing balance in a child with cerebral palsy: a single-subject design. *Phys Ther.* 1986;66:663-667.

7   Riddle DL, Freeman DB. Management of a patient with a diagnosis of bilateral plantar fasciitis and Achilles tendinitis: a case report. *Phys Ther.* 1988;68:1913-1916.

8   Rothstein JR, Echternach JL. Hypothesis-oriented algorithm for clinicians: a method for evaluation and treatment planning. *Phys Ther.* 1986;66:1388-1394.

9   Sackett DL, Straus SE, Richardson WS, et al. *Evidence-Based Medicine: How to Practice and Teach EBM.* 2nd ed. New York, NY: Churchill Livingstone; 2000.

10 Rothstein JM. Thirty years later...[editor's note]. *Phys Ther.* 2000;80:6-7.

11 Parker MJ. Managing an elderly patient with a fractured femur. *Br Med J.* 2000;320:102-103.

12 McEwen IR, Karlan GR. Case studies: why and how. *Augmentative and Alternative Communication.* 1990;6:69-75.

13 Beattie P. The use of an eclectic approach for the treatment of low back pain: a case study. *Phys Ther.* 1992;72:923-928.

14 Henson KT. Case study in teacher education. *The Educational Forum.* 1988;52:236-241.

15 Ready RK. The case study II. Letter to the editor. *The Journal of Applied Behavioral Science.* 1968;4: 232-235.

16 DeBakey L, DeBakey S. The case report, I. Guidelines for preparation. *Int J Cardiol.* 1983;4:357-364.

17 Petrusa ER, Weiss GB. Writing case reports: an educationally valuable experience for house officers. *J Med Educ.* 1982;57:415-417.

18 Roland CG. The case report. *JAMA.* 1968;205:83-84.

19 Heriza CB. Implications of a dynamical systems approach to understanding infant kicking behavior. *Phys Ther.* 1991;71:222-235.

20 Kaltenborn FM. *Mobilization of the Extremity Joints.* Oslo, Norway: Olaf Norlis Bokhandel Universitetsgaten; 1980.

21 Lazarus AA, Davison GC. Clinical innovation in research and practice. In: Bergin AE, Garfield SL, eds. *Handbook of Psychotherapy and Behavior Change: An Empirical Analysis.* New York, NY: John Wiley & Sons Inc; 1971:196-213.

22 McClure PW, Flowers KR. Treatment of limited shoulder motion: a case study based on biomechanical considerations. *Phys Ther.* 1992;72:929-936.

23 Lister MJ, ed. *Contemporary Management of Motor Control Problems: Proceedings of the II STEP Conference.* Alexandria, Va: Foundation for Physical Therapy Inc; 1991.

24 Carmick J. Clinical use of neuromuscular electrical stimulation for children with cerebral palsy, part 1: lower extremity. *Phys Ther.* 1993;73:505-513.

25 Carmick J. Clinical use of neuromuscular electrical stimulation for children with cerebral palsy, part 2: upper extremity. *Phys Ther.* 1993;73:514-527.

26 Pape KE. Caution urged for NMES use. Letter to the editor. *Phys Ther.* 1994;74:265-266.

27 Head J, Patterson V. Performance context and its role in treatment planning. *Am J Occup Ther.* 1997;51:453-457.

28 Guide to Physical Therapist Practice. 2nd ed. *Phys Ther.* 2001;81:9-744.

29 Moyer PA. *Guide to Occupational Therapy Practice.* Bethesda, Md: American Occupational Therapy Association; 1999.

Chapter 2

Choosing a Case to Report

Cases do not have to be unusual or unique to be published in *Physical Therapy* or in many other journals. Some medical journals are interested in publishing reports only of new phenomena or new approaches to diagnosis and management,[1,2] but that's probably because some areas of medicine are much older and have a large cache of case reports and other professional literature from which to draw.

How do you decide whether a case is worth reporting? Case reports involving patients, for instance, should illustrate elements of patient/client management that have not yet been well described in the professional literature. Because of the overall lack of case reports in rehabilitation, a well-reasoned and clearly presented report of almost any type of patient would meet this criterion! Nonetheless, a literature search—described in detail in **Chapter 3**—is necessary to determine whether a number of case reports or research reports already have been published on your topic. Even if the answer is "yes," you shouldn't automatically give up on your idea. The search results may tell you that your case report has a different angle that would make it something "new."

To get the most out of your literature search, you need to answer an important question before you begin: What's the general focus of the case report that has been waiting, half-formed, in the back of your mind?

Your case does not have to be unusual or unique to contribute to the body of knowledge.

The Essentials

A case report involving a patient or a group of patients should address all of the essential elements of patient/client management (examination, evaluation, diagnosis, prognosis, and intervention) and outcomes, but the case report may *focus* on one or more of them.[3] The essential elements of patient/client management provided by physical therapists are defined by the *Guide to Physical Therapist Practice*[4] (See **Chapter 6** for more).

Keeping the elements of patient/client management in mind, how might you focus your case report? You might—

■ **Select a patient whose diagnosis was difficult to make.** Focus your report on your decision-making processes related to the examination, evaluation, and diagnosis. The rich description of this process could then be followed by a briefer, but replicable, description of the intervention (if any) and the outcomes.

■ **Describe changes in one or more patients with chronic conditions over an extended period of time.** This is what Dal Bello-Haas and colleagues[5] did when they described a patient's physical therapy through the six stages of amyotrophic lateral sclerosis. Another case report might focus on the management and ambulation outcomes of several children with spastic diplegia from 1 year to 15 years of age. Such a longitudinal, multiple-patient case report could help other clinicians better predict the changing ambulation abilities of children with certain characteristics, given certain interventions. It also would help develop hypotheses for future research.

■ **Report on two or more patients with similar characteristics who received different interventions and had different outcomes.** The details of all of the patient/client management elements would be of interest to clinicians and researchers. Clinicians would probably attempt to replicate the case, and researchers could use it to identify variables for future research.

■ **Report on the atypical management of patients with common problems.** Perhaps you believe that a certain test helps you classify patients with low back pain so that you can target the intervention to their problem more effectively; perhaps you have developed an innovative exercise program for patients with traumatic brain injury that seems to achieve better outcomes than do other interventions. A case report about the patients with low back pain might emphasize the examination element of patient/client management, and a case report about patients with traumatic brain injury might emphasize the intervention. Both case reports would have to provide some information about the other elements in order to make the entire clinical decision-making process explicit and to enable replication by other clinicians.

■ **Report on unusual patients.** Again, although case reports don't have to involve "unique" cases, reports of patients with unusual problems or unusual responses to intervention can contribute to our clinical knowledge base. Documentation of unusual cases could be helpful to other clinicians who encounter similar situations for the first time, and documentation of several cases may help identify a previously unknown condition or lead to better classification of patients with unexpected responses to an intervention.

■ **Apply theory to patient/client management.** Have you used motor learning theory or dynamic systems theory as a basis for one or more elements of patient/client management? If you have, other clinicians and researchers want to know about it! Although motor learning theory has been a popular conference and continuing education topic, few illustrations of the application of motor learning theory to the treatment of actual patients—particularly those with motor control problems—exist in the literature. Case reports can show how to apply theory to patient/client management and also can help researchers identify testable hypotheses that reveal more about a theory's usefulness.

■ **Report on an administrative or academic experience.** Perhaps you've had an experience as an administrator that could save others time and effort if you shared the experience by writing a case report. With just a little modification, the patient/client management elements can be used to decide on a focus and content for your case. The "examination" would be the process of gathering data related to your administrative issue or problem. Many sources of information and methods to collect data might be used, such as observations, written reports, surveys, and interviews. The "evaluation" would be the analysis of the initial data and any subsequent information to arrive at a "diagnosis" of the problem and a "prognosis" for improvement. The "intervention" could be anything from a modified work schedule to installation of a distance learning network. The "outcome" could include prevention and management of the problem; consequences of the problem; cost-benefit analysis; and consumer, student, or employee satisfaction.

Don't Shy Away From Negative Outcomes

All clinicians plan for and want to report positive patient outcomes, but not all patients get better. Some patients even get worse, despite competent management. It is important to report negative outcomes, particularly when patient/client management has been brilliant (or even good). Just as our professional literature has little information about what is effective for which patients, it has little information about what is *not* effective for which patients. If careful application of specific motor learning principles was ineffective with a patient who had certain characteristics following traumatic brain injury, for instance, a case report still would be valuable to the reader:

■ **"Applying those motor learning principles didn't work for that patient— but it might work for mine."** Even though the intervention was not effective for the patient described in the case report, other practitioners might find it effective for other patients. A clear description of how motor learning princi-

> **The physical therapy professional literature offers little information about what is effective for which patients—let alone about what is *not* effective.**

ples were used in an intervention would be helpful to clinicians struggling to create ways to apply the theory to practice.

■ **"I'm applying those principles, and my patients aren't progressing either."** The case report would be informative to therapists using the same approach with similar patients, particularly if the patients also are not progressing. A clear description of elements of even the "typical" management of patients who don't get better would help clinicians identify where clinical decision making is breaking down. Are the tests and measures failing to identify critical patient characteristics? Is the evaluation disregarding important information? Is the diagnosis incomplete? Is the prognosis incorrect? Was too little of the intervention applied too quickly, or would another intervention be more effective, given a more complete evaluation? Was the outcome measure used capable of identifying meaningful change? Professional dialogue and examination of practice resulting from such case reports could lead to more effective patient/client management and improved outcomes.

■ **"I'm applying those principles, and my patients are progressing."** If other therapists using the same approach with similar patients have found that their patients *are* making progress, the case report may inspire them to write their own case reports to describe any differences in interventions or patients to help determine what works for whom. Through this process, useful hypotheses can be developed for research to further clarify combinations of patient and intervention characteristics that result in desirable (or undesirable) outcomes.

Prospective, Retrospective, or Both?

If you determine on the first visit that a patient may be a potential focus for a case report, you can plan ahead for a prospective report and gather necessary documentation over the course of intervention. If you decide after the fact that something might be worth reporting, you can review available documentation to prepare a retrospective report. Some case reports include information gathered both retrospectively and prospectively: A therapist who treats a patient over a long period of time may decide to write a case report while the patient still is receiving physical therapy.

Given the incomplete state of many patient records, prospective case reports are likely to provide more accurate and complete information than retrospective reports do. It is possible, however, to prospectively plan for retrospective case reports by making certain that histories, tests and measures, decision-making rationale, interventions, and outcomes are clearly and completely documented for all patients. If good information is available, retrospective case reports are especially useful for accumulating information across several patients. In medicine, combing patient records for common signs, symptoms, and outcomes has identified many conditions.

Patient Consent and Institutional Approval

Is patient consent needed specifically for the writing of a case report? The *Uniform Requirements for Manuscripts Submitted to Biomedical Journals*,[6] which was developed by a group of editors of general medical journals ("Vancouver Group"), contains the following statements regarding the protection of patients' rights to privacy:

> Patients have a right to privacy that should not be infringed without informed consent. Identifying information should not be published in written descriptions, photographs, and pedigrees unless the information is essential for scientific purposes and the patient (or parent or guardian) gives written informed consent for publication. Informed consent for this purpose requires that the patient be shown the manuscript to be published.

> Identifying details should be omitted if they are not essential, but patient data should never be altered or falsified in an attempt to attain anonymity. Complete anonymity is difficult to achieve, and informed consent should be obtained if there is any doubt. For example, masking the eye region in photographs of patients is inadequate protection of anonymity.

> The requirement for informed consent should be included in the journal's instructions for authors. When informed consent has been obtained it should be indicated in the published article.[6]

More than 500 journals have adopted the Uniform Requirements, which means that when you submit your case report to a journal, you may be required to obtain written informed consent from the patients who are described in your report. *Physical Therapy* currently is considering asking authors to obtain patient consent *if* the case is unusual enough that (1) the patient would recognize himself or herself or (2) the patient's acquaintances would be able to identify the patient. Remember that patient consent always is required to use photographs or any other material that reveals identity. As noted by the Vancouver group, tape placed across the eyes of a patient in a photograph does not conceal identity.[6]

When it comes to case reports, the Uniform Requirements specify that "informed consent" includes *showing* the manuscript to the patient. Some writers also have the patient review a draft of the case report for accuracy and detail before writing the final draft for submission for publication.[7] Many case reports could benefit from patient input and review. *Physical Therapy*'s Information for Authors states that "authors are encouraged to allow participants (subjects or patients) to see manuscripts of all types whenever the authors believe that the participant can assist in making the paper credible, in verifying the content of the paper, and in ensuring that participant confidentiality is maintained" (**Appendix 1**).

An important step in finalizing your choice of a case is to obtain institutional approval. In most cases, it won't be necessary to obtain approval of an institutional review board or human subjects committee (as would be required for research); however, the hospital or facility still may want to review and approve the case report before it is submitted for publication. A phone call is usually all it takes to find out.

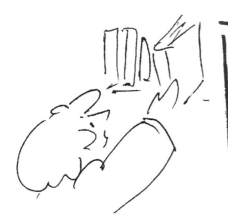

Next: What Does the Literature Say?

Once you have a good idea about the kind of case report you want to write, it's time to conduct a literature search to determine whether your case has something new to offer and to learn what authors have said about your topic. A search can be both low tech (using printed sources) and high tech (using computerized databases). Either way, locating information isn't as difficult as you might think!

References

1 Squires BP. Case reports: what editors want from authors and peer reviewers. *CMAJ*. 1989;141:379-380.

2 Riesenberg DE. Case reports in the medical literature. *JAMA*. 1986;255:2067.

3 Rothstein JM, Delitto A. Writing case reports. Presentation: Joint Congress of the Canadian Physiotherapy Association and the American Physical Therapy Association; June 4-8, 1994; Toronto, Ontario, Canada.

4 Guide to Physical Therapist Practice. 2nd ed. *Phys Ther*. 2001;81:9-744.

5 Dal Bello-Haas V, Kloos AD, Mitsumoto H. Physical therapy for a patient through six stages of amyotrophic lateral sclerosis. *Phys Ther*. 1998;78:1312-1324.

6 Uniform Requirements for Manuscripts Submitted to Biomedical Journals. *Ann Intern Med*. 1997;126:36-47. Document is available at: http://www.icmje.org. Accessed May 8, 2001.

7 Bergsjø P. On case reports. *Acta Obstet Gynecol Scand*. 1992;71:257-258.

Chapter 3

Searching the Literature

More than likely, nothing exactly like your case has been reported in the literature; however, a literature search is necessary to verify that a number of similar case reports or research reports on the same topic have not been published. Even if you find that a similar or identical report has been published, your case still may be publishable—if you acknowledge similarities to the previous report and can make a convincing argument that your case adds something important to the literature. Your search also will serve other purposes. It will help you understand more about your particular case, and, if you decide to write a report, it will help you prepare the introduction. The introduction is the section of the case report that shows how existing research, theory, and opinion support the need for your case report and justify your patient/client management.

Literature review for case reports is much less extensive than that for research reports, and the sources are accessible. You just need to know where to look!

What Types of Source Material Should You Use?

The information for your case report should come from credible published sources, not through personal communication or from course notes.

In the introduction to their case report on the management of a 14-year-old boy with tarsal coalition, a relatively uncommon pathological condition of the foot, Kelo and Riddle[1(p521)] described the literature search that they conducted in relation to their case:

We began our literature review by examining the work of Jahss.[14] We found that the diagnostic term "tarsal coalition" has essentially replaced the term "peroneal spastic flatfoot" in more recent literature. We therefore conducted a MEDLINE search using the key words "peroneal spastic flatfoot" and "tarsal coalition" for the years 1970 to present. We used the reference lists of articles found in the MEDLINE search to identify additional relevant literature. We also used the 3-volume series on the foot and ankle by Jahss[14] to identify additional references.

In their search, Kelo and Riddle found two types of credible published sources: *primary* sources and *secondary* sources. Both types can be either peer-reviewed or non–peer-reviewed.

Primary sources. Firsthand accounts of research procedures and results are "primary sources" of information and constitute the strongest support for your case report. Use primary sources of information whenever possible. If you were to write a case report on serial casting of a patient's ankle, for instance, citing journal articles that described basic research on the effects of prolonged stretch on soft tissue structures would help support your intervention and help explain your patient's outcome. If your patient is an adult with head injury, and no research on serial casting has been carried out with similar patients, you also might look at related research. You could review research about effects of similar procedures, such as splinting, or effects of serial casting with other types of patients, such as children with cerebral palsy.

How can you tell if an article is a primary source of information? If you have the article, the easiest way is to see whether it's organized like most research reports—with a methods section (subjects, procedures, and data analysis) and a results section. Often this information also is in the abstract. If you look for articles by reading reference lists or find an article in a database that doesn't give much information about the article's content, the title may indicate whether it's a primary source that's worth pursuing. If the title is something like "Effect of serial casting on heel-strike in children with spastic diplegia," the article probably is a research report and a primary source. If it's "Serial casting for children with cerebral palsy" (a general topic with no independent variable stated), it's probably not a primary source—but the reference list of that article may *lead* you to primary sources.

In your literature search, you might come across a meta-analysis. A *meta-analysis* is a statistical compilation of the results of several studies that address the same topic. Although the authors of the meta-analysis did not carry out the experimental studies themselves, you can consider the results of the meta-analysis to be a primary source of research, because combining the results of several studies generates new information. The reference list of a meta-analysis can be a valuable source of primary research articles on a topic. Make sure that you read the articles yourself and don't just repeat what the authors of the meta-analysis said about them! You usually can identify a meta-analysis by the use of the term "meta-analysis" in the title or abstract.

Secondary sources. Secondary sources of information are reports by authors who performed a literature review and abstracted or synthesized the work of others. Often they combine this information with their own opinions. Review articles, textbooks, and reference manuals may provide excellent summaries of existing literature. Kelo and Riddle[1] used a secondary source, Jahss's *Disorders of the Foot and Ankle: Medical and Surgical Management*, to find primary sources that were not identified in their database search. Use of secondary sources is an efficient way to identify primary sources; however, you should not assume that they are an accurate account of the original work until you have consulted the primary source to verify accuracy. The primary source always should be cited.

On reference lists or in databases, secondary sources often can be identified by their titles or the type of publication. "Review," "perspective," "update," and similar words in the title are clues that the article probably is a secondary source. Books and book chapters also are likely to be secondary sources—primary research articles usually are published in journals.

The importance of using peer-reviewed sources. Using material published in peer-reviewed journals ensures that the information has been subjected to a peer-review process, which lends credibility.

Peer review represents the "collective wisdom" of a profession. This collective wisdom makes peer review "the 'gold standard' for scholarly work, and peer review can only get more important as we increasingly face the task of separating signal from noise in the tidal wave of electronic information."[2(p68)]

When a paper is peer-reviewed, it is reviewed by people who are experts on the paper's subject matter and who have a record of publication in the subject area. They examine the methods, research design, organization, writing, and content relevance, and they comment on the paper's strengths and weaknesses. When an article appears in a peer-reviewed publication, it has reached a standard of quality, and its authors have addressed the weaknesses pointed out by the peer reviewers.[3]

Newspaper and magazine sources are not peer reviewed and should not be included in your literature search. Examples of non–peer-reviewed rehabilitation publications include *Advance* (for several professions), *PT—Magazine of Physical Therapy*, *OT Week*, and *Rehab Management*. Articles in these publications can be used to identify sources, but they should not be cited. You might want to contact a course instructor or an author who has published in a non–peer-reviewed publication to ask for references to support the concepts communicated during a lecture or within an article.

How can you tell whether a journal is peer-reviewed? Some journals will say so in the front part of each issue, in the section that contains the basic information about the editor, subscriptions, and where the journal is indexed. *Physical Therapy*, for example, has the following editorial statement: "*Physical Therapy*...is a scholarly, refereed journal..." ("refereed" and "peer-reviewed" mean the same thing). Like many journals, the *American Journal of Occupational Therapy* does not say that it is peer-reviewed, but its instructions for authors indicate a peer-review process. Most professional journals (but not magazines or newsletters) are peer-reviewed.

Another way to verify whether a journal is peer reviewed is to check whether it is listed in *Index Medicus* or its electronic counterpart MEDLINE. Being peer reviewed is one of the requirements for a journal to be listed in *Index Medicus*/ MEDLINE. Many peer-reviewed journals that are of interest to rehabilitation professionals are not listed in *Index Medicus*/MEDLINE, however. Just because a journal is not listed in *Index Medicus*/MEDLINE does not mean that it is not peer reviewed.

The same rules for credibility apply to material obtained from Web sites. Much of the material on the Web is not peer-reviewed; however, more and more peer-reviewed journals are becoming available online and are just as credible as their print counterparts.

Starting Your Search

Starting a literature search may seem intimidating, given the vast amount of biomedical literature available. Your first step, however, can take place in your own home. You might already have a great deal of information in your home library—textbooks, issues of *Physical Therapy*, bibliographies from continuing education courses, or readings from school. You can start your search by reading textbook chapters to find primary sources (either references to specific articles or to frequently cited journals).

After combing your own resources for references or articles, you are ready for the next step: a trip to the local library. Reference materials at most libraries are available to the public. Your best bet for a successful literature search would be at an academic or health sciences library, such as those affiliated with colleges of health sciences, medical schools, law schools, or programs in sociology, psychology, education, or engineering. These libraries will have the best access to print indexes, databases, and the specialized biomedical literature. Public libraries provide access to common publications and government documents, and they might have online access to biomedical databases and journal Web sites; however, they might not have the journals or textbooks that you require.

For assistance in locating an academic library, consult the *American Library Directory*,[4] which lists US libraries and the services they provide. The National Network of Libaries of Medicine (NN/LM) (www.nnlm.nlm.nih.gov), part of the National Library of Medicine, also can help locate a nearby medical library. The NN/LM has established a network of several regional libraries, more than a hundred resource libraries (primarily at medical schools), and more than 4,500 primary-access libraries (usually at hospitals).

Reference librarians can help you find the appropriate print indexes or databases; instruct you in the use of databases; suggest appropriate search terms; and, if the library does not have a particular reference work in its collection, help you with other options such as interlibrary loans.

Journal indexes. Because you know your topic, you also may be familiar with the professional journals that publish information relevant to your case. Most professional journals, such as *Physical Therapy*, provide an annual index by subject and author. Some journals, including *Physical Therapy*, also publish cumulative author and subject indexes that cover several years, which can help speed up your research. If your case report is on the effects of an orthosis on a patient's gait pattern, for instance, you might refer to the index that appears in every December issue of *Physical Therapy*; ask an orthotist to lend you index issues of *Orthotics and Prosthetics*; or go to your local health sciences or university library, which might have *Orthotics and Prosthetics* index issues.

Multiple-journal indexes. You may need to search material from a number of professional sources. Information about orthoses, for example, is published in the physical therapy, occupational therapy, orthotic, engineering, and medical literature. Multiple-journal indexes are an efficient way to search several bodies of literature simultaneously. Each of these indexes provides a listing of articles related to particular disciplines and can be searched using keywords to identify articles written on a given topic. You can either identify the terms yourself or use the list of subject headings that are specific to each index. Your terms can be broadened or narrowed using other terms provided by the index.

Print versus electronic indexes. The development of CD-ROMs (compact disc read-only memory) and high-speed processors and the growth of the Internet have led to important changes in library reference collections. Because CD-ROMs and Internet databases have a large storage capacity, are easy to search, and take up less space than print indexes, many libraries have "gone digital" with their reference collections, using electronic indexes, or databases, instead of continuing to subscribe to print indexes.[5] Why then are print indexes still important? Some publishers may have decided not to incorporate older references into their databases. A literature search on a given database therefore may retrieve references that only go back as far as 1980, for instance—in which case, you would need to consult the print index to find older references. **Figure 3** lists examples of print indexes that may be useful for literature searches related to physical therapy. (All of these print indexes also are available electronically.) For more information, ask your librarian, or consult reference books such as *Information Industry Directory*.[6]

Databases. Databases—on CD-ROM, on the World Wide Web—have revolutionized the literature search process. Many libraries have converted their card catalog to an electronic catalog, which can make your search for texts and government documents more efficient.

Databases and Web sites offer important advantages, such as the ability to conduct searches that are more thorough than those conducted with print indexes, the ability to combine or separate search terms, and sometimes the ability to read full-text articles without digging through the library stacks. A database may not include older material, however, and the quality of the information found on the Internet is highly variable and depends on the source of the information. Beware of Web sites that make unsubstantiated claims!

Databases, many of which correspond to a print index, are available at almost every university library. Some public libraries have access to these databases through online commercial services such as DIALOG and DataStar. (You may have to make an appointment with a librarian to use these services.) Some computer searches may use CD-ROMs, which contain enormous amounts of information, including bibliographies, abstracts, and sometimes full-text articles and reports

Print Indexes

Most print indexes include tables of contents and author information; many contain abstracts. All of the following have an electronic or Internet version.

- Index Medicus
- Cumulative Index of Nursing and Allied Health Literature (CINAHL)
- Current Contents
- Current Index to Journals in Education (CIJE)
- Resources in Education
- Psychological Abstracts
- Social Sciences Citation Index (SSCI)
- Biological Abstracts
- Dissertation Abstracts International

Figure 3. *Examples of print indexes that may be useful for literature searches related to physical therapy and other rehabilitation disciplines.*

from additional sources that are not found within the library. Some databases are now available from the home or clinic via the Internet. (**Figure 4**.)

Databases allow you to combine and separate terms. For instance, if a serial casting case report involved a patient with traumatic brain injury, the search could be narrowed to "prolonged muscle stretch and soft tissue structures and traumatic brain injury." The search could be further narrowed by requesting only those articles written in English, those written during a particular time period, or those written by a particular author. The search could be narrowed yet again by using other search terms based on diagnosis or outcome measures. For an orthosis case report involving a patient with diabetes, the terms "orthosis," "orthotic," and "molded shoe insert" could be used for a broad search; then the search could be narrowed by adding such terms as "diabetes" for diagnosis or "ulcer healing" for outcome measure.

The most difficult part of the search is not in using the computer, but in manipulating terms to find exactly what you want. In this way, electronic searching is no different from print searching! Database search screens differ, but they all have basic similarities. For instance, some may use the term "subject," "subject word," "query word," or "keyword" to refer to search words. In database searches, you have to use the keywords that are used by that particular program, and it can be frustrating to look for information that is not listed under the terms you use. Even so, the search will identify at least a few key articles whose reference lists you then can use to find more articles on your topic. In addition, the abstracts of these articles may provide more appropriate keywords to use in your search.

Before you begin using a database, make certain that it covers the years you need for your search, find the proper search terms using its subject headings list (if it has one), and examine which parts of the citation it searches. Many databases can be found on the Internet, allowing you to conduct a literature search from your home or office; however, they may charge a fee. Before going online to use an unfamiliar database, ask a reference librarian to demonstrate how to use it.

© 1996 Sidney Harris

IF THERE WERE COMPUTERS IN GALILEO'S TIME

Computerized Databases

Most of the resources below are available through university and college libraries; via the Internet; or, for a fee, through commercial services such as Ovid Online, DataStar, and DIALOG.

BIOETHICSLINE

Ethics and public policy issues in health care and research, available through Internet Grateful Med: igm.nlm.nih.gov

CANCERLIT

A bibliographic database with more than 1.5 million citations and abstracts from more than 4,000 journals, books, theses, and other sources.
www.cancernet.nci.nih.gov/
overview.html

CINAHL Database

Computerized version of the print index, *Cumulative Index of Nursing and Allied Health Literature*. www.cinahl.com

The Cochrane Library

An electronic publication containing systematic reviews of the effects of health care, principally randomized controlled trials; critical assessments and structured abstracts of systematic reviews published elsewhere; and bibliographic information on controlled trials.
hiru.mcmaster.ca/cochrane/cdsr.htm

Current Contents Search

Tables of contents from leading journals in the sciences, social sciences, arts, and humanities; computerized equivalent of *Current Contents*. www.isinet.com

DIRLINE: Directory of Health Organizations

Contains location and descriptive information about resources providing health and biomedical information services, including organizations, research resources, projects, and databases. dirline.nlm.nih.gov

EMBASE

More than 13 million abstracts and citations to international literature on drugs, pharmacology, and human medicine, including European and Asian publications; 1966 to present. Electronic equivalent of *Excerpta Medica*. www.embase.com

ERIC: Educational Resources Information Center

A compilation containing education information. Includes *Resources in Education*, *Current Index to Journals in Education*, and child educational resources. www.accesser-ic.org/home.html

HealthSTAR

Citations to published literature on health services, technology, administration, and research, with a focus on both clinical and nonclinical aspects of health care delivery. Available through Internet Grateful Med:
www.cdlib.org/guides/medline

HISTLINE: HISTory of Medicine OnLINE

Resources for historical scholarship in medicine and related sciences. Available through Internet Grateful Med:
igm.nlm.nih.gov

HSRProj (Health Sciences Research Projects in Progress)

Descriptions of health services research projects, including health technology assessment and development and use of clinical practice guidelines. Available through Internet Grateful Med:
igm.nlm.nih.gov

IAC Health Periodicals Database

Wide range of health and specialized medical topics; selected full text.

IAC Health & Wellness Database

Broad coverage in the areas of health, medicine, fitness, and nutrition for health professionals and consumers; selected full text.

Institute for Scientific Information (ISI) Biochemistry and Biophysics Citation Index

Bibliographic data and abstracts to more than 3,600 journals with content applicable to medicine and health care.
www.isinet.com

MEDLINE

International biomedicine literature; electronic equivalent of *Index Medicus*. (See "What Is MEDLINE?" on page 30)

OT Search

Bibliographic data and abstracts on occupational therapy and related subjects such as rehabilitation, education, psychiatry, psychology, and health care delivery or administration. Includes monographs, proceedings, reports, doctoral disertations, master's theses, journals, and newsletters.
www.aota.org/otbibsys/index.asp

PEDro: The Physiotherapy Evidence Database

Abstracts to randomized controlled trials and systematic reviews in physical therapy, compiled by the Centre for Evidence-Based Physiotherapy.
ptwww.cchs.usyd.edu.au/pedro/

PsycINFO

Contains more than 1.5 million references to the international literature of psychology and related behavioral and social sciences, emphasizing original research. Electronic equivalent of *Psychological Abstracts*. For more information:
www.apa.org

REHABDATA

A literature database on disability and rehabilitation produced by the National Rehabilitation Information Center (NARIC). Its main file includes more than 12,000 research reports, books, journal articles, and audiovisual materials from 1993 to the present. www.naric.com

Social SciSearch

An international, multidisciplinary database to the social, behavioral, and related sciences. It contains all the records published in the *Social Sciences Citation Index*.
www.isinet.com

Figure 4. *Some of the computerized databases that may be useful in conducting a literature search.*

What Is MEDLINE?

MEDLINE is the electronic equivalent of *Index Medicus*, a print index that is maintained through the Literature Selection Technical Review Committee, an advisory committee chartered by the National Institutes of Health (NIH). This database offers the best access to the core physical therapy literature.[1] More than 4,000 journals are indexed in *Index Medicus*. MEDLINE currently includes more than 10 million references to articles covering all medical topics; new records are added almost daily. Years indexed in MEDLINE are 1966 to present. It contains some articles for the years 1960 through 1965, but they are few in number.

Data from MEDLINE can be accessed in several ways. Some involve a fee for use, and others are available free:

- University and health service libraries may have either online access to MEDLINE or CD-ROM disks.

- Grateful Med, a software package available from National Technology Information Services (NTIS), allows users to access the MEDLINE database via modem. Users must establish an account with the National Library of Medicine (NLM) in Bethesda, Maryland. At press time, its toll-free telephone number is 888/346-3656.

- Internet Grateful Med and PubMed allow users to conduct a MEDLINE search via the World Wide Web free of charge. Go to the NLM Web site at www.nlm.nih.gov, click on the **Free MEDLINE** button, and select either Internet Grateful Med or PubMed. (To see some key features of PubMed, refer to the following pages.) Some databases, including DIRLINE, HealthSTAR, HISTLINE, and HSRPROJ, are available for free only on Internet Grateful Med.

- Several commercial database services, such as DIALOG and DataStar, allow access to MEDLINE for a fee.

[1] Wakiji EM. Mapping the literature of physical therapy. *Bull Med Libr Assoc*. 1997;85:284-288.

The most challenging part of a search is in manipulating the key words to find exactly what you want.

Using MEDLINE: Step by Step

Imagine you are writing a case report on the use of weight-bearing exercise in the management of a 66-year-old woman with osteoporosis. You first need to search for case reports that may have been written on this topic (and for articles that provide the theory that supports your intervention program). Because MEDLINE offers the best access to the core physical therapy literature,[7] you decide to use an online version of MEDLINE called PubMed (www.ncbi.nlm.nih.gov/PubMed).

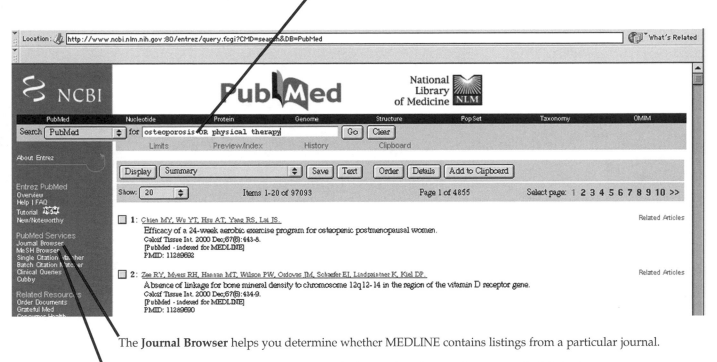

osteoporosis OR physical therapy

The **Journal Browser** helps you determine whether MEDLINE contains listings from a particular journal.

Use the **MeSH Browser** to search the National Library of Medicine's thesaurus—the Medical Subject Headings directory. This is a great way to find the proper terms to use when starting your search.

Step 1: Identify keywords. To help you find the proper terms to use in your search, PubMed has a browser that accesses the National Library of Medicine's thesaurus—the Medical Subject Headings (MeSH) directory. (MeSH is also included in the MEDLINE software, and it is published in a print version.) You click on the MeSH Browser link to begin your search for proper terms.

In the MeSH browser, you enter the term **rehabilitation** in the query box, and click on the **Go** button. The browser finds this term in three places on the MeSH category tree: under "Therapeutics," under "Physical Medicine," and under "Health Services." Based on these search results and the definition of "Rehabilitation" provided by the browser, you determine that this term is too general for you to use in the search. The term "Physical Therapy," however, is part of the "Therapeutics" branch and is listed under "Rehabilitation." You click on its link and find that the definition of "Physical Therapy" includes exercise. After deciding that "Osteoporosis" and "Physical Therapy" are appropriate search terms, you are ready to begin your search, and you exit the browser.

Step 2: Begin your search. In the PubMed query box, you type **osteoporosis OR physical therapy** and click on the **Go** button. (**Figure 5**) (In PubMed, operators such as "AND" or "OR" must be capitalized in order for the search to work.) PubMed then searches for these terms in the title, abstract, and MeSH categories of each citation—and produces more than 97,000 matches! This means that your search was too wide and included articles on such topics as low back pain and other subjects unrelated to your topic.

Figure 5. *Beginning your search. Note: The PubMed screens in this chapter appear courtesy of the National Library of Medicine. Remember that screens may look somewhat different depending on the online service or browser that is being used.*

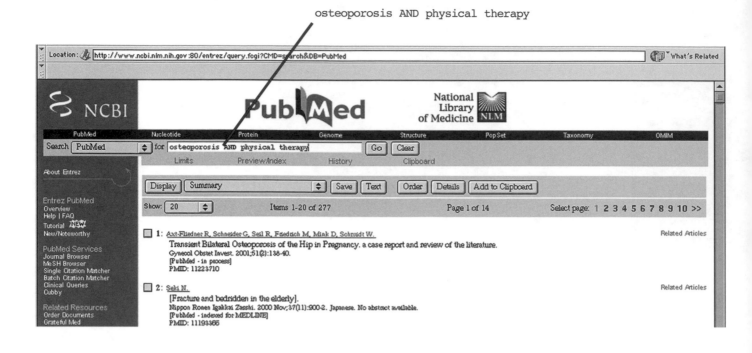

osteoporosis AND physical therapy

Figure 6. *Narrowing your search. By changing OR to AND, you narrow your search to citations that have both of these keywords.*

Step 3: Narrow your search. As your first step in refining your search, you change your operator from **OR** to **AND** in order to find articles with both keywords (**Figure 6**). This change results in 277 matches. To search for case reports that are similar to your case, however, you will need to conduct a further winnowing process.

PubMed offers a number of different options to narrow your search. First, you can set some limits on the types of articles that PubMed looks for. On the Features bar, you click on the Limits link. PubMed displays a number of different options in dropdown menus that you can use to set limits on your search: fields within the citation (eg, title, journal, MeSH heading), publication type (eg, clinical trial, review, randomized clinical trial, meta-analysis), language, age group, human or animal study, gender, citations with abstract only (a check box), and publication date (**Figure 7**). You select English and check the "Abstracts Only" box. After you click on the **Go** button, PubMed limits the search based on your criteria.

PubMed produces 138 citations. You then decide to add another search term— "case report"—to your search. In the query box, you add parentheses around your original search combination to restrict the search to the citations that PubMed has already found. You then type **AND case report** after the combination (**Figure 8**). PubMed displays 17 citations. When you find a particularly relevant article, you click on the Related Articles link to find similar articles.

You can limit your search to certain types of publications, such as review articles, or to sex or certain patient populations (in this case, you might select "Female" and "Aged: 65+ years") by clicking on the Limits link. To find articles written by a particular author, you clear the query box and type in the author's last name followed by first and middle initial, and PubMed then pulls up every article in the database written by that author. (Be aware that PubMed can list the same

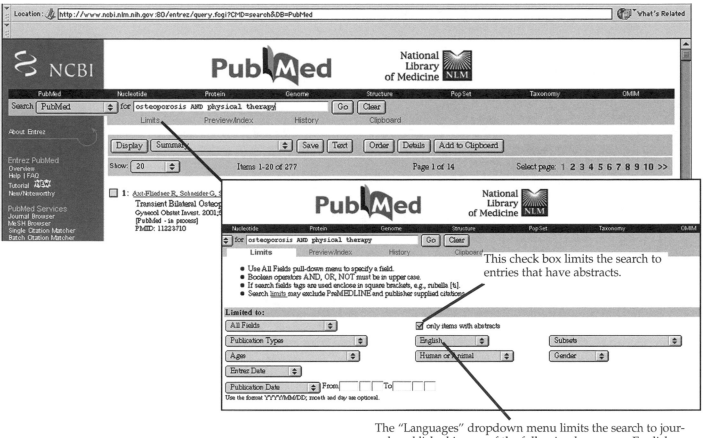

The "Languages" dropdown menu limits the search to journals published in one of the following languages: English, French, German, Italian, Japanese, Russian, or Spanish.

author using one or two initials, depending on the publication. This may affect the result of your author search.) If you find a citation of another article, you can use the Single Citation Matcher—located under the link to the MeSH browser—to find that article. You can also find out if a particular journal is listed in MEDLINE by clicking on the Journal Browser link under "PubMed Services" (**Figure 9**).

Step 4: Select the articles you need. Now that your search has been narrowed, you review the citations from the list produced by PubMed. The default setting for the list is "Summary," which provides the author name, title, and bibliographic information for each citation. For each abstract, the list of authors is shown as a link. To view the abstract for a citation, you click on the author names.

As you review the abstracts, you select those articles that you believe are more pertinent to your case report. You then print out your selections, so you don't have to worry about errors you might make in copying the information by hand. You take the printout directly to the stacks to find the journals that you need.

If you decide that you want to conduct several different searches of the literature in one session, you can click on the **Add to Clipboard** button, and PubMed will save your selections for up to one hour of inactivity, enabling you to conduct other searches. This function will also help you if you choose to order copies of these articles through the Loansome Doc service of PubMed.

Figure 7. *When you click on the* Limits *link on the Features bar, PubMed displays a number of different options (inset) that you can select to limit your search. In our example, you check the "only items with abstracts" box and select English from the "Languages" dropdown menu.*

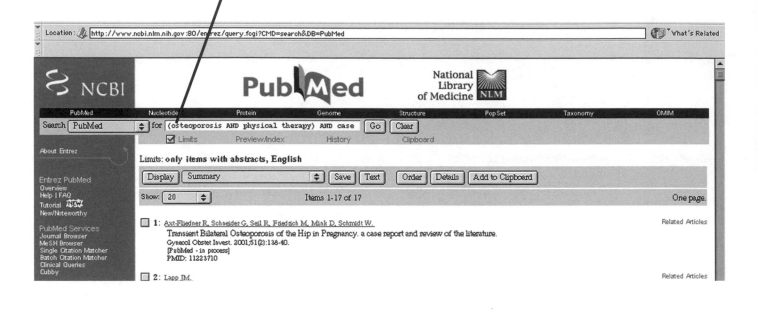

`(osteoporosis AND physical therapy) AND case report`

Figure 8. *Narrowing your search to case reports. To further narrow the search to case reports in your original search combination, you add another keyword—**case report**—but first you put parentheses around your original search combination to make sure that PubMed searches only those entries.*

The introduction section of a case report written by Vance et al[8(p1004)] reveals the process of a typical literature search. It begins:

> A MEDLINE search encompassing the period 1966 to June 1995 yielded no research reports relating to the use of diathermy for primary dysmenorrhea. A search using the key words "primary dysmenorrhea and TENS" yielded five articles.[4-8] All of these articles described studies of patients with primary dysmenorrhea using TENS and ibuprofen compared with ibuprofen only.... Using the key words "diathermy and pelvic inflammatory disease," a second MEDLINE search yielded only one reference....

It is not necessary to write about your literature search in the way that these authors wrote about theirs; in fact, it may be preferable not to. As you read other published case reports, note the different ways in which authors incorporate the results of their literature searches.

PubMed's default display setting is "Summary." To view the abstracts or citations of all the items retrieved by your search, select "Citation" or "Abstract" from this dropdown menu and click on the **Display** button next to the list. To view the abstract of a particular citation, click on the author names that are underlined and highlighted in blue; this link will bring you into the record.

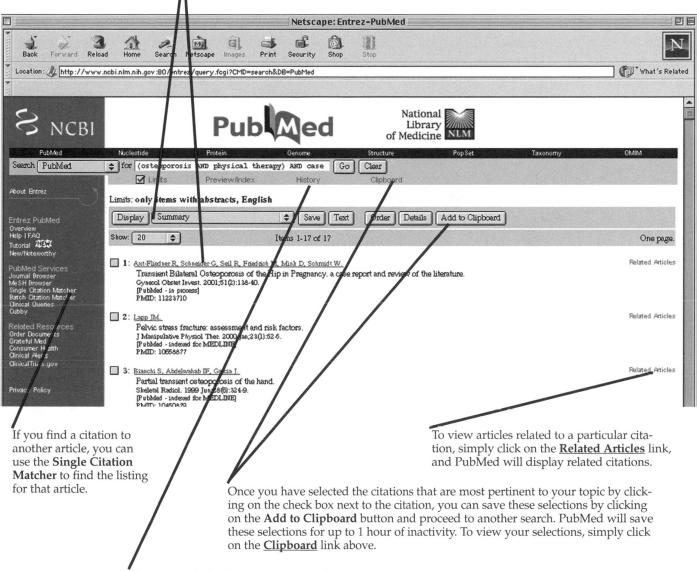

If you find a citation to another article, you can use the **Single Citation Matcher** to find the listing for that article.

To view articles related to a particular citation, simply click on the **Related Articles** link, and PubMed will display related citations.

Once you have selected the citations that are most pertinent to your topic by clicking on the check box next to the citation, you can save these selections by clicking on the **Add to Clipboard** button and proceed to another search. PubMed will save these selections for up to 1 hour of inactivity. To view your selections, simply click on the **Clipboard** link above.

The **History** link allows you to go back to previous searches.

Figure 9. *The PubMed main screen. This figure displays your completed search for case reports on physical therapy and osteoporosis. It highlights other options that you can use to search the database as well as handy tools to make the search speedy and efficient.*

Obtaining the Articles

The library where you conducted your search may store textbooks in the stacks; journals in a special periodicals room, in the stacks, or on microfiche or microfilm; and government documents grouped together in a special location. Consult the library's card catalog or electronic catalog to find the call number of a particular item. If you have problems locating an item, a librarian can help.

If the library does not have the item you need, you can request an interlibrary loan. The librarian can locate the journal or book using the citation you provide. Other libraries (in the same city or in a different state or region) will lend you a book or send you a copy of the article. The interlibrary loan may require a fee to cover the costs of copying and postage.

If you use MEDLINE, PubMed, or Internet Grateful Med to conduct your literature search, you can order the full text of articles through the National Library of Medicine's Loansome Doc service. If the library where you conducted you search does not offer Loansome Doc, you can contact a participating library in the National Network of Libraries of Medicine (NN/LM) and set up an account. For a list of list of libraries that provide Loansome Doc service, call NN/LM at 800/338-7657. More information about Loansome Doc, including questions that you should ask your provider, is available online at www.nnlm.nlm.nih.gov/nnlm/docdel/loansome.html. Other document delivery services include those operated by The UnCover Company and Bell & Howell Information and Learning (formerly UMI).

The Internet is another source for full-text articles. Many journals have a home page where you can access full-text articles, and PubMed and Internet Grateful Med have links to some journal Web sites. With some rare exceptions, you will have to pay a fee to access or download an article. Your library, however, might subscribe to the journal, and you could log on to the Web site from the library. Check with your librarian.

If an article is fairly recent, you may be able to contact the author for a reprint. If the article was published several years ago, however, you may not be able to locate the author.

Remember: Don't forget the obvious! Ask your colleagues if they have access to a particular publication.

Next: You've Chosen a Case—Are You Ready to Write?

You've reviewed the literature and found no case reports or research articles on your exact topic. You've even found the literature to support the importance of your topic and the credibility of your patient/client management. You're almost ready to start writing! But first, you have some important "almost-writing" tasks. You need to think about operational definitions—and reliability and validity of measurements.

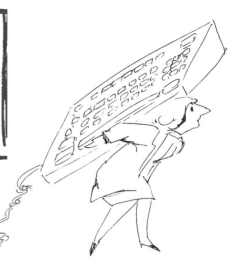

References

1 Kelo MJ, Riddle DL. Examination and management of a patient with tarsal coalition. *Phys Ther*. 1998;78:518-525.

2 Davidoff F. Masking, blinding, and peer review: the blind leading the blinded [editorial]. *Ann Intern Med*. 1998;128:66-68.

3 Rothstein JM. Peer review [editor's note]. *Phys Ther*. 1991;71:88-89.

4 *American Library Directory*. 51st ed. New Providence, NJ: RR Bowker's Database Publishing Group; 1998.

5 Hardesty L. Do we need academic libraries? A position paper of the Association of College and Research Libraries (ACRL). Available at: www.ala.org/acrl/academiclib.html. Accessed April 6, 2000.

6 *Information Industry Directory*. 21st ed. Detroit, Mich: The Gale Group; 1999.

7 Wakiji EM. Mapping the literature of physical therapy. *Bull Med Libr Assoc*. 1997;85:284-288.

8 Vance AR, Hayes SH, Spielholz NI. Microwave diathermy treatment for primary dysmenorea. *Phys Ther*. 1996;76:1003-1008.

Suggested Readings

Bailey DM. Reviewing the literature. *Research for the Health Professional: A Practical Guide*. 2nd ed. Philadelphia, Pa: FA Davis Co; 1997.

Currier DP. Literature review. *Elements of Research in Physical Therapy*. 3rd ed. Baltimore, Md: Williams & Wilkins Co; 1990.

Domholdt E. Locating the literature. *Physical Therapy Research: Principles and Applications*. 2nd ed. Philadelphia, Pa: WB Saunders Co; 2000:379-393.

Chapter 4

Defining and Measuring

Have you ever read patient charts and wondered what the treating therapist meant when describing the patient, an examination, or an intervention procedure? Part of the problem is that therapists often use jargon or ambiguous terms. We use these terms because we think that "everyone knows what they mean." But "everyone" doesn't know what those terms mean! Does "moderate assistance" really indicate how much you have to help the patient? When you read, "I cleared the patient's neck," do you know what procedures were used? If treatment is said to include "balance training," will you be able to replicate it? Exactly what is "neurodevelopmental treatment"? How would another clinician replicate and recognize "capsular end feel"?

Everyone *doesn't* know what you mean! Make certain that others will be able to replicate what you did.

Operationalize!

Because a case report is the purest description of how we practice, operational definitions are an essential ingredient. No matter what topic the case report covers, the interactions between the author and the patient (or other entity) must be "operationalized." Operational definitions traditionally have been viewed as descriptions of what to look for, what to do, and how to obtain a measurement. When we operationally define something, we describe all of the steps involved in completing a task.

Operational definitions allow us to replicate and interpret the measurements of others—and ourselves. For example, if we all take a measurement in the same way—that is, if we all follow the same operational definition—we get the same result (or almost the same result). In the absence of operational definitions, however, each of us may use a different set of rules to take a measurement, greatly

A Tower of Babel?

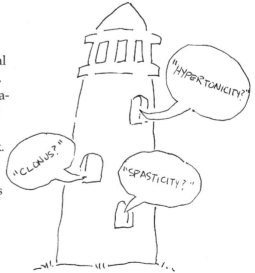

increasing the chances for error. The position of the patient, for example, can make a difference in a range-of-motion measurement. Time of day, type of floor surface, type of footwear, and medication all are factors that can affect the distance that a patient walks or the amount of assistance that a patient needs for getting dressed. Clear descriptions of these and any other relevant conditions reduce the chances of measurement error.

For the purpose of case reports, the classic term "operational definition" should be broadened to apply not only to measurements but to histories, interventions, and outcomes. The reader should be able to:

- Identify patients who have characteristics that are similar to those of the patient in the case report.

- Replicate the procedures for the examination (history, systems review, and tests and measures).

- Replicate the intervention.

- Assess the outcome of the intervention in a similar way.

- Understand the author's clinical reasoning process.

Tips on providing operational definitions will be given throughout this manual. This chapter focuses on measurement reliability and validity—the "two-headed monster" that is closely related to operational definitions.

What Constitutes a Measurement?

To describe patient examinations and outcomes—and sometimes interventions—clinicians have to take measurements. APTA's *Standards for Tests and Measurements in Physical Therapy Practice*[1] defines "measurement" as "the numeral assigned to an object, event, or person or the class (category) to which an object, event, or person is assigned according to rules." This definition implies that any time a therapist assesses something based on a set of rules or steps, the therapist has taken a measurement.

It is especially important that the therapist (and the reader) have confidence that the measurements in case reports accurately reflect the patient's condition.

What constitutes a measurement can be very subtle. When you determine the extent of assistance that a patient requires to dress, you are taking a measurement. When you assess the magnitude of a patient's report of pain, you are taking a measurement. When you observe and subsequently describe a patient's gait pattern, you are taking a measurement. In a case report, these and all other types of measurements must meet at least minimal requirements of reliability and validity. Why? In case reports, measurements are taken for only one patient or a few patients at a time, unlike studies with large numbers of subjects. It is especially important that the therapist (and the reader) have confidence that the measurements accurately reflect the patient's condition.

The *reliability* of the measurement indicates how much error exists in the measurement. All measurements have at least a little error, but too much error makes a measurement meaningless. Where does error come from? A variety of sources:

Examiner error. Examiners contribute error to a measurement when they do not follow the operational definition of the examination procedure. When a therapist measures the range of motion at a joint but does not align the goniometer properly, for example, error occurs. Error also occurs when a therapist does not follow the instructions for administering a standardized test.

Instrument error. How many times have you measured range of motion with a goniometer that had a loose hinge that prevented you from reading the angle properly? Instruments aren't limited to devices or machines; they also can be the written instructions (operational definitions again) that must be used to obtain a measurement, such as a set of rules to classify a patient's movement pattern. When the set of rules is not understandable (operational), it can be considered to be faulty and may add error to the assessment.

Patient error. The patient as a source of error in clinical practice may be a difficult concept to understand. If you assess the force production of a patient's biceps muscle 3 hours postsurgery and compare that measurement with one taken the next day, the two measurements will be different. The difference, however, doesn't represent true change in the force-producing capacity of the biceps muscle. Changes in force-production capability can take weeks to occur. The difference may relate to the fact that the patient still was experiencing effects from the anesthesia during the first test. When patient-related factors such as this one influence a measurement, error results.

Measurement error can be minimized *only when* therapists do everything they can do to eliminate the possible sources of error. The higher the reliability for a single measurement—that is, the more assured we are that there is no examiner, instrument, or patient error—the more likely the measurement is to represent the true status of the patient. High reliability is particularly important when repeated measurements are taken over time to assess change in a patient's status. Small changes in highly reliable measurements are likely to indicate a real change in the patient's condition, whereas small changes in lower-reliability measurements are likely to indicate error.

What Constitutes "Real" Change?

You can never be absolutely certain that measurements over time represent real change in the variable being measured. There always is an element of uncertainty in dealing with reliability, just as there is uncertainty in most other aspects of practice. But in a case report you must provide *some* evidence that the measurements adequately reflect the status of the patient and not measurement error—that is, you must show that the measurements have an acceptable level of reliability.

The word "acceptable" requires clarification. Reliability coefficients often are used to indicate the degree of agreement between measurements. Coefficients can be calculated using a variety of statistics, but the resulting numbers generally are interpreted in the same way. These numbers can represent agreement between measurements taken by different testers (*intertester reliability*) or by the same tester (*intratester reliability*). A reliability coefficient is a number between 0 and 1.0, with 0 indicating no agreement and 1.0 indicating perfect agreement. Numbers that are closer to 1.0, such as .95, indicate better agreement than do numbers that are lower, such as .65. Portney and Watkins[2] recommended a general guideline for interpreting coefficients:

0 to .50 = poor reliability

.50 to .75 = moderate reliability

.75 to 1.0 = good reliability

What is an acceptable level of agreement for a case report? Portney and Watkins suggested that most clinical measurements should have a reliability of at least .90. Acceptable reliability depends on how precisely the variable can be measured and how the measurement will be interpreted and used. Remember that these estimates are only guidelines. For instance, if the reliability coefficient for a measure were .95, you could be reasonably confident that relatively small changes represent real change. If the coefficient were .70, however, relatively large changes would have to occur to indicate real change.

Here is a more specific example to help clarify this issue. If you state in a case report that a 2-degree change in ankle dorsiflexion indicates a meaningful change in range of motion, you have to provide some evidence that this small change represents a real change (and also that it means something to the patient's care or recovery). If you rely on the literature to support an argument for acceptable measurement reliability for a patient, you will find the following: If the same tester repeats the measure, a 2-degree change in dorsiflexion range of motion represents real change for many patients with limited dorsiflexion; however, if different therapists take the measurements, a 2-degree change is likely to be attributable to measurement error.[3,4] You also find that for this measure of range of motion, the intraclass correlation coefficient (ICC)—a statistic that indicates the degree of agreement between two or more measurements—is on the order of .90 when the same therapist repeats the measure (high intratester reliability). It is .50 or less when a different therapist repeats the measure (low intertester reliability). This suggests that small changes, such as 2 degrees, represent measurement error. If the measurement changed by 8 degrees, however, you could make a strong argument—based on the literature—that this change represents a real change in dorsiflexion range of motion. With a change as large as 8 degrees, it does not matter whether the same therapist or different therapists took the repeated measurements.

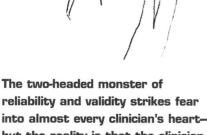

The two-headed monster of reliability and validity strikes fear into almost every clinician's heart—but the reality is that the clinician deals with that monster every day.

On the other hand, if the patient in the case is a child with spastic quadriplegic cerebral palsy, a change of 8 degrees may not represent real change. Harris et al[5] found that both intratester and intertester reliability showed wide daily variations; they concluded that even a change of 10 to 15 degrees probably does not represent real change.

How Can You Show That Your Measurements Are Reliable?

Strategy 1: Reference previously published reliability studies. This may be the most common and most sound way of providing evidence for acceptable reliability of measurements in a case report. Reliability studies usually are designed with large numbers of patients and therapists, which enhances the generalizability of the findings. Therapists who use measurements that have a pre-established level of reliability can be reasonably certain that their measurements are reliable, assuming that they followed the operational definitions or standardized procedures for the measurement. If you cite a previously published study to support the reliability of the measurements you obtained, make certain you explain how you followed the operational definitions or standardized procedures. It is also important to ensure that the measurements were taken by therapists who have been trained similarly to those who took the measurements in the previously published reliability study. As illustrated in the example above, the pertinent characteristics of the patient or patients in the case report also should be similar to those of the subjects in the reliability study.

Crum[6(p133)] described the incidence of temporomandibular joint (TMJ) dysfunction in a group of four patients who were wearing halo braces following a spinal cord injury. Here's how she supported the notion that the reliability of her measurements was adequate:

> Some other clinically meaningful observations are apparent in these four subjects. Agerberg established that vertical displacement changes of 4 mm and horizontal displacement changes of 2 mm should be the minimum amount of variation from previous measurements in order for clinicians to evaluate the response of the TMJ to treatment.[6]

Watson and Schenkman[7(p198)] referenced the literature to support the notion that the shoulder range-of-motion measurements obtained in their case report were reliable. The following excerpt from their case report also exemplifies the practical and clinical importance of differentiating between intratester and intertester reliability:

> Active range of motion (AROM) and passive range of motion (PROM) were measured using a universal goniometer. Goniometric measurements of shoulder PROM have high intratester reliability.[25] Boone and colleagues[26] concluded that the intratester reliability of goniometric measurements of upper-extremity AROM is higher than intertester reliability. As a result, they suggest that when more than one tester measures the same upper-extremity motion, changes in ROM should exceed 5 degrees in order to demonstrate improvement.[26] Intertester reliability is relevant, as this case report describes a patient who relocated to another state during the course of his treatment. His first 5 months of physical therapy measurement and treatment was done by one therapist, and the last 3 months was done by a second therapist.

Knowledge of the normal curve (**see opposite**) can help us understand how Harris and colleagues[8(p609)] provided evidence to support the reliability of measurements obtained using developmental indexes on five children exposed to alcohol prenatally:

> Both the Mental Developmental Index (MDI) and the Psychomotor Developmental Index (PDI) of the Bayley Scales have a mean of 100 and a standard deviation of 16.[13] The standard errors of measurement (68% confident intervals) for the MDI and PDI vary, depending on the infant's age at testing....

The authors subsequently reported the standard error of measurement (SE_{meas}) to substantiate the usefulness of the developmental measurements. The SE_{meas} is a reliability measure of response stability.[2] If a person is measured an infinite number of times, all of the measurements will not be exactly the same because measurement error always exists. The SE_{meas} provides a range of measurements within which the "real" score lies. If the SE_{meas} for a goniometric measurement were 5 degrees and the author obtained a measurement of 100 degrees, for instance, the therapist could be reasonably confident (68% of the time, which relates to ± 1 standard deviation) that the real measurement lies between 95 degrees and 105 degrees. The therapist could be 96% confident (± 2 standard deviations) that the real measurement lies between 90 degrees and 110 degrees. If the therapist repeated the measurement 2 weeks later and the motion increased to 125 degrees, the therapist could be confident, at both the 68% and 96% confidence intervals, that the change was real and not due to error. The SE_{meas}, then, allows the therapist to make decisions about whether measured change is likely to represent real change.

If the therapist wants to derive the error associated with a change score (eg, the difference between a preintervention and a postintervention measurement), the SE_{meas} value must be multiplied by the square root of 2 because both measurements contribute error to the change score.[9] If the SE_{meas} in the above example were 5 degrees and the therapist took two measurements and found a change of 5 degrees, this change would probably be due to error because both measurements contribute error to the change score.

Unfortunately, with the exception of norm-referenced scales for children, the SE_{meas} has not been documented extensively in our literature, so therapists do not have many opportunities to use it. Future research should determine the SE_{meas} for the measures commonly used in clinical practice.

You can find published reliability studies through a literature search. To give you a head start, **Appendix 2** provides references for some of the studies that have been published on the reliability of many measurements used with a variety of patients.

Strategy 2: Conduct a mini-reliability study. When measures have not been adequately studied previously for reliability, you can do a mini-reliability study as part of the case report. When Gross and Schuch[10(p74)] examined the usefulness of a strengthening exercise program for a patient with a diagnosis of post-polio syn-

Using "The Curve"

Remember worrying about being graded "on the curve" at school? The curve also is important for understanding a standard error of measurement (SE_{meas}), such as the one that Harris et al[1] reported for the Bayley Scales. The "normal" curve is a distribution of measurements in which most of the people have the middle measurement and fewer people have the lower and higher measurements. In physical therapy, such distributions of measurements are most often found for developmental tests used with children. If measurements are taken on enough subjects, however, a distribution of measurements could be derived for anything—scores of 6-month-old infants on a motor development test, 50-yard dash times of junior high boys, or hip abduction range of motion. (For more information about distributions of measurements, refer to the hip abduction example in the *Primer on Measurement*,[2] an excellent resource for case report writers.)

When measurements are normally distributed, the familiar bell-shaped curve results. In our example, the mean (average) measurement is 100. The curve also shows that the mode (the most frequently occurring measurement) and the median (the middle measurement) of a normal distribution are the same as the mean.

Another measurement concept that is important to understand is the standard deviation of a distribution of measurements. The standard

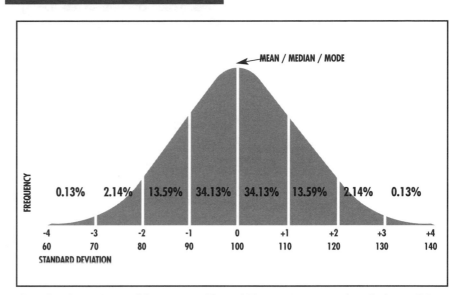

Adapted with permission of the American Physical Therapy Association from Rothstein JM, Echternach JL. *Primer on Measurement: An Introductory Guide to Measurement Issues.* Alexandria, Va: American Physical Therapy Association; 1993.

deviation tells us how variable the measurements are within the distribution. If, for example, we know that a mean measurement is 100 and we have a patient who measures 90, is 90 within the "normal" range or not? We can't tell without knowing about how much the distribution of scores varied. The curve above shows a theoretical mean of 100 and a standard deviation of 10. Knowing that the standard deviation is 10 allows us to interpret the patient's measurement. We know that approximately 68% (34.13% + 34.13%) of all measurements of the population from which the measurements were derived will be between 1 standard deviation below the mean (-1 on the chart) and 1 standard deviation above the mean (+1

on the chart). If the mean is 100 and the standard deviation is 10, then 68% of measurements were between 90 and 110. Looking at it another way, a score of 90 is 1 standard deviation below the mean, which means that it is higher than 15.86% (0.13% + 2.14% + 13.59%) of measurements and lower than 84.14% (34.13% + 34.13% + 13.59% + 2.14% + 0.13%) of measurements.

References

1 Harris SR, Osborn JA, Weinberg J, et al. Effects of prenatal alcohol exposure on neuromotor and cognitive development during early childhood: a series of case reports. *Phys Ther.* 1993;73:608-617.

2 Rothstein JM, Echternach JL. *Primer on Measurement: An Introductory Guide to Measurement Issues.* Alexandria, Va: American Physical Therapy Association; 1993:42.

drome, they performed a mini-reliability study and successfully provided evidence of adequate reliability:

> One of the authors (MTG) has evaluated the reliability of this testing protocol for another investigation (in progress). Six subjects were tested twice with the previously described protocol, with two days separating the testing sessions. Each subject provided an extension and a flexion peak torque measurement for each leg at both test velocities, for a total of eight observations per subject. The Pearson product-moment correlation coefficient for 48 repeated measurements of peak torque was .93 and the mean difference between repeated measurements was 6.1 ft·lb....

Reliability estimates from mini-reliability studies are more limited than those from larger reliability studies, and the number of subjects in a mini-reliability study is usually too small to generalize to other settings. Whenever possible, therefore, larger reliability studies still should be referenced.

A mini-reliability study is not difficult to do. It just takes some time to set up the study and to obtain and analyze the repeated measurements. The purpose of the mini-reliability study is to determine the consistency of measurements taken more than once by the same clinician (intratester reliability) or taken by two or more clinicians (intertester reliability).

When two sets of measurements are taken by one tester, it is important to "mask" the results from the tester if remembering the measurement could cause bias. When measuring range of motion, for example, tape can be placed over the numbers on the side of the goniometer visible to the tester, and another clinician can read and record the results. Some measurements are difficult or impossible to mask and easy to remember. In these cases, the better course of action might be to determine intertester reliability. Intertester reliability should also be determined when more than one clinician is taking measurements throughout a patient's course of care.

The type of statistical analysis used depends on the type of data and other factors that are too numerous to explain in this manual. The book by Portney and Watkins[2] is one good source of information about reliability studies and should be useful for clinicians who have minimal background in research design and statistics. Other research and statistics texts also can give good advice. If you don't feel up to dealing with a mini-reliability study on your own, don't hesitate to ask for help from local university faculty or other colleagues with knowledge in this area.

Strategy 3: Make a presumptive argument. With this strategy, the author essentially develops a theoretical argument that supports the notion that the measurement adequately represents the variable of interest and has an acceptable level of reliability. This method should be the method of last resort, however, and should be used only when published reliability studies do not exist and it is not possible to do a mini-reliability study (eg, when reporting a case retrospectively).

Selby[11(p1922)] made a presumptive argument for the reliability of her measurements of a child's gait pattern:

> Heel contacts were at first assessed by observation of the child's gait and by calculating the ratio of the number of heel contacts to the number of steps. This method proved fairly difficult and unreliable, so videotapes were taken of the child from a sagittal view with a video camera placed in a fixed position on a tripod. The videotaped portion of the child's 30-ft walk gathered data for between three and four steady-state steps of the entire walk. Samplings from three of the child's walks were recorded for three conditions: 1) barefoot, 2) wearing sneakers, and 3) wearing orthoses and sneakers. To avoid the possibility of the child introducing artificial attempts to attain or not attain heel strike, attention was not called to the video camera or to the section of the walk recorded on the videotape. The recording of a walk was considered usable if the child was not skipping, running, or performing any other form of play.

Selby operationally defined what constituted an acceptable trial by stating that trials in which the child was running or skipping were not analyzed. She theorized that because the video system was nonintrusive and was used to gather multiple samples of the child's true gait, the measurements were likely to be reliable and reflective of the child's true gait pattern.

Presumptive arguments for reliability were also made in a case report written by Watson and Schenkman,[7(p198)] who made two presumptive arguments to support the use of manual muscle testing and videotaping for a patient with paralysis of the serratus anterior muscle:

> Manual muscle testing (MMT) was performed using the system described by Daniels and Worthingham.[23] The reliability of MMT grades has not been well established.[24] Manual muscle testing, however, is an integral part of the physical examination and provides information that is useful in the diagnosis, prognosis, and treatment of neuromuscular disorders.[19]

> Visual observation was used for assessment of general muscle symmetry and to assess the movement of this patient's scapula specifically. Goniometric measures were not used because it is difficult to reproduce the reference point on which to measure scapular motion.[27] The patient's active shoulder flexion and abduction were also videotaped during his second and seventh visits to physical therapy. Videotaping made it possible to slow down the motion for more accurate visualization of the shoulder biomechanics and to record the subtle changes in scapular AROM [active range of motion] on film.

An acceptable presumptive argument often is simply an explanation of what you do in the clinic to ensure that measurement error is minimized. Depending on the type of measurement and your knowledge of likely sources of measurement error, you could explain how you ensured that the patient was positioned in the same way each time, was always measured at the same time of day, or was measured by the same therapist each time (intratester reliability is usually higher than intertester reliability) using written operational definitions of the measurement procedure. Most presumptive arguments simply describe good clinical measurement practices.

If a strong case can be made for the reliability of the measurements, the validity of the measurements is the next issue to be faced. It's important to remember that measurements can be reliable even if they are not valid, but they cannot be valid if they are not reliable. Validity of measurements in a case report, like reliability of measurements, can usually be handled adequately by descriptions of sound practice and clinical reasoning.

Validity: Using Measurement in Clinical Decisions

The concept of validity may seem elusive, but all it really means is how a measurement is used in making clinical decisions.

The validity of a measurement can be an elusive concept to understand. *Standards for Tests and Measurements in Physical Therapy Practice*[1] defines validity as the "degree to which a useful (meaningful) interpretation can be inferred from a measurement." The concept of validity relates to what the measurement is used for and how it is used in making decisions. There are two broad types of validity: criterion-based and theory-based (**Table 2**).

Criterion-based forms of validity. This type of validity relates to the direct testing of how well a measurement reflects what it is designed to reflect. Does a test purported to measure balance, for example, produce measurements that reflect the construct of balance, or do the measurements *really* reflect a patient's ability to understand instructions? Does a test developed to identify newborn infants who will later be diagnosed as having cerebral palsy succeed in this prediction? Does performance on a functional limitation test in the clinic relate to a patient's performance at home? **Table 2** includes definitions of some types of criterion-based validity (concurrent validity, predictive validity, and prescriptive validity). These and other forms of criterion-based validity are discussed thoroughly in the *Primer on Measurement*[12] and in other references.

The criterion-based forms of validity are studied directly in research by comparing the measurement of interest to an already validated measurement, or the *criterion measurement*. The extent of validity of the measurement is assessed by determining how well the measurement of interest correlates with the criterion measurement. The correlation coefficients are interpreted in the same way that reliability coefficients are interpreted, with correlations closer to 1.0 indicating a stronger relationship between the measurement of interest and the criterion measurement. If, for example, children's scores on a new quick test of motor development had a correlation coefficient of .90 with an established test of motor development, the quick test would have strong concurrent validity with the criterion test and might be used in place of it. On the other hand, if the correlation between the height of basketball players' vertical jump on one foot and the number of rebounds during the season was .25, vertical jump would have poor predictive validity for number of rebounds.

Table 2. Definitions and Examples of Types of Validity[a]

Criterion-Based Forms of Validity		Theoretical Forms of Validity	
Concurrent validity:	Inferred interpretations are justified by comparing a measurement with supporting evidence that was obtained at approximately the same time that the measurement being validated was obtained. If measurements using a simple and inexpensive test to detect balance problems could be shown to be related to measurements using sophisticated and expensive equipment, the simple test then could be used in place of and interpreted like the expensive test because the tests have good *concurrent validity*.	**Construct validity:**	The conceptual (theoretical) basis for using a measurement to make an inferred interpretation. Knowledge of reflexes, the nervous system, and neuropathology could provide a theoretical basis for the development of both a testing procedure (eg, the reflex hammer) and a measurement (eg, the reflex response). This knowledge, a theoretical underpinning, is the *construct* on which the test and measurement are developed.
Predictive validity:	Inferred interpretations are justified by comparing a measurement with supporting evidence obtained at a later point in time. That is, *predictive validity* involves the justification of the use of a measurement to say something about future events or conditions. We frequently base our decisions on tests that we assume predict the future, but little evidence exists to support the predictive validity of many of these tests. Do preseason screenings of football players, motor assessments of infants, and preemployment tests actually predict later performance or injury?	**Content validity:**	A theoretical form of validity that deals with the extent to which a measurement is judged to reflect the meaningful elements of a construct and not any extraneous elements. Content validity is closely related to construct validity. The "construct" of balance could be defined with knowledge of structures and mechanisms believed to contribute to balance. The *content validity* of a test to measure balance would then be judged by its ability to measure the relevant structures and mechanisms, and not extra elements that don't relate to balance or conflicting elements, such as a patient's ability to follow instructions.
Prescriptive validity:	Inferred interpretation of a measurement is the determination of the form of intervention that a person is to receive. That is, *prescriptive validity* is justified based on the successful outcome of the chosen intervention. If results of a test to determine the cause of patients' low back pain led to a specific intervention that resulted in patients' return to work, the test would have prescriptive validity.		

[a]Information adapted from Rothstein JM, Echternach JL. *Primer on Measurement: An Introductory Guide to Measurement Issues.* Alexandria, Va: American Physical Therapy Association; 1993.

The research literature supporting the criterion-related forms of validity is, for the most part, lacking. Most authors of case reports therefore have addressed validity by either referencing the theories of others or by discussing the theoretical bases for the meaningfulness of the measurements used in the report.

Theoretical arguments for why a measurement is useful. The theory that supports the use of a measurement may be based on anatomical, biomechanical, physiological, or psychological concepts. The two theoretical forms of validity are construct validity and content validity (**Table 2**). Construct validity and content validity are so closely related that case report authors can often address both forms of validity by describing the theoretical basis of the tests and then clearly relating the testing procedures to that theoretical basis.

Discussions of the theoretical forms of validity of measurements obtained in a case report may appear in the introduction to the case. Anderson and Tichenor[13] described the theoretical bases supporting the construct validity for upper-limb tension tests, a series of tests used to determine if the cervical nerve roots and peripheral nerves are contributing to the patient's complaints. The authors then operationally defined the tests that were used to collect data on a patient with a diagnosis of de Quervain tenosynovitis. The operational definitions gave support for the content validity of the tests, which were logically related to the theoretical basis of the construct being tested.

In the introduction of their case report, McClure and Flowers[14] discussed what they perceived to be flaws in the theoretical bases for measurements of accessory motion in joints. They used their theoretical arguments to serve as the basis for recommending an alternative examination and intervention program for a patient with limited motion of the shoulder.

Authors also may reference the work of others when addressing the validity of a measurement. Gill-Body and colleagues[15(p130)] dealt with both the theoretical and criterion-based forms of validity of some of their measurement procedures:

> The medical workup for each patient just prior to physical therapy consisted of a neurological examination by a neurologist... and posturography testing utilizing the Equitest™ system.[15,16] Each patient also underwent a three-dimensional movement analysis in our biomotion laboratory. A full-body kinematic and kinetic analysis of key activities of daily living (ADLs) (standing, free and paced gait, walking in place, ascending steps, and rising from a chair) was completed.[17,18]

Although the types of validity that the authors supported by citing the work of others is not entirely clear, it appears that the two references following mention of the equipment support the theoretical basis (construct validity and content validity) for the posturography test and that the other two references support the criterion-based validity of the kinematic and kinetic analysis. The type of criterion-based validity is not clear unless the reader looks up the references.

Malouin et al[16(p782)] referenced the work of others to substantiate the theoretical and criterion-based forms of validity of two of the measurements used in their case report. They examined the usefulness of an intensive gait training program for a series of 10 patients diagnosed with an acute cerebrovascular accident:

> The functional level and the sensorimotor performance of the patients, as measured 5 to 7 days after stroke with the Barthel Index[13] and Fugl-Meyer stroke assessment scale,[14] are reported in Table 1. On the basis of the scores obtained from the initial Barthel Index evaluation, the patients were placed in either a poor (score <20) or a good (score ≥20) prognosis group.

Presumptive arguments for why a measurement has validity. Just as presumptive arguments can be given for reliability, they can be given for validity. In a case report describing a task-oriented approach to the rehabilitation of a patient with left-sided hemiplegia, Flinn[17(p563)] wrote:

> Although the validity of manual muscle testing (MMT) (Daniels & Worthingham, 1980) in cases of central nervous system deficit has been questioned in the presence of abnormal tone (Bobath, 1990; Daniels & Worthingham, 1980; Davies, 1985), there is support for using MMT as one component of evaluation for clients with central nervous system dysfunction (Bohannon, 1989). MMT was used in this case because weakness was hypothesized to be the critical control parameter for this client's function. Therefore, some measurement of that critical control parameter was essential.

The author of a case report may deal with both reliability and validity in the same discussion. When Watson and Schenkman[7] argued for the use of videotaping the shoulder range of motion of the patient with paralysis of the serratus anterior muscle, they based their argument on issues related to both reliability and validity, suggesting that the videotape data were more reliable than goniometric measurements and stating that the videotape data better reflected the variable of interest (movement of the scapula).

What Outcome Measurements Should You Report?

A discussion of validity in a case report would not be complete without addressing this question. When an author describes the patient's outcome in a case report, the strongest argument the author can make to support the possible value of the intervention is to thoroughly describe the changes in the patient's functional abilities. Descriptions of changes in impairments (eg, range of motion, force production, pain level) alone should not be used to measure patient outcomes. Measurements of impairment may have changed but may not be related to functional gains (ie, may not have concurrent validity with functional ability); functional gains measured in the clinic may not predict performance at home (ie, may have poor predictive validity). In a case report, it can be important to report changes that relate to patients' impairments—but it is even more important to report changes in functional limitations and disability. (For more on this, see **Chapter 5**.)

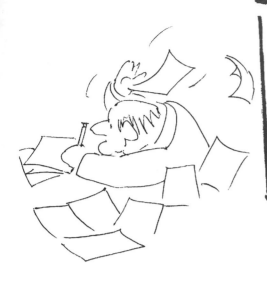

Next: Putting Words on Paper

You've chosen your case, thought out your focus, operationalized your definitions, considered issues of reliability and validity. Now it's time to write! The hardest part about writing is getting started, and nothing creates writer's block more than when you sit down to begin at the beginning. Words that once flowed so effortlessly through your mind may disappear when you are faced with a blank first page. This manual starts with the introduction because it comes first in the manuscript. But feel free to begin writing wherever you like.

References

1 *Standards for Tests and Measurements in Physical Therapy Practice.* Alexandria, Va: American Physical Therapy Association; 1991.

2 Portney LG, Watkins MP. *Foundations of Clinical Research: Applications to Practice.* 2nd ed. Upper Saddle River, NJ: Prentice Hall Health; 2000.

3 Elveru RA, Rothstein JM, Lamb RL. Goniometric reliability in a clinical setting: subtalar and ankle measurements. *Phys Ther.* 1988;68:672-677.

4 Youdas JW, Bogard CL, Suman VJ. Reliability of goniometric measurements and visual estimates of ankle joint range of motion obtained in a clinical setting. *Arch Phys Med Rehabil.* 1993;74:1113-1118.

5 Harris SR, Smith LH, Krukowski L. Goniometric reliability for a child with spastic quadriplegia. *J Pediatr Orthop.* 1985;5:348-351.

6 Crum NA. Signs of temporomandibular joint dysfunction in spinal cord injured patients wearing halo braces: a clinical report. *Phys Ther.* 1990;70:132-137.

7 Watson CJ, Schenkman M. Physical therapy management of isolated serratus anterior muscle paralysis. *Phys Ther.* 1995;75:194-202.

8 Harris SR, Osborn JA, Weinberg J, et al. Effects of prenatal alcohol exposure on neuromotor and cognitive development during early childhood: a series of case reports. *Phys Ther.* 1993;73:608-617.

9 Ottenbacher KJ, Johnson MB, Hojem M. The significance of clinical change and clinical change of significance: issues and methods. *Am J Occup Ther.* 1988;42:156-163.

10 Gross MT, Schuch CP. Exercise programs for patients with post-polio syndrome: a case report. *Phys Ther.* 1989;69:72-76.

11 Selby L. Remediation of toe-walking behavior with neutral-position, serial-inhibitory casts: a case report. *Phys Ther.* 1988;68:1921-1923.

12 Rothstein JM, Echternach JL. *Primer on Measurement: An Introductory Guide to Measurement Issues.* Alexandria, Va: American Physical Therapy Association; 1993.

13 Anderson M, Tichenor CJ. A patient with de Quervain's tenosynovitis: a case report using an Australian approach to manual therapy. *Phys Ther.* 1994;74:314-326.

14 McClure PW, Flowers KR. Treatment of limited shoulder motion: a case study based on biomechanical considerations. *Phys Ther.* 1992;72:929-936.

15 Gill-Body KM, Krebs DE, Parker SW, Riley PO. Physical therapy management of peripheral vestibular dysfunction: two clinical case reports. *Phys Ther.* 1994;74:129-142.

16 Malouin F, Potvin M, Prévost J, et al. Use of an intensive task-oriented gait training program in a series of patients with acute cerebrovascular accidents. *Phys Ther.* 1992;72:781-793.

17 Flinn N. A task-oriented approach to the treatment of a client with hemiplegia. *Am J Occup Ther.* 1995;49:560-569.

Part 2

START WRITING!

"Writing is a rough trade. *D'abord, il faut durer.*

[Above all, hang in there]."

Ernest Hemingway

Chapter 5

"The Introduction": Making the Case for Your Case

The introduction is the first part of a case report, after the title and abstract (more about titles and abstracts later—they're easier to write once you've written the rest of the case report). The introduction is followed by the case description (**Chapter 6**), the outcomes section (**Chapter 7**), and the discussion (**Chapter 8**). For a detailed checklist of the important components of a case report, refer to **Appendix 3**. Using the checklist will help you keep on track as you write your report.

The introduction of a case report sets the stage. Not only does it "introduce" the topic of the case and explain why the case is important, but it communicates to the reader that there is sufficient support or rationale for the management aspects of the case. Clear and credible rationale is needed—regardless of whether the purpose of the report is to describe an unusual case, share information about an intervention, or cast doubt on a theory. The introduction should clearly explain:

■ Why the topic is important

■ What is known—and not known—about the topic

■ The theoretical context for the case

■ The support that exists for the management aspects of the case

■ The gap in the literature that the case report will fill

■ The purpose of the case report

How long should the introduction be? Most case reports are about 15 typed double-spaced pages in length, or approximately 3,700 words. As a rough guide-

Just as mystery writers supply motives for what their characters do, case report writers should supply a rationale for what the therapist does.

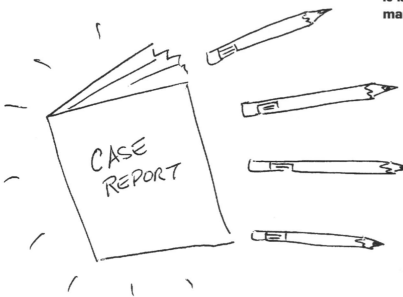

Introduction:

Introduces the topic of the case and states why it is important, citing literature to support the management of the case.

Case Description:

Includes information about the patient, situation, or other entity; the examination; the hypothesis about cause; and the intervention.

Outcomes Section:

Describes the status of the patient, situation, or other entity after the intervention.

Discussion:

Reflects on possible explanations for what happened and gives suggestions for future research.

line, allow 800 to 1,300 words for the introduction, 1,500 to 2,000 words for the case description, 250 to 500 words for the outcomes section, and 800 words for the discussion. The actual length of each section will depend, of course, on the amount of material that has to be covered for the purposes of your case report.

Start With Your Knowledge of Practice

Most introductions start by clearly explaining why the topic is an important one. In a case report on an intervention for motion sickness, Rine and colleagues[1] made an immediate, focused argument about the lack of information on management of motion sickness:

> Investigations that have examined the symptoms, predictors, and causes of motion sickness and the underlying mechanisms involved in motion sickness have revealed that a conflict of visual and vestibular information, as it relates to postural control and visual stabilization, is a critical factor.[1-8] Despite these reports and recent interest in postural control and clinical intervention for individuals with dizziness or vertigo,[5,7,8] little information exists about evaluation or effective treatment to ameliorate the symptoms of motion sickness, except as it relates to astronauts and pilots.[3,6,9-13]

In the first few sentences of their introduction, Rine et al accomplished two tasks: They gave a rationale for the importance of their topic (lack of information about examination, evaluation, and intervention for motion sickness), and they set the stage for their subsequent discussion of the definition of motion sickness, the

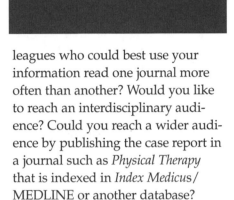

Who's Your Audience?

Where do you want to publish? It may seem premature to ask this question, but it's not. Different journals have different audiences and different requirements, and that has a bearing on how you write your case report. Find out which journals publish case reports, then read several reports in each journal to determine whether your case is more like those published in one journal than in another. *Physical Therapy*, for instance, publishes case reports across the broad spectrum of physical therapist practice; other journals may be more specialized. Do the colleagues who could best use your information read one journal more often than another? Would you like to reach an interdisciplinary audience? Could you reach a wider audience by publishing the case report in a journal such as *Physical Therapy* that is indexed in *Index Medicus/MEDLINE* or another database?

Once you have decided on a journal, you can "customize" your report according to the style and readership of that journal. Obtain a copy of the journal's instructions for authors, and follow them carefully. Most journals, including *Physical Therapy* (**Appendix 1**), publish instructions for authors on a regular basis. Instructions also can be obtained by contacting the journal's editorial office, which usually is listed on the masthead page of each issue, or by accessing the journal's Web site. Instructions include referencing style, limitations on the number of pages, formats for tables and figures, how to write the cover page, and requirements for the abstract.

mechanisms involved in motion sickness, and the support for their own examination, evaluation, and intervention procedures. The authors' approach is clear and direct—and it is very likely to capture the attention of readers who work with patients who have motion sickness.

The background and justification of your case come in part from your knowledge of practice. That knowledge is shaped by a process of trial and error—as you observe what goes wrong and what works—and by a process of inquiry, which begins when you ask yourself such questions as, "*Why* is there no change with this intervention?" and "*Why* did this particular way of stretching make such a difference in this patient's pain and function?" The inquiry process continues when you share your observations with colleagues and try to find explanations for what you have seen. But even though sharing anecdotes in the clinic can help stimulate ideas about how to introduce your case, those ideas cannot stand alone.

A Critical Review of the Literature

The trial-and-error process and the intuition of the clinician are extremely important sources of knowledge for understanding practice and for building a foundation for future research. An even more highly valued source of knowledge comes from research using the scientific method.[2] If knowledge derived from trial and error and intuition is to make a meaningful contribution to the professional knowledge base, it must be placed in the context of existing literature—preferably the research literature. A common saying among investigators in many fields is that "one must stand on the shoulders of giants to see farther." The scientific literature provides the "shoulders" on which the evidence base of practice can be built.

Case reports start with a "clinical claim." You've already searched the literature to determine whether your case can contribute something new to the profession; now you must go one step further to find out what is known or not known about your clinical claim. Based on their clinical experience, Riddle and Freeman[3] made the following claim in a case report:

> A major problem when treating aerobic dancers is identifying the underlying cause for the development of their symptoms. We believe that the reason for the development of the symptoms must be identified before an effective treatment can be initiated. The purpose of this report is to describe the method we used in determining when orthoses might be an effective treatment modality for a patient with a diagnosis of bilateral plantar fasciitis and Achilles tendinitis.

Riddle and Freeman did not stop there. They went on to explain and support their claim with knowledge reported in the literature. The literature that they needed to cover is clear from their claim: They needed support for the likely cause of their patient's symptoms, support for the use of examination procedures to identify the cause, and rationale for the use of orthoses to treat the cause.

Even if you find cases similar to yours in the literature, you may have different outcomes to report or another clinical claim or perspective to offer. In an introduction to multiple-patient case reports, for example, Harris et al[4(p609)] stated, "Although a number of published studies have described neonatal behavioral differences in infants with FAS [fetal alcohol syndrome][3-5] as well as developmental motor outcomes...none of these reports have provided assessment data collected at repeated intervals...." After making this claim, Harris et al had to report the literature describing neonatal behavioral differences and developmental motor outcomes in infants with FAS and the literature supporting the need for repeated assessment data.

In the literature review incorporated into the introduction of a case report on postoperative management of flexor pollicis longus tendon laceration, Ahlschwede[5] provided a table that contained a summary comparison of protocols that had been published in the literature (**Table 3**). As you'll see in subsequent chapters, tables (and figures) can be a useful way to convey information in case reports.

You may envision long hours in the library trying to uncover everything that has been written on your topic, but, as shown in **Chapter 3**, that isn't the purpose of a case report's literature review. The introduction should simply provide evidence of the process of inquiry that you used to enhance your understanding of your particular case.

Table 3. Example of a Tabular Summary of Literature Review Findings[a]

Comparison of Flexor Tendon Protocols

No. of Weeks After Repair	Protocol			
	Immobilization	Duran[b]	Kleinert[c]	Washingtor[d]
1	Immobilization in cast—moderate flexion	Dorsal block splint—wrist 20°, MP 45°, IP neutral, passive ROM to affected digit	Dorsal block splint—wrist 45°, MP 50°, IP relaxed, active extension against traction	Dorsal block splint—wrist 45°, MP 40°, IP 0°, active extension against traction, protected passive ROM to affected digit
3	Discontinue cast, begin active ROM	Continue same	Passive ROM if contracture	Continue same
4	Continue active flexion and extension	Begin active ROM in splint	Allow more wrist extension in splint	Continue same
5	Passive extension as tolerated, no splint	Discontinue splint	Discontinue splint, add wrist cuff	Discontinue traction, full active ROM in splint
6	Dynamic splint for more extension, if needed	Continue active exercise	Unrestricted active ROM	More wrist extension
7	—	—	—	Discontinue splint, allow light use
8	—	Strengthening	Strengthening	Blocking, graded resistance
12	Full, normal activity	Full, normal activity	Full, normal activity	Full, normal activity

Note. MP = metacarpophalangeal joint; IP = intercarpophalangeal joint; ROM = range of motion.

[a]Reprinted with permission of the American Occupational Therapy Association from Ahlschwede K. Postoperative management of flexor pollicis longus laceration in two cases. *Am J Occup Ther*. 1991;45:361-365.

[b](Duran, Houser, Coleman, & Stover, 1984) [c](Jaeger & Mackin, 1984). [d](Chow et al., 1987).

The process of inquiry involves critically reviewing the literature—with the emphasis on *critically*. Depoy and Gitlin[6] recommended using three questions to assist in a critical review of the literature:

1. What work has already been done on this topic or related topics? Is that work relevant to your case?

2. How has the existing knowledge been generated (eg, research versus someone's opinion)? How strong is the evidence for the truth of the knowledge?

3. What theory exists to provide a framework for the case?

Let's look at how these questions may apply in real life. Imagine that you are Anderson and Tichenor[7] and that you believe that a particular manual therapy approach to a patient with de Quervain tenosynovitis and carpal tunnel syndrome is worth reporting. As you prepare to "make your case for your case," you must critically review the literature.

Question #1:
What Work Has Already Been Done—and Is It Relevant?

The first step in any literature review is to identify the key topic areas. Depending on the patient's problem, several topics may apply, and there may be a large amount of supporting literature—or no literature at all. Begin by setting some parameters.

Posterior Thigh Pain in a Patient With Low Back Pain

Introduction of the Topic and Statement of Its Importance

Consider the following statement:

> Patients with leg pain are commonly treated in the clinic. Some of these patients benefit from stretching exercises to break adhesions in scar tissue that prevent nerve structures from gliding. Therefore, therapists need to incorporate stretching exercises in programs for patients with leg pain.

What does this statement tell you? Based on this statement, can you determine that the focus of the case report will be on patients with back pain who also have leg pain? Is it clear that there may be a variety of treatment approaches to consider, and that identifying the source of the problem is an important factor in selecting interventions? Compare with this statement:

> Patients with low back pain report a variety of symptoms. Complaint of pain in the thigh is often one of the problems. Patients who report pain in the thigh as part of their back problem may require different forms of treatment depending on the factors that are thought to be responsible for the thigh pain. Developing a hypothesis for why the thigh pain exists, based on examination findings, may help guide intervention decisions and improve treatment effectiveness for these patients.

The above statement expresses the importance of the case report, that is, that individuals with back pain may also have leg pain and that there may be a variety of ways to manage the patient, depending on the source of the leg pain.

Anderson and Tichenor[7] identified several key topics for their literature review. They started by citing data from the US Department of Labor Statistics to support the importance of de Quervain tenosynovitis and carpal tunnel syndrome as patient problems. They then reviewed literature on 1) clinical signs, symptoms, and pathophysiology of de Quervain tenosynovitis; 2) pathophysiology and diagnostic tests; and 3) clinical signs and symptoms and pathophysiology of carpal tunnel syndrome. Next, the authors used the literature to support their opinion that entrapment of a nerve may make it susceptible to further injury at sites either proximal or distal to the entrapment. This claim was followed by literature citations that built a case for using upper-limb tension tests in examination and intervention for patients with de Quervain tenosynovitis and carpal tunnel syndrome. Finally, the authors described how to administer and interpret the upper-limb tension tests. (Tests may be described in the introduction when, as in this case report, the examination is one of the case report's focuses. Otherwise, tests usually are included in the case description.)

Posterior Thigh Pain in a Patient With Low Back Pain

Literature Review

In the introduction, the writer must develop a theoretical argument for why tests that examine the patient's response to stretching of tissues are important. As this author's outline shows, the complete literature review would include:

- Review of previously published literature that has described these tests for the lower extremity.
- Review of literature examining the reliability and validity of these tests for the lower extremity.
- Description of how the theoretical basis for tests that examine the patient's response to stretching guides treatment decisions, using references as bases for a discussion of the following:
  - how tissue injury could lead to shortened connective tissue structures.
  - how shortened connective tissue could result in functional limitation or disability.
  - how controlled forces applied for a predetermined period of time (treatment) could have a beneficial effect on the shortened structures.

The literature review would be incomplete or inadequate when:

The theoretical basis for the case is discussed only by the use of secondary references. When reviewing a textbook, for instance, the writer may find that a research report was cited to support a given issue. The research report would be the primary reference and the textbook would be the secondary reference. When possible, it is the primary reference that should be cited.

The cited literature does not relate to the case. A lengthy discussion on the incidence of low back pain and various causes of low back pain may include many references, but all the references in the world cannot make the literature review better if they do not relate to the purpose of the case report (in this case, treating leg pain associated with low back pain).

The theoretical basis for the examination or intervention is not discussed. Examination procedures and interventions are described without justifying the reasons for selecting these procedures and interventions.

Note that Anderson and Tichenor covered literature that related directly to their topic. They did not include irrelevant or marginally relevant information. They didn't review the research on surgical approaches, for example, or even the research on other physical therapy approaches. Although such information is related to the topic, the authors didn't need to include it to achieve their stated purpose of illustrating "the interrelationship among examination, assessment, and treatment response in the Australian approach to manual therapy"[7(p314)] for patients with de Quervain tenosynovitis and carpal tunnel syndrome.

Again, you don't have to cite every article or book chapter related to your topic, but you should give a fair overview of the most recent and credible work. Identifying the key concepts will help you to develop the rationale for your case, regardless of how much or how little is known. For instance:

■ In a case report on aerobic exercise for a patient with chronic multiple impairments, Kinney LaPier et al[8] provided a "light" review of the literature in their introduction. Because almost no literature existed on their topic, their introduction included summary statements about the literature that was relevant to 1) deconditioning associated with chronic disorders, 2) intensity, duration, and frequency of exercise required to produce a training effect in people who are deconditioned, and 3) adaptation of exercise for people with disabilities. The authors then proceeded to state the purpose of their case report, which was to "illustrate the process used to develop an exercise prescription to enhance aerobic capacity in a patient with chronic multisystem impairments."[8(p418)]

■ In a case report on a patient with limited shoulder motion, McClure and Flowers[9] wrote a "heavy" literature review. Their case report had two purposes: 1) to describe the management of the patient and 2) to cast doubt on a frequently applied theory—the concave-convex rule in arthrokinematic movements. The second purpose required a comprehensive literature review, one in which the authors discussed in detail the specific studies that supported their criticism of the theory.

As you read various journals, note that the extent of the literature review varies among case reports. Remember that, regardless of length, the purpose of the introduction is to provide the rationale and foundation that underlie the purpose of your case report.

Question #2:
How Has the Existing Knowledge Been Generated?

In your search of the literature, have you found case reports, people's opinions, or research? The more credible your sources of information, the more credible your introduction will be. Although case reports and people's opinions can stimulate and provide some support for your ideas, they are not highly credible sources of knowledge. Research is by far the best source of knowledge. Not all research is equal, however; the credibility of research and the ways in which it can be interpreted depend on the type and quality of the research design.

How can a clinician with minimal research background make decisions about the quality of research design during a literature search? Ask yourself this key question: Is the research descriptive or explanatory? *Descriptive* studies, as explained in Chapter 1, disclose existing conditions or examine relationships among variables without manipulating them. *Descriptive studies cannot identify cause-and-effect relationships.* These studies often use only descriptive statistics (eg, means, standard deviations, frequency, minimum, and maximum) or tests of association (eg, correlation or regression). In interpreting these studies, the following caution for statistics students can be helpful to clinicians as well: Correlation does not equal causality! For instance, just because a study finds a statistically significant negative correlation between body weight and amount of exercise—with people who weigh more doing less exercise than people who weigh less—we can't say that weight causes people to exercise less or that more exercise causes less weight.

Explanatory studies, on the other hand, are experimental studies in which the researcher manipulates the experimental variables while controlling potentially confounding variables. Experimental studies therefore can determine cause-and-effect relationships. The strength of the evidence is stronger for studies that randomly assign subjects to intervention and comparison groups than it is for studies that do not use random assignment. You may be able to tell whether a study is explanatory by the types of statistical tests that are used, such as *t* tests and analyses of variance (ANOVAs).

Another easy way to address the quality of the design without knowing much about research is to answer a related question: Is the study published in a peer-reviewed journal, or is it published in a professional magazine or journal that is not peer reviewed? Articles in peer-reviewed journals are critically reviewed both by reviewers who have expertise in the topic area and by journal editors (see **Chapters 3 and 10**). That is not to say that the research published in peer-reviewed journals never has design flaws—most research does. But when an article has passed peer review, you can expect that the flaws are not so serious that they would jeopardize the credibility of the study.

As part of your evaluation of the literature, be sure to read the discussion sections of research articles, in which the authors often identify the design flaws for you and discuss how those flaws affect interpretation of the results.

In their case report, Anderson and Tichenor cited several journal articles in the description and diagnosis of de Quervain tenosynovitis and carpal tunnel syndrome. Because upper-limb tension testing was a relatively new examination and intervention procedure, however, description and support of the procedure had to come from *generalizing literature* on the examination of the lower quarter (straight leg raising), books, and conference proceedings. The credibility of the case report would have been stronger if the authors had been able to support their approach with good-quality research articles. As is often the case in rehabilitation, however, such research was not available.

How did Anderson and Tichenor handle this? Following their review of the literature to support their beliefs about proximal and distal consequences of nerve entrapment, they acknowledged that the cited literature was not research-based. If research-based literature to support their opinion had existed, they would have cited it. And if they had found research reports that did *not* support their opinion, they would have been obligated to explain to the reader why they thought their opinion was viable in light of the conflicting evidence.

When writing the introduction, then, be sure to clearly differentiate information that is research-based from information that is an opinion or a conclusion. Using such words as *found, revealed,* and *identified* leads the reader to believe that the information is the result of primary research. *Concluded, believed,* and *attributed* are words that suggest the information is not a primary research finding. An author you are citing might have drawn a conclusion or proposed an explanation based on research findings; if this is the case, be sure to say so, to avoid suggesting that the author's conclusion or proposal is a research finding when it is not.

Consider an example from a case report by Blanton and Wolf[10(p848)] on the use of upper-extremity constraint-induced movement therapy for a patient with stroke: "Tower[4] noted that following unilateral lesions of the pyramidal tract at the spinal cord level, monkeys would fail to use the affected side." Use of the verb *noted* in the last sentence suggests that Tower made the observation during a research study. On the other hand, the verb *explained* in the following sentence from Blanton and Wolf does *not* suggest a primary research finding: "Traub et al[5] explained the learned nonuse behavior as resulting from the animals' inability to move the deafferented extremity due to the presence of a shock-like condition that persists weeks or months after removal of sensory input through all cervical dorsal roots."

As emphasized in **Chapter 3**, primary sources of research usually provide the most credible support for a case report—when they're available. Make certain that your introduction clearly indicates which information is based on primary research and which information is not.

Question #3:
What Theory Exists to Provide a Framework for the Case?

Much has been written about the importance of linking theory to practice. Academicians have been criticized for being "too theoretical," whereas clinicians have been criticized for being "too practical." The reality is that both groups need each other. Practitioners are action-oriented and may be most interested in theory for how it helps them manage patients. The fact that there are many ambiguous and lengthy definitions of *theory* contributes to the myth that theory is "old," is difficult to understand, and has nothing to do with the real world.[11] But as Tammivaara and Shepard[12] explained it, theory "encompasses two concepts: contemplation and observation," both of which are central to day-to-day practice.

"THE BEAUTY OF THIS IS THAT IT IS ONLY OF THEORETICAL IMPORTANCE, AND THERE IS NO WAY IT CAN BE OF ANY PRACTICAL USE WHATSOEVER."

Think of theory as a framework for organizing information into a larger scheme that allows prediction across specific cases. Clinicians manage patients according to implicit theories that they hold about the nature of normal function and dysfunction (eg, the basis of typical movement and the causes of movement abnormalities). These theories usually stem from their analysis of what has worked with their patients.[13] Although individualized theories can be useful in practice, in a case report it is important to contribute to the professional knowledge base by showing how individual observations support or refute the established theory that is found in the professional literature. In their case report, for instance, Malouin et al[14] described the application of an intensive task-oriented training for patients who had had acute cerebrovascular accidents and who were relearning how to walk. The intervention was based in motor learning principles that suggest the best way to learn a task is to practice the task rather than to focus on presumed components of the task, such as balance or weight shifting.

The dynamic nature of theory allows us to challenge the use of a given theory. We have many "theories" about the application of certain clinical techniques or approaches, theories that were based on some literature and that were quickly applied to practice. Instead of challenging these theories as we gain new insights and understandings, however, we may continue to use them as a way to explain what we do. The case report on intervention for limited shoulder motion written by McClure and Flowers[9] challenged the concave-convex theory of arthrokinematic motion,[15] which is the theoretical underpinning of many clinicians' understanding of joint motion. The authors proposed an alternative theory, based on current research on humeral head motion.

The theoretical basis for patient/client management in your case may not be clear or may not exist; if so, it will be necessary for you to acknowledge that. Or the theory may exist, but your case might not contribute anything new to the understanding or application of that theory. Your case still may be worth publishing, however, if you use broad conceptual models or frameworks to show how your case fits with the existing literature.

Two types of models may be particularly useful for organizing case reports: disablement models, such as those adapted from Nagi,[16-18] and the hypothesis-oriented algorithm for clinicians (HOAC).[19]

Disablement Models

The use of a conceptual model of the "disablement process," a term used by Verbrugge and Jette,[20] has important applications to practice in general and to the writing of case reports in particular. Conceptual models are based on partial knowledge, and they change as new knowledge is added.[21] Case reports can provide real-life examples of the conceptual elements and can help guide research to support, modify, and expand the conceptual model. Jette[22] summarized the uses of a conceptual model of disablement:

1. Postulate the potential effects of disease, injury, or congenital abnormalities on the functioning of specific organs or body systems, on basic physical and mental actions, and on individual behavior or roles in daily life.

2. Describe the various personal and environmental factors that can accelerate or retard the disablement process. These factors include predisposing risk factors that propel disablement as well as interventions applied to avoid, retard, or reverse the disablement process.

All functional limitations and disabilities are associated with impairments, but not all functional limitations lead to disability. In case reports that use disablement models, clinicians can "tease out" these complex interrelationships.

Table 4. Some Disablement Models[a]

Nagi Scheme

Active Pathology	→	Impairment	→	Functional Limitation	→	Disability
Interruption or interference with normal processes, and efforts of the organism to regain normal state		Anatomical, physiological, mental, or emotional abnormalities or loss		Limitation in performance at the level of the whole organism or person		Limitation in performance of socially defined roles and tasks within a sociocultural and physical environment

WHO—International Classification of Impairments, Disabilities, and Handicaps (ICIDH) (1980)

Disease	→	Impairment	→	Disability	→	Handicap
The intrinsic pathology or disorder		Loss or abnormality of psycho-logical, physiological, or anatomical structure or function at organ level		Restriction or lack of ability to perform an activity in normal manner		Disadvantage due to impair-ment or disability that limits or prevents fulfillment of a normal role—depending on age, sex, sociocultural factors— for the person

National Center for Medical Rehabilitation Research Classification (1992)

Pathophysiology	→	Impairment	→	Functional Limitation	→	Disability	→	Societal Limitation
Interruption with normal physiological develop-mental processes or structures		Loss or abnormality of cognitive, emotional, physiological, or anatomical structure or function		Restriction or lack of ability to perform an action in the manner or range consistent with the purpose of an organ or organ system		Limitation or inability in performing tasks, activi-ties, and roles to levels expected within physical and social contexts		Restriction attributable to social policy or barriers that limit fulfillment of roles

[a]Adapted with permission of the American Physical Therapy Association from Guide to Physical Therapist Practice. 2nd ed. *Phys Ther.* 2001;81:28 and from Jette AM. Physical disablement concepts for physical therapy research and practice. *Phys Ther.* 1994;74:381.

In 1965, sociologist Saad Nagi proposed a disablement model based on the concepts of active pathology, impairment, functional limitation, and disability[16-18] (**Table 4**). Several similar schemes have been proposed since then, including the World Health Organization's (WHO) *International Classification of Impairments, Disabilities, and Handicaps* (ICIDH-1)[23] (**Table 4**), the WHO's proposed *International Classification of Impairments, Activities, and Participation* (ICIDH-2),[24] and the evolving version of ICIDH-2, the *International Classification of Functioning, Disability, and Health*[25]; the National Center for Medical Rehabilitation Research (NCMRR) model[26] (**Table 4**); and the Institute of Medicine models,[21,27] including the enabling-disabling model[21] shown in **Figure 10**. Any of these models could serve as a theoretical framework for a case report. (For example, see the way in which Hakim et al[28] used the ICIDH-1 model in their case report on outcomes of patients with pelvic-ring fractures managed by open reduction internal fixation.)

The Enabling–Disabling Process

Transitional Factors

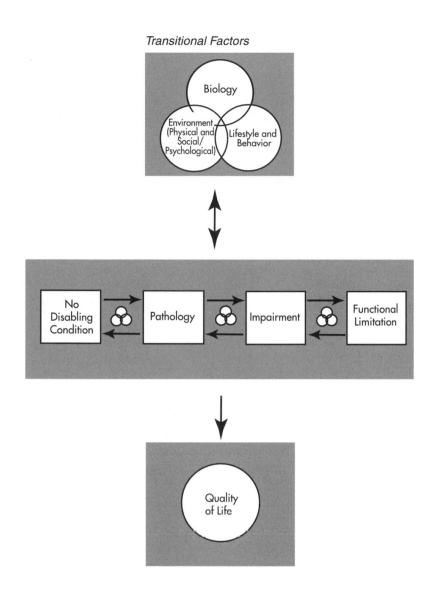

Figure 10. *The enabling-disabling model. "The state of 'disability' does not appear in this model since it is not inherent in the individual but, rather, a function of the interaction of the individual and the environment."*[21(p7)] Reprinted with permission of the Institute of Medicine from Brandt EN Jr, Pope AM, eds. *Enabling America: Assessing the Role of Rehabilitation Science and Engineering.* Washington, DC: National Academy Press; 1997:68.

The *Guide to Physical Therapist Practice*[29] uses an expanded disablement model[30,31] that "provides both the theoretical framework for understanding physical therapist practice and the classification scheme by which physical therapists make diagnoses."[29(p27)] The Guide[29(p27-28)] uses the following definitions, which are based on the Nagi model:

■ *Active pathology is the interruption of or interference with normal processes and the simultaneous efforts of the organism to restore itself to a normal state by mobilizing the body's defense and coping mechanisms.* Pathologies are commonly known as disease, injury, or congenital or developmental conditions. The patient's medical diagnosis usually defines the pathology. Examples of pathologies are the diagnoses of osteoarthritis, fractured femur, and cerebral palsy.

■ *Impairment is the loss or abnormality of anatomical, physiological, mental, or psychological structure or function.* Examples of impairments are decreased vital

Table 5. Examples of the Disablement Process Using the Nagi Model[a]			
Active Pathology	**Impairment**	**Functional Limitation**	**Disability**
Parkinson disease	Rigidity	Shuffling gait	Unable to attend church
	Tremor	Slow getting out of chair	Unable to visit friends
	Poor balance		
Herniated nucleus pulposus	Decreased spinal motion	Unable to sit without pain	Unable to work
	Low back pain	Unable to bend forward	Unable to golf

[a]Adapted with permission from Jette AM. Design and Management of Outcomes Effectiveness Research in Physical Therapy [course notes], Alexandria, Va: American Physical Therapy Association; 1992.

capacity, pain, lost motion at a joint, or a weakened muscle group. Impairments are distinguished from pathology in that impairments typically result from pathology; however, impairments can occur in the absence of pathology.

■ *Functional limitation is a restriction of the ability to perform a physical action, task, or activity in an efficient, typically expected, or competent manner at the level of the whole organism or person.* Verbrugge and Jette[20] emphasized the word "action" because it implies the "situation-free" nature of functional limitations. That is, functional limitations are not associated with a social context. When a person's ability to perform an action (walking, rising to a standing position, climbing steps) is affected, a functional limitation exists.

■ *Disability is the inability to perform—or a limitation in the performance of—actions, tasks, and activities usually expected in specific social roles that are customary for the individual or expected for the person's status or role in a specific sociocultural context and physical environment.* Verbrugge and Jette[20] emphasized "activity" in identifying disabilities because an activity is done in a given social situation. Inability to return to work and inability to participate in a community softball league are examples of disabilities.

Two examples of the disablement process using the Nagi model are shown in **Table 5**.

The Guide to Occupational Therapy Practice[32(p7)] incorporates a different model—the WHO's *International Classification of Impairments, Activities, and Participation.*[24] This model also has four dimensions, which *The Guide to Occupational Therapy Practice* links to occupational therapy terminology and intervention:

■ *"Disease" or "disorder" is defined as pathological changes, symptoms and signs, and health condition.* The corresponding occupational therapy terms are "biological," "cognitive," "psychological," and "social potential." The aim of occupational therapy intervention is remediation/restoration.

Posterior Thigh Pain in a Patient With Low Back Pain

Statement of Purpose

Consider the following statement:

> The purpose of this report is to describe a patient with lower-extremity pain.

What does this statement tell you? Not much. It does not help the reader determine the focus of the report. Is the report simply describing patient characteristics, or is it describing examination, interventions, and decision making? Compare it with the following:

> The purpose of this report is to describe how the theoretical basis for tests that examine the patient's response to passive stretching of tissues can be used to guide decisions about intervention selection and progression for a patient with low back pain who has posterior thigh pain.

By explaining the examination and intervention approaches used with this patient, the above statement may help other therapists deal with patients with similar problems.

■ *"Impairments" are defined as loss or abnormality of body structures or of a physiological or psychological function.* Impairments relate to occupational therapy "performance components," and the aim of intervention is remediation/restoration.

■ *Activity limitations indicate the nature and extent of functioning at the level of the person. Activities associated with everyday life may be limited in nature, duration, and quality.* Activity limitations relate to "performance areas" (eg, activities of daily living [ADL], work and productive activities, and play or leisure activities). Intervention focuses on compensation/adaptation.

■ *Participation restrictions indicate the nature and extent of a person's involvement in life situations in relation to impairments, activities, health conditions, and contextual factors. Participation may be restricted in nature, duration, and quality.* Corresponding occupational therapy terms are "performance context" (temporal and environmental aspects) and "roles"; intervention includes compensation/adaptation, supportive services, and advocacy.

Another important model was developed in 1997 by the Committee on Assessing Rehabilitation Science and Engineering, which was convened by the Institute of Medicine.[21] The committee modified the Nagi[16-18] and 1991 Institute of Medicine[27] model by retaining the Nagi nomenclature to describe the elements of the model but increasing the emphasis on the interaction between the person and the environment in determining whether disability occurs. The Committee also added the concept of the "enabling-disabling" process. The disabling process occurs when a person is removed from the social and physical environment; the enabling (rehabilitative) process provides environmental modification and restoration to reintegrate the person into the environment. The enabling-disabling process is illustrated in **Figure 10**.

In any of the models, pathology is associated with impairments—but some impairments are not associated with pathology. All functional limitations and disabilities are associated with impairments, but not all functional limitations necessarily lead to disability. The enabling-disabling model "suggests a bidirectional interaction among the components, in which improvement in one component has an effect on the development or progression of a preceding component" and "recognizes that functional limitations and disability may be reversed."[21,29(p32)] The interrelationships among the four concepts can become quite complex. The case report is one forum that authors can use to attempt to tease out these complex relationships.

Disablement models provide a "pathway" with logical connections, through which therapists can better understand how and why interventions may have an impact on a patient's ability to function. In fact, case reports are an excellent format for illustrating the impact of therapy on the disablement process.

Beattie[33] used a disablement framework for his case report on the use of an eclectic approach for low back pain in a pole vaulter. In his introduction he defined "impairment" and "disability" according to the disablement model he was using. (Including definitions of these terms in a case report is important because the models do not always use the same terms or define terms in the same way.) Beattie then stated that one of the purposes of the case report was "to describe an examination approach that relates identification of an impairment to a disability."[33(p923)] In this case, the patient's *impairment* was decreased lumbar range of motion, which the author linked to the patient's inability to compete as a pole vaulter—which was the patient's *disability*.

The terms used to describe the four concepts in the Nagi model are used throughout this manual to provide the reader with consistent terminology. The examples taken from the case report literature also illustrate the use of disablement terms when describing patients. As Verbrugge and Jette[20] pointed out, communication is made difficult when undefined terms are used to describe the disablement process. By using one model as a framework for clearly describing patient/client management and outcomes, the case report writer provides another set of operational definitions that can help others understand and replicate the case.

The Hypothesis-Oriented Algorithm for Clinicians (HOAC)

Several theorists and researchers have described conceptual models of the clinical problem-solving process.[19,34,35] The HOAC (**Figure 11**) is a step-by-step description of a procedure designed to guide the process of examination, evaluation, and intervention[19] and for that reason may be particularly useful in writing case reports.

Riddle and Freeman[3] used the HOAC as a framework for their case report about a patient with bilateral plantar fasciitis and Achilles tendinitis. In their introduction, they clearly stated that "the hypothesis-oriented algorithm for clinicians (HOAC) was used as a model for determining the treatment."[3(p1913)] They then referred to the steps of the model in subsequent sections of the report as they described their management and outcomes.

It is important to note that in the introduction of this 1988 case report, the authors mentioned the HOAC in just one short sentence, followed by a reference so that readers wanting more information could look up an article describing the model. Today, reviewers and editors would ask the authors to briefly describe the model so that readers who are not familiar with the HOAC could understand the report without having to find and read the original article on the HOAC. This is a good example of how standards for writing case reports have changed. Although published case reports can give potential authors ideas about how to present a case, none should be viewed as a "perfect" model.

The Purpose Statement

The review of related literature should lead clearly and logically to the purpose of the case report, which usually is stated explicitly at the end of the introduction. In their case report on resumption of occupational therapy for a patient 5 years after traumatic brain injury, Nelson and Lenhart[36(p223)] wrote:

> Recent case reports on brain injury in the *American Journal of Occupational Therapy* have focused on patients with relatively severe disabilities requiring residential care (Katzmann & Mix, 1994; Pulaski & Emmet, 1994; Sandler & Harris, 1992; Sladyk, 1992; Toglia, 1991). The present report is unique in that it describes (a) an outpatient method of delivery; (b) the resumption of occupational therapy several years after discharge; (c) a focus on naturalistic occupation in community settings; and (d) reports of occupational therapy efficacy by the referral source, the client's family, and, most importantly, the client herself.

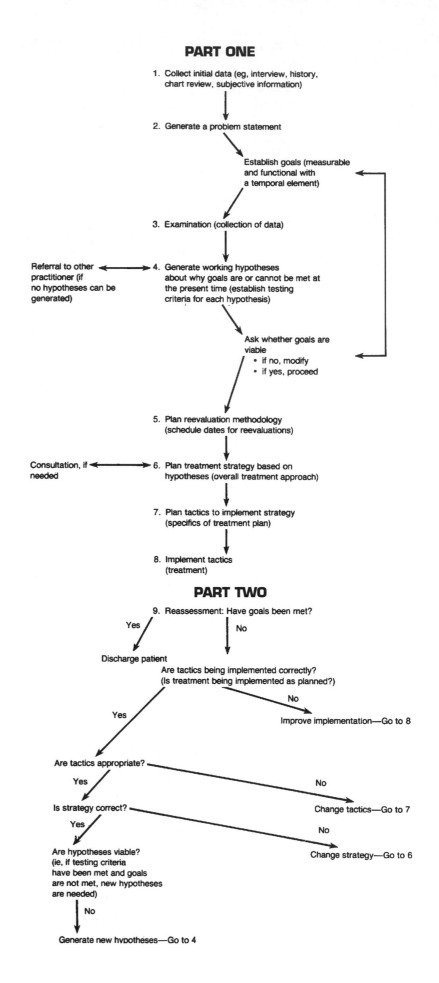

PART ONE

1. Collect initial data (eg, interview, history, chart review, subjective information)

2. Generate a problem statement

Establish goals (measurable and functional with a temporal element)

3. Examination (collection of data)

Referral to other practitioner (if no hypotheses can be generated) ← 4. Generate working hypotheses about why goals are or cannot be met at the present time (establish testing criteria for each hypothesis)

Ask whether goals are viable
- if no, modify
- if yes, proceed

5. Plan reevaluation methodology (schedule dates for reevaluations)

Consultation, if needed ← 6. Plan treatment strategy based on hypotheses (overall treatment approach)

7. Plan tactics to implement strategy (specifics of treatment plan)

8. Implement tactics (treatment)

PART TWO

9. Reassessment: Have goals been met?

Yes → Discharge patient

No → Are tactics being implemented correctly? (Is treatment being implemented as planned?)

No → Improve implementation—Go to 8

Yes → Are tactics appropriate?

No → Change tactics—Go to 7

Yes → Is strategy correct?

No → Change strategy—Go to 6

Yes → Are hypotheses viable? (ie, if testing criteria have been met and goals are not met, new hypotheses are needed)

No → Generate new hypotheses—Go to 4

Figure 11. *The Hypothesis-Oriented Algorithm for Clinicians.*[19] *Part 1 contains guidelines for evaluation and treatment planning. Part 2 is a branching program.*

Next: Who (or What) Is Your Focus?

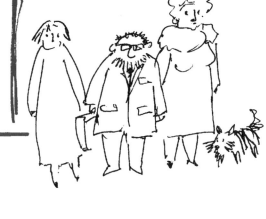

The purpose statement in the introduction helps to focus readers' attention as they begin to read the next section—the case description. Of all the components of the case report, this may be the one that comes easiest to you, because often it focuses on what therapists know best: the patient.

References

1 Rine RM, Schubert MC, Balkany TJ. Visual-vestibular habituation and balance training for motion sickness. *Phys Ther*. 1999;79:949-957.

2 Polit D, Hungler B. *Nursing Research: Principles and Methods*. 4th ed. New York, NY: JB Lippincott Co; 1991:15-27.

3 Riddle DL, Freeman DB. Management of a patient with a diagnosis of bilateral plantar fasciitis and Achilles tendinitis: a case report. *Phys Ther*. 1988;68:1913-1916.

4 Harris SR, Osborn JA, Weinberg J, et al. Effects of prenatal alcohol exposure on neuromotor and cognitive development during early childhood: a series of case reports. *Phys Ther*. 1993;73:608-617.

5 Ahlschwede K. Postoperative management of flexor pollicis longus laceration in two cases. *Am J Occup Ther*. 1991;45:361-365.

6 Depoy E, Gitlin L. *Introduction to Research: Multiple Strategies for Health and Human Services*. St Louis, Mo: CV Mosby Co; 1993:61-77.

7 Anderson M, Tichenor CJ. A patient with de Quervain's tenosynovitis: a case report using an Australian approach to manual therapy. *Phys Ther*. 1994;74:314-326.

8 Kinney LaPier TL, Sirotnak N, Alexander K. Aerobic exercise for a patient with chronic multisystem impairments. *Phys Ther*. 1998;78:417-424.

9 McClure PW, Flowers KR. Treatment of limited shoulder motion: a case study based on biomechanical considerations. *Phys Ther*. 1992;72:929-936.

10 Blanton S, Wolf SL. An application of upper-extremity constraint-induced movement therapy in a patient with subacute stroke. *Phys Ther*. 1999;79:847-853.

11 D'Onofrio CN. Theory and the empowerment of health education practitioners. *Health Educ Q*. 1992;19:385-403.

12 Tammivaara J, Shepard KF. Theory: the guide to clinical practice and research. *Phys Ther*. 1990;70:578-582.

13 Shepard K. Theory: criteria, importance and impact. In: Lister MJ, ed. *Contemporary Management and Motor Control Problems: Proceedings of the II Step Conference*. Alexandria,Va: Foundation for Physical Therapy; 1991:5-10.

14 Malouin F, Potvin M, Prévost J, et al. Use of an intensive task-oriented gait training program in a series of patients with acute cerebrovascular accidents. *Phys Ther*. 1992;72:781-793.

15 Kaltenborn FM. *Mobilization of the Extremity Joints*. Oslo, Norway: Olaf Norlis Bokhandel Universitetsgaten; 1980.

16 Nagi SZ. Some conceptual issues in disability and rehabilitation. In: Sussman MB, ed. *Sociology and Rehabilitation*. Washington, DC: American Sociological Association; 1965:100-113.

17 Nagi S. *Disablity and Rehabilitation: Legal, Clinical, and Self-Concepts and Measurements*. Columbus, Ohio: Ohio State University Press; 1969.

18 Nagi S. Disability concepts revisited: implications for prevention. In: Pope AM, Tarlov AR, eds. *Disability in America: Toward a National Agenda for Prevention*. Washington, DC: National Academy Press; 1991.

19 Rothstein JM, Echternach JL. Hypothesis-oriented algorithm for clinicians: a method for evaluation and treatment planning. *Phys Ther*. 1986;66:1388-1394.

20 Verbrugge LM, Jette AM. The disablement process. *Soc Sci Med*. 1994;38:1-14.

21 Brandt EN Jr, Pope AM, eds. *Enabling America: Assessing the Role of Rehabilitation Science and Engineering*. Washington, DC: National Academy Press; 1997.

22 Jette AM. Physical disablement concepts for physical therapy research and practice. *Phys Ther*. 1994;74:380-386.

23 *ICIDH-1: International Classification of Impairments, Disabilities, and Handicaps*. Geneva, Switzerland: World Health Organization; 1980.

24 *ICIDH-2: International Classification of Impairments, Activities, and Participation.* Geneva, Switzerland: World Health Organization; 1997.

25 *ICIDH-2: International Classification of Functioning, Disability, and Health.* Geneva, Switzerland: World Health Organization; 2000.

26 *National Advisory Board on Medical Rehabilitation Research, Draft V: Report and Plan for Medical Rehabilitation Research.* Bethesda, Md: National Institutes of Health; 1992.

27 Pope AM, Tarlov AR, eds. *Disability in America: Toward a National Agenda for Prevention.* Washington, DC: National Academy Press; 1991.

28 Hakim RM, Gruen GS, Delitto A. Outcomes of patients with pelvic-ring fractures managed by open reduction internal fixation. *Phys Ther.* 1996;76:286-295.

29 Guide to Physical Therapist Practice. 2nd ed. *Phys Ther.* 2001;81:9-744.

30 Guccione AA. Arthritis and the process of disablement. *Phys Ther.* 1994;74:408-414.

31 Guccione AA. Physical therapy diagnosis and the relationship between impairments and function. *Phys Ther.* 1991;71:499-504.

32 Moyers PA. *Guide to Occupational Therapy Practice.* Bethesda, Md: American Occupational Therapy Association; 1999.

33 Beattie P. The use of an eclectic approach for the treatment of low back pain: a case study. *Phys Ther.* 1992;72:923-928.

34 Rogers JC, Holm MB. Occupational therapy diagnostic reasoning: a component of clinical reasoning. *Am J Occup Ther.* 1991;45:1045-1053.

35 Jones MA. Clinical reasoning in manual therapy. *Phys Ther.* 1992;72:875-884.

36 Nelson DL, Lenhart DA. Resumption of outpatient occupational therapy for a young woman five years after traumatic brain injury. *Am J Occup Ther.* 1996;50:223-228.

Chapter 6

Describing the Patient or Other Entity

Descriptions of the patient (or patients), the examination, the evaluation, the process used to decide on an intervention, and the intervention itself fall under the heading of "case description." Some case reports describe approaches to patient/client management; others describe such entities as an ethical issue or the interactions between students and instructor in a classroom.

Remember that a case report is not written like a clinic note. When writing a case description, be sure to use complete sentences, and avoid simply *listing* elements the way you might do in a patient's chart.

In case reports that involve patients, it is important to remember that the "case" is not the patient. The case is the patient's condition, including the therapeutic and personal consequences of that condition. Making this distinction avoids the dehumanizing aspects of the word "case," a word that implies the patient is a clinical problem rather than a human being who has an essential role in decision making and outcomes.[1,2]

Avoid cluttering your case report with information that is not relevant. You can demonstrate your clinical judgment by selecting only the important factors. The detailed birth history of a child with cerebral palsy, the record of a patient's performance on every item of a comprehensive test of activities of daily living (ADL), or the use of a dozen orthopedic tests probably is not necessary.

Your patient or situation and your interventions are what you know best. Your challenge is to describe them in a way that allows others to recognize similar patients or situations.

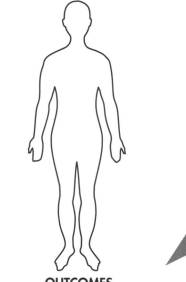

DIAGNOSIS
Both a process and a label. Process includes integrating and evaluating examination data, which the physical therapist organizes into defined clusters, syndromes, or categories to help determine the prognosis (including the plan of care) and the most appropriate intervention strategies. Physical therapists use diagnostic labels that identify the impact of a condition on function at the level of the system (especially the movement system) and at the level of the whole person.

EVALUATION
A dynamic process in which the physical therapist makes clinical judgments based on data gathered during the examination. This process also may identify possible problems that require consultation with or referral to another provider.

**PROGNOSIS
(Including Plan of Care)**
Determination of the level of optimal improvement that may be attained through intervention and the amount of time required to reach that level. The plan of care specifies the interventions to be used and their timing and frequency.

EXAMINATION
The process of obtaining a history, performing a systems review, and selecting and administering tests and measures to gather data about the patient/client. The initial examination is a comprehensive screening and specific testing process that leads to a diagnostic classification. The examination process also may identify possible problems that require consultation with or referral to another provider.

INTERVENTION
Purposeful and skilled interaction of the physical therapist with the patient/client and, if appropriate, with other individuals involved in care of the patient/client, using various physical therapy procedures and techniques to produce changes in the condition that are consistent with the diagnosis and prognosis. The physical therapist conducts a reexamination to determine changes in patient/client status and to modify or redirect intervention. The decision to reexamine may be based on new clinical findings or on lack of patient/client progress. The process of reexamination also may identify the need for consultation with or referral to another provider.

OUTCOMES
Intended results of patient/client management, which include the impact of physical therapy interventions in the following domains: pathology/pathophysiology (disease, disorder, or condition); impairments, functional limitations, and disabilities; risk reduction/prevention; health, wellness, and fitness; societal resources; and patient/client satisfaction.

Figure 12. *The five elements of patient/client management. Adapted with permission of the American Physical Therapy Association from Guide to Physical Therapist Practice. 2nd ed. Phys Ther. 2001;81:43.*

As part of the operational definition of the history and other components of their examination, authors should clarify for the reader the sources of data reported in the case report. Remember that one goal of your description is replicability. After reading your case report, other therapists with similar professional experience should be able to collect the same type of information about a patient with a similar problem.

A good way to avoid omitting important steps in the clinical process is to follow a guide for patient/client management. Depending on the target audience for your case report, the *Guide to Physical Therapist Practice*[3] or the *Guide to Occupational Therapy Practice*[4] would be good sources of information about processes and terminology as they have been described and defined by the American Physical Therapy Association and the American Occupational Therapy Association, respectively. **Figure 12** defines the five elements of patient/client management from the *Guide to Physical Therapist Practice.*[3] Figure 13 illustrates the occupational therapy process.[4] Although the terminology and emphases differ somewhat, the overall processes are similar.

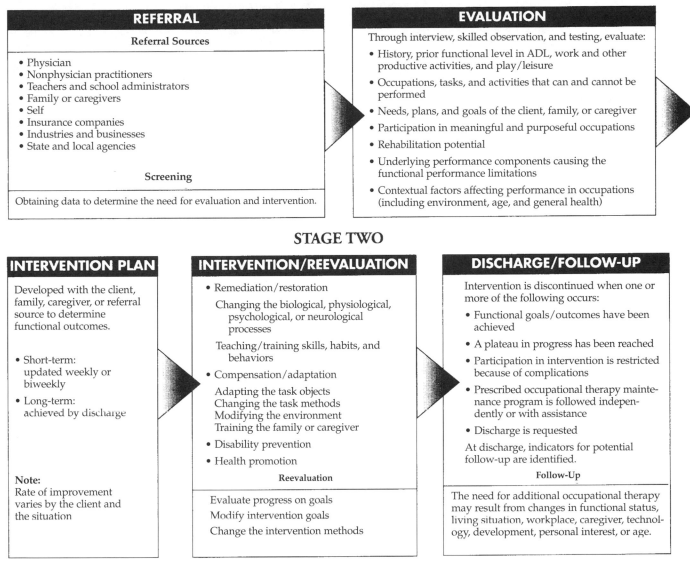

STAGE ONE

REFERRAL

Referral Sources

- Physician
- Nonphysician practitioners
- Teachers and school administrators
- Family or caregivers
- Self
- Insurance companies
- Industries and businesses
- State and local agencies

Screening

Obtaining data to determine the need for evaluation and intervention.

EVALUATION

Through interview, skilled observation, and testing, evaluate:

- History, prior functional level in ADL, work and other productive activities, and play/leisure
- Occupations, tasks, and activities that can and cannot be performed
- Needs, plans, and goals of the client, family, or caregiver
- Participation in meaningful and purposeful occupations
- Rehabilitation potential
- Underlying performance components causing the functional performance limitations
- Contextual factors affecting performance in occupations (including environment, age, and general health)

STAGE TWO

INTERVENTION PLAN

Developed with the client, family, caregiver, or referral source to determine functional outcomes.

- Short-term: updated weekly or biweekly
- Long-term: achieved by discharge

Note:
Rate of improvement varies by the client and the situation

INTERVENTION/REEVALUATION

- Remediation/restoration

  Changing the biological, physiological, psychological, or neurological processes

  Teaching/training skills, habits, and behaviors
- Compensation/adaptation

  Adapting the task objects
  Changing the task methods
  Modifying the environment
  Training the family or caregiver
- Disability prevention
- Health promotion

Reevaluation

Evaluate progress on goals
Modify intervention goals
Change the intervention methods

DISCHARGE/FOLLOW-UP

Intervention is discontinued when one or more of the following occurs:

- Functional goals/outcomes have been achieved
- A plateau in progress has been reached
- Participation in intervention is restricted because of complications
- Prescribed occupational therapy maintenance program is followed independently or with assistance
- Discharge is requested

At discharge, indicators for potential follow-up are identified.

Follow-Up

The need for additional occupational therapy may result from changes in functional status, living situation, workplace, caregiver, technology, development, personal interest, or age.

When the Focus Is Your Patient: The History

In case reports involving people, the first subheading under "Case Description" usually is "Patient," "Client," "Child," "Student," or another term that is appropriate for the case. The patient description often includes such information as age, sex, history, and any other relevant background information that could have contributed or did contribute to the clinical reasoning process. In the *Guide to Physical Therapist Practice*, this type of information is included in the patient/client history; in the *Guide to Occupational Therapy Practice*, this information is included in stage one, referral and evaluation.

The patient is a common source of information. Other sources may include the patient's physician, the patient's family or friends, and the patient's medical chart. **Figure 14** gives a comprehensive list of the types of information that may be obtained in taking a history. Obviously, not all of the information is relevant for all patients. An important contribution of a case report is to show what pieces of infor-

Figure 13. *The occupational therapy process. Adapted with permission from* The Guide to Occupational Therapy Practice. *Bethesda, Md: American Occupational Therapy Association; 1999.*

mation are important for particular patients with particular characteristics and how that information informs the decision-making process.

Be sure to say why you chose this patient for the case report, especially when the case is not unusual. For instance, were particular patients with carpal tunnel syndrome selected because they got better and others did not? Unless the patient is obviously unusual or unique, clearly state your selection criteria. When describing more than one patient, describe the first patient thoroughly, adding only important differences for the other patients.[5] Throughout the description, be careful to disguise the patient's identity, even when you have the patient's permission to write the case report.

In most published case reports dealing with patients, the patient and the interview data are described in the text of the report; however, as shown by examples later in this chapter, tables and figures also can be useful when the history is lengthy or complex.

The patient's symptoms, reason for seeking care, and desired outcomes typically are included, using descriptions that delineate the patient's functional limitations and disabilities. History information that is considered to be relevant also should be reported, including a chronologically based description of symptoms.

Patient's reason for seeking care. The interview data reported by Anderson and Tichenor[6(p318)] elucidated the patient's reason for seeking care (she was diagnosed with de Quervain tenosynovitis) and indicated the extent of the patient's functional limitations and disability:

> The patient was a 41-year-old right-handed bookkeeper. At work in the morning, she sat at a desk and rotated her upper trunk toward a table on her left to count bills and receipts with her left hand....

> The patient...complained of a constant, deep left wrist pain that radiated anteriorly up the forearm to the cubital fossa. After flipping and filing pages or counting bills with her left hand for half an hour, her wrist would throb and give occasional sharp, shooting pains to the cubital fossa. There was intermittent sharp, shooting pain at the carpometacarpal joint of the thumb, radiating proximally along the lateral aspect of the radius of the mid-forearm. She reported needing to stop for 5 to 10 minutes to alleviate the shooting pain. She needed to stop every half hour for relief of symptoms.

Similarly, Watson and Schenkman[7(p197)] described the functional limitations and disabilities reported by their patient with an isolated paralysis of the serratus anterior muscle:

> On his initial visit to physical therapy, the patient's chief complaint was difficulty in using his arm overhead. He gave the specific examples of inability to lift his child onto his shoulders, inability to use his right

upper extremity for lifting even light weights over shoulder height, and restricted ability to reach objects over shoulder height. He also noted "a funny feeling with lifting like my shoulder joint is sliding out of place," but denied having any shoulder pain at this point in time.

Sometimes people seek care for another person. Dunbar[8(p231)] described a child's behaviors that led others in the child's environment to refer her for occupational therapy:

> The teacher reported that Sara had frequent tantrums and was unable to maintain attention to tabletop tasks. She threw toys at other children and frequently ran around the room when the teacher asked her to stay in her chair. Sara's mother reported that Sara exhibited daring behaviors in the home setting, including jumping from high counters and purposely running into walls. The speech-language pathologist treating Sara for expressive language delays in the school setting recommended occupational therapy to enhance Sara's ability to tolerate the school environment.

History of other interventions. Many patients, particularly those with lengthy or chronic problems, have a history of intervention before the episode of care that is the focus of the case report. Did your patient previously receive therapy? If so, describe the intervention as clearly as you can. If the information is based on patient report, that's fine; just be sure to state the source of your information, regardless of what or who it is. Similarly, be sure to report previous medications, surgery, or other interventions, along with the patient's opinion of their effectiveness.

Chronology. A case report written by Gross and Schuch[9(p73)] illustrates the importance of clear chronology when describing the temporal elements of a patient's problem. The authors' purpose was to describe the effect of an exercise program on the force-production capability of a patient with a diagnosis of post-polio syndrome. The description of the patient's condition as it changed over time helps other clinicians identify patients with similar characteristics:

> The patient was a 59-year-old male who contracted poliomyelitis in 1944 at the age of 16 years, with an initial loss of all active movement in the left lower extremity.... The patient did not use any orthosis and walked with a compensatory foot-drop pattern that was discernible to the acute observer. The patient resumed vigorous athletic activity between 1945 and 1948, including football, basketball, baseball, volleyball and tennis. Although he was unable to run as quickly as he had before contracting poliomyelitis, his only complaint was difficulty in walking over irregular surfaces. The patient's pattern of physical activity since 1973 involved playing tennis three times weekly, in addition to a usual amount of walking and stair-climbing activities.

> In 1978, at the age of 50 years, the patient noted some deterioration of muscle strength and endurance in the left lower extremity, with a noticeable effect on gait. He became more fatigued when walking lengthy distances, and there was an appreciable increase in the frequency

General Demographics
- Age
- Sex
- Race/ethnicity
- Primary language
- Education

Social History
- Cultural beliefs and behaviors
- Family and caregiver resources
- Social interactions, social activities, and support systems

Employment/Work (Job/School/Play)
- Current and prior work (job/school/play), community, and leisure actions, tasks, or activities

Growth and Development
- Developmental history
- Hand dominance

Living Environment
- Devices and equipment (eg, assistive, adaptive, orthotic, protective, supportive, prosthetic)
- Living environment and community characteristics
- Projected discharge destinations

General Health Status (Self-Report, Family Report, Caregiver Report)
- General health perception
- Physical function (eg, mobility, sleep patterns, restricted bed days)
- Psychological function (eg, memory, reasoning ability, depression, anxiety)
- Role function (eg, community, leisure, social, work)
- Social function (eg, social activity, social interaction, social support)

Social/Health Habits (Past and Current)
- Behavioral health risks (eg, smoking, drug abuse)
- Level of physical fitness

Family History
- Familial health risks

Medical/Surgical History
- Cardiovascular
- Endocrine/metabolic
- Gastrointestinal
- Genitourinary
- Gynecological
- Integumentary
- Musculoskeletal
- Neuromuscular
- Obstetrical
- Prior hospitalizations, surgeries, and preexisting medical and other health-related conditions
- Psychological
- Pulmonary

Current Condition(s)/ Chief Complaint(s)
- Concerns that led the patient/client to seek the services of a physical therapist
- Concerns or needs of patient/client who requires the services of a physical therapist
- Current therapeutic interventions
- Mechanisms of injury or disease, including date of onset and course of events
- Onset and pattern of symptoms
- Patient/client, family, significant other, and caregiver expectations and goals for the therapeutic intervention
- Patient/client, family, significant other, and caregiver perceptions of patient's/client's emotional response to the current clinical situation
- Previous occurrence of chief complaint(s)
- Prior therapeutic interventions

Functional Status and Activity Level
- Current and prior functional status in self-care and home management, including activities of daily living (ADL) and instrumental activities of daily living (IADL)
- Current and prior functional status in work (job/school/play), community, and leisure actions, tasks, or activities

Medications
- Medications for current condition
- Medications previously taken for current condition
- Medications for other conditions

Other Clinical Tests
- Laboratory and diagnostic tests
- Review of available records (eg, medical, education, surgical)
- Review of other clinical findings (eg, nutrition and hydration)

Figure 14. *Types of data that may be generated from the history. For the purposes of a case report, describe only the data that influenced your clinical decision making or that you believe may have had an effect on the outcomes. Adapted with permission of the American Physical Therapy Association from Guide to Physical Therapist Practice. 2nd ed.* Phys Ther. 2001;81:44.

- **Why did the patient receive physical therapy?** Only the relevant details of the history should be included in the case report. The complete prenatal and birth history of a person with cerebral palsy, for instance, usually isn't necessary; note only the reason for the current episode of physical therapy. Do include the physician's diagnosis (if any) and any other diagnoses or history that could influence the course of physical therapy or the outcomes. Current medication, previous surgery, and prior physical therapy for other problems are examples of information that could be important in understanding your case.

- **What patient behaviors and social and environmental factors may have affected physical therapy and outcomes?** Physical therapists are becoming increasingly aware of the importance of psychological, social, and environmental factors as we learn to predict outcomes more precisely in managed care environments. Although it is beyond our scope of practice to diagnose psychological or social problems, we *can* describe patient behaviors and social and environmental factors that may affect physical therapy and outcomes. A supportive family, the desire to go back to school, the rewards of workers' compensation, a home with architectural barriers—these are just a few examples of the countless factors that enter into the clinical decision-making process and that may have a critical influence on outcomes.

- **Did the patient receive other services?** Physical therapy may not be the only intervention that patients receive, particularly if the problem is long-standing or if the patient has multiple problems. A patient with neck pain, for instance, may have seen other health care professionals before arriving in your clinic. A patient with a stroke could be receiving occupational therapy, speech-language pathology services, rehabilitation nursing, and therapeutic recreation services. Although case reports cannot sort out the relative contribution of physical therapy and other services to outcomes, case reports *should* describe the other services as part of the "package" of patient care.

- **Were there any other problems that could have influenced the anticipated goals and expected outcomes and the means used to achieve them?** Was the patient grossly overweight? Did the patient have seizures? Did the patient have a serious cognitive deficit? These and other comorbidities could influence physical therapy and outcomes.

- **How well did the patient understand the problem?** The patient's understanding can influence physical therapy and outcomes. In general, patients who have a good understanding of their condition are likely to have better outcomes than those who do not.

- **What did the *patient* want to accomplish?** The *Guide to Physical Therapist Practice* and APTA's *Guidelines for Physical Therapy Documentation*[1] emphasize that patients/clients and their significant others should participate in establishing the anticipated goals and expected outcomes and that these goals and outcomes should be "stated in measurable terms." The goals of both the patient and the people who are important in the patient's life must drive physical therapy. Functional outcomes can usually be identified by listening to what the patient wants to be able to do, such as, "I want to be able to work all day," "I want to play in the first game of the season," or "I want to be able to walk to the bathroom by myself." Measurement of the level of achievement of goals should be included in case reports.

References

1 Guidelines for Physical Therapy Documentation. BoD 03-01-16-51. Alexandria, Va: American Physical Therapy Association; 2001.

of catching his toe on objects with the affected left leg. The patient began to use a polypropylene ankle-foot orthosis [AFO] in 1980, primarily when he anticipated walks exceeding 0.25 mile or walked over irregular surfaces. The patient reported that the use of the AFO increased ankle stability and enabled him to ambulate at a more rapid rate with less expenditure of energy. The patient limited his use of the AFO because he feared becoming totally dependent on the orthosis.

In 1986, the patient noted a continued and somewhat more pronounced diminution of muscle strength and endurance. He, therefore, decided to wear the AFO more frequently. By 1987, the patient perceived a further decline in the strength and the endurance of the left hamstring muscle group, and occasionally developed cramping during recreational activities. The patient decided to attempt to increase his strength through a regular exercise program to prevent greater dependence on the AFO.

In this description of a history, the reader is able to clearly follow the temporal sequence of the patient's condition. The progressive nature of the impairments and functional limitations also is described clearly.

When describing the temporal sequence of events in a case report, authors typically have used two strategies. The first—as used by Gross and Schuch—is to report chronology by giving the dates for important health-related historical events that are associated with the patient's condition. The other strategy is to reference health-related events to the amount of time passed since the onset of symptoms or the current episode of care, as Beattie[10(p924)] did: "The patient first noticed this pain and stiffness approximately 1 year prior to his initial physical therapy visit.... Approximately 1 month following the onset of LBP and stiffness he began receiving treatments of chiropractic manipulation."

Dunbar[8(p232)] explained the chronology of concern about the child in her case report in this way: "The mother reported that Sara was always an active child and that she did not suspect that Sara's behavior was unusual until Sara entered a preschool program.... Sara had attended preschool for approximately 6 months before the referral to occupational therapy. Her mother reported that the teacher had expressed concerns from the first month."

Perhaps the best way to determine whether you have captured the chronology of your case report is to have a colleague read the report. Your colleague should be able to report back to you the temporal sequence of the pertinent events prior to and after referral for therapy. It is usually easier to grasp the chronology of events when the amount of time since the most relevant event (eg, injury or referral for therapy) is reported, rather than reporting dates from which the reader then has to calculate. When the time span of your case does not cover several years, use the amount of time since onset to describe the temporal sequence.

Systems Review

The systems review is defined by the *Guide to Physical Therapist Practice* as "a brief or limited examination of (1) the anatomical or physiological status of the

Posterior Thigh Pain in a Patient With Low Back Pain

Description of the Patient

In the description below, some information about pain, the association of back injury with the current complaint, past treatment, and medical diagnostic tests is given; however, other information that contributed to the therapist's decision making is not included:

> The patient was a 33-year-old man with a chief complaint of left posterior thigh pain that has gotten progressively worse in the past 6 months. He reported he also had experienced low back pain intermittently for the last several years. His most recent bout of low back pain was 1 year ago when he was loading a truck at work following an especially busy day. He did not see a physician for the problem. The low back pain resolved after 2 weeks of taking nonsteroidal anti-inflammatory agents and using a hot pack at home. The patient had a magnetic resonance imaging (MRI) test of the lumbar spine approximately 3 weeks prior to our examination. The MRI was judged to be normal.

Compare with the description below, which includes pain location and behavior, mechanisms for symptom reproduction, occupational and recreational activities that may either relate to the problem or indicate the level of disability, history of problems that may be related to the present case, past medical treatment, and results of medical diagnostic tests:

> The patient was a 33-year-old man with a chief complaint of inability to work full time driving a truck. Specifically, he reported that he had pain in his left posterior thigh when pushing on the clutch with his left foot. He first noticed the pain approximately 6 months prior to our examination, after driving for several hours. The posterior thigh symptoms resolved a few hours after getting out of the sitting position. Over the past month, he had posterior thigh pain within 30 minutes of driving his truck. He stated that the posterior thigh symptoms increased when he pushed down on the clutch pedal and when he got in and out of his truck.
>
> The patient's recreational activities also are affected by the problem. He is unable to play soccer during the weekends because of severe pain in the posterior thigh when sprinting or when trying to kick the ball with his left foot. The patient is concerned about this problem because he fears it may get worse. The patient was asked about any previous bouts of low back symptoms. He reported that he has experienced low back pain intermittently for the last several years. His most recent bout of low back pain was 1 year ago. He reported that last year he was loading a truck at work and had several days of severe low back pain following an especially busy day. He did not see a physician for the problem. The low back pain resolved after 2 weeks of taking nonsteroidal anti-inflammatory agents and using a hot pack at home. The patient had a magnetic resonance imaging (MRI) test of the lumbar spine approximately 3 weeks prior to our examination. The MRI was judged to be normal.

cardiovascular/pulmonary, integumentary, musculoskeletal, and neuromuscular systems and (2) the communication ability, affect, cognition, language, and learning style of the patient." The findings of the systems review can be noted in the case report to show how they guided the selection of specific tests and measures.

The literature shows that effective practitioners collect only the data they need for deciding what to do next.

Tests and Measures

When the focus of a case report is a patient or client, the "tests and measures" section begins with an analysis of the information obtained from the interview, chart, other sources of initial data, and the systems review. Based on this information, the therapist selects procedures that are most likely to shed light on the patient's problem. If the focus of the report is a clinic, an education program, or another "nonpatient" entity, the analysis will vary. But regardless of the type of case report, you should clearly explain not only what you did to examine the problem, but *why* you did it. Clinical decisions are difficult to put into words because many times these decisions seem almost reflexive. Nonetheless, the decision-making process must be made explicit for the reader.

The literature shows that effective practitioners collect only the data they need for deciding what to do next. Elstein and colleagues[11] and Payton[12] demonstrated that, early on, when taking the history, clinicians determine what problems are important, what types of examination data are needed, and what interventions may be useful. Excerpts from a published case report show how a clinician focused the examination—directly and indirectly—on the history, symptoms, and goals.

'SCIENCE IS NOTHING BUT TRAINED AND ORGANIZED COMMON SENSE.' THOMAS HUXLEY, 1825-1895

NONSENSE. 'SCIENCE IS ORGANIZED KNOWLEDGE.' HERBERT SPENCER, 1820-1903

© 1996 Sidney Harris

Linking patient information with the examination. Beattie[10] reported on the management of a patient with low back pain who was unable to compete in a pole vault competition. Beattie clearly linked his approach to the patient's history and goals and decided, based on the location of symptoms and the movements associated with the problematic activity, that spinal motion should be examined:

The patient's complaints were most noticeable during the take-off phase of pole vaulting. This activity requires that the individual assume a position of spinal extension, with side-bending and rotation of the trunk to the right.[2] The central location of the patient's pain and stiffness suggested that "local" limitation of spinal movement[16] (ie, limited motion in the midlumbar spinal segments) may have been related to his inability to pole vault. Thus, the initial problem statement was that the patient's midlumbar symptoms were associated with an abnormality of spinal motion, which prevented him from pole vaulting.

The Nonpatient

Case reports that deal with entities other than patients (eg, administrative issues) also should describe the entity clearly, include all pertinent information, and reveal the sources of all data. There is a wide variety of cases, and it is not possible to give guidelines for describing all of the possible entities, but you should use the same general guidelines that apply to case reports on patients: Describe the case in such detail that the reader could recognize it or could identify cases that are similar.

When describing a clinical practice, for example, it may or may not be important to describe such diverse characteristics as the square footage of the department, the salary of employees, the elements of the quality improvement program, the program goals, the years of experience therapists have had, the number of patients seen daily, the ethnic makeup of the department staff, or the status of therapist-administrator relations. In general, identify and report the characteristics and infor-

mation that went into decision making and that could be related to outcomes, regardless of the type of entity being described.

Hazari's case report on the design and implementation of a local area network (LAN)[1] describes a university program:

> Over the past five years computers had been regularly installed to support instruction. All labs and department offices within the school had their own workstations and peripherals. With a critical need to exchange data, share expensive resources such as plotters and printers, and communicate using electronic mail, it was only a matter of time before the need for a LAN was identified.

It was determined that the network would help support the school's long-term goals as outlined in the Strategic Plan, which emphasized distinction in undergraduate education, plus excellence in teaching, research, and creative activity. Priorities for Action in the plan called for integrating information technology in courses to improve learning.

The case report goes on to describe other characteristics of the program and how they related to the decisions that were made about the LAN's design and implementation. The information about the Strategic Plan and Priorities for Action is an example of the type of detail that could be important information for others trying to develop a similar system.

Reference

1 Hazari S. Multi-protocol LAN design and implementation: a case study. *Technological Horizons in Education Journal.* 1995;22(9):80-85.

Most of the data collected during the course of a patient's care are obtained for a reason. Therapists do not have time to do a thorough systems review or to measure everything that can be measured during a patient's course of care—nor would they want to do so, because that information would be of little or no use for the decisions they have to make.

When writing a case report, explain why you examined each system or performance component, why you used each test and measure, and what the information from each test and measure contributed to your clinical reasoning. A laundry list of tests and measures, without an explanation of why you did them or what they contributed, is a sure way to get a letter saying that the case report you submitted for publication is rejected!

Posterior Thigh Pain in a Patient With Low Back Pain

Examination

When you read the excerpt below, think about what information is missing. Are descriptions of test methods used in the examination and evidence for measurement reliability provided? Note that the examiner's interpretation of the tests is stated without actually describing the results of the tests. It is unclear how the examiner came to conclusions based on the test results.

Pain intensity level: The patient reported increased pain after 30 minutes of driving.

Lower-quarter screening examination: Negative for neurological involvement.

Range of motion of the trunk: Patient was limited in forward bending. Repeated motion tests in forward bending did not increase symptoms in the posterior thigh. All other trunk motions are within normal limits.

The SLR test: The SLR test was positive at 50% of full range.

Observational gait analysis: The patient demonstrated an abnormal gait pattern. The step length was asymmetrical. Open-chain phase of stair climbing increased pain.

Below, in an elaborated (though still abbreviated) examination portion of the case description, each method of testing is referenced, and, where possible, evidence for reliability of measurements is also referenced. Although no data are provided from the sensory examination, a presumptive argument is made for reliability and validity of these measurements. Descriptions of the test results help the reader understand how the tests were interpreted. Notice that the description makes it clear why the examination procedures were chosen when the link between a procedure and the initial data is not obvious. The inadequate description does not make this link.

Pain intensity level: A 10-mm visual analogue scale was used to quantify pain intensity.[1] The patient reported a pain intensity level of 4 after 30 minutes of driving. The pain symptom reached a level of 7 when he pushed in the clutch and when he got in and out of his truck.

Sensation testing and myotomal testing: Testing was done as described by Magee.[2] Sensation was intact, and no deficits were found with myotomal testing. No data exist to support the reliability of these assessments, but we believe that the assessments were still meaningful. The patient did not report that he had a sensation loss and reported no deficit in the use of his muscles. We therefore believe our assessments reflected the status of the patient's nervous system.

Range of motion of the trunk: Forward bending was assessed using the fingertip-to-floor method, a procedure that has been shown to provide highly reliable measurements.[3] The measurement of forward bending was 18 in. The patient reported thigh pain at the end-range of forward bending. A series of five repeated forward-bending motion tests were done to determine whether repeated movements worsened the pain. Repeated motion testing helped us determine intervention intensity. If the symptom intensity had remained the same with repeated movements, our intervention would have been more aggressive than if the symptom intensity had increased with subsequent repeated movements.

Straight-leg-raise (SLR) test: The SLR test was done as described by Magee.[2] The reliability of SLR test measurements was demonstrated by McCombe et al.[4] The patient reported that pain occurred in the left posterior thigh at a 45-degree angle. The addition of neck flexion or ankle dorsiflexion to the SLR to 45 degrees increased the intensity of the symptoms above the level reported during the SLR test alone. The SLR test on the right side was to 80 degrees. The patient reported a stretching sensation near the end-range during the SLR test on the right.

Observational gait analysis: The patient's gait was assessed while he ambulated at a "self-selected pace." No deviations in step length were observed. When the patient was instructed to walk rapidly, he was observed to have a shorter step length on the left compared with the right. The patient had no pain in the left lower extremity when he stepped up one 8-in step, but he reported posterior thigh pain when stepping up two steps.

References

1 Price DD, McGrath PA, Rafii A, Buckingham B. The validation of visual analogue scales as ratio measures for chronic and experimental pain. *Pain.* 1983;17:45-56.

2 Magee DJ. *Orthopedic Physical Assessment.* 2nd ed. Philadelphia, Pa: WB Saunders Co; 1992.

3 Gauvin MG, Riddle DL, Rothstein JM. Reliability of clinical measurements of forward bending using the modified fingertip-to-floor method. *Phys Ther.* 1990;70:443-447.

4 McCombe PF, Fairbank JCT, Cockersole BC. Reproducibility of physical signs in low back pain. *Spine.* 1989;14:908-918.

Operational definitions. Operational definitions of the procedures that were used to obtain examination data also must be included in case reports. (Refer to **Chapter 4** for more on operational definitions.) Operational definitions can be accomplished in a variety of ways. Some authors have operationally defined the procedures that they used, whereas others have referenced the operational definitions that were used and published by others. Beattie[10] used a combination:

> The patient's AROM [active range of motion] was normal, as defined by Magee[25] and Hoppenfeld.[26] The straight-leg-raising (SLR) test was performed as described by Hoppenfeld.[26] The patient's SLR was 90 degrees bilaterally, and no pain was elicited during this procedure. Manual muscle testing was performed using the "break test" by requesting the patient to perform each of the eight movements against manual resistance that I applied.[29] No muscular force deficits were noted in the lower extremities. I performed sensory testing, using a light brushing motion with my hands over the dermatomes that correspond to L2 through S2, to determine the presence and symmetry of the patient's light touch sensation.[25,26]

> Palpation of the posterior trunk was performed as follows. The patient lay on a treatment table in the prone position. The paravertebral soft tissues were examined using fingertip palpation. Pain was elicited with palpation unilaterally, 1 cm to the right of the spinal segmental levels of L2-4....

Gill-Body and colleagues[13(p132)] relied on operationalizing their "clinical balance assessment" of a patient with unilateral vestibular dysfunction:

> Clinical balance assessment revealed that the patient could stand with her eyes closed and her feet together for 60 seconds (measured with a digital stopwatch), but it demonstrated a significantly increased ankle sway (sway was observed and not measured). Unilateral stance with eyes open could be performed for 7 seconds, and the patient was unable to perform unilateral stance with her eyes closed. The patient could perform tandem stance for 60 seconds with her eyes open and for 5 seconds with her eyes closed. Stance on foam with eyes open could be performed for 60 seconds without difficulty; with eyes closed, stance on foam could be performed for 20 seconds with a marked ankle sway.... Gait was wide based and characterized by an immobile trunk, no arm swing, and gaze fixation on the floor. The patient was unable to ambulate in a straight line at any speed; rather, she moved in a side-to-side path (to both sides) as she moved forward. Turns (90°) were performed slowly and with multiple small steps. During attempts to ambulate while rotating her head from side to side, the patient's speed of gait decreased and she crossed one foot over the other repeatedly.

The above description defines for the reader what variables the clinicians observed and characterized. Because the authors provided thorough descriptions of what they did and observed, other therapists can replicate the procedures.

Depicting Patient Data

Figures and tables can be used to supplement the text and to summarize some of the patient data. Canélon[14] included a table that provided "patient profiles" in a three-patient case report on job-site analysis and work reintegration. The table also contains a summary of outcomes (**Table 6**). Gross and Schuch[9] used a table to summarize the manual muscle test findings for a patient with a diagnosis of post-polio syndrome (**Table 7**).

Harris and colleagues[15] summarized the characteristics of a group of children exposed to alcohol prenatally (**Table 8**). Toth-Fejel et al[16] used a table (**Table 9**) to show changes in physical measures of a woman with cubital tunnel syndrome at baseline, following 10 weeks of Standard Hand Rehabilitation Protocol, and after Standard Hand Rehabilitation Protocol with use of an experience sampling method.

To their case report, Anderson and Tichenor[6] added a figure of the body chart used to identify the anatomical location of the patient's reported pain (**Figure 15**).

Table 6. Patient Profiles and Outcomes[a,b]

Variable	Case 1	Case 2	Case 3
Age (years)	25	43	45
Gender	Female	Female	Male
Marital status	Single	Divorced	Married
Diagnosis	(R) Stroke	Subarachnoid hemorrhage	(R) Distal ulna fracture
Onset	6/26/91	5/29/91	4/1/92
Dominance	Right	Right	Right
Initial outpatient presentation	8 weeks	3 weeks	10 weeks
Occupation	Assembly worker	Policy clerk	Dry end assistant
Time of job site analysis[a]	16 weeks	7 weeks	52 weeks
Physical demands	Light	Sedentary	Very heavy
Time of return to work[a]	24 weeks	17 weeks	59 weeks
Outcome	Job rotation	Previous job	Reassignment

[a]After onset of illness.

[b]Reprinted with permission of the American Occupational Therapy Association from Canélon MF. Job site analysis facilitates work reintegration. *Am J Occup Ther.* 1995;47:461-467.

Table 7. Strength of Affected Musculature in Left Lower Extremity Three Years After Onset of Poliomyelitis[a,9]

Muscle or Muscle Group	Muscle Strength Grade (%)
Hip flexors	90
Hip extensors	80
Hip abductors	80
Hip adductors	80
Knee flexors	70
Knee extensors	90
Tibialis anterior	20
Tibialis posterior	10
Peroneals	80
Gastrocnemius	0
Soleus	20
Toe flexors	5
Toe extensors	0

[a]Manual muscle testing performed according to procedure of HO Kendall, FP Kendall, and GE Wadsworth, *Muscles: Testing and Function*, ed 2, Baltimore, MD, Williams & Wilkins, 1971.

Table 8. Characteristic Features of Prenatal Alcohol Exposure and Their Presence in the Five Infants Studied.[a,15]

Characteristic	Infant No. 1	2	3	4	5
Growth retardation (<10th percentile)	+	−	−	−	−
Characteristic facial features	+	+	+	+	+
Cognitive delay	+	+	−	+	±
Motor delay	+	+	±	+	±
Generalized hypotonia	+	+	−	+	±
Feeding/oral-motor concerns	+	+	−	−	−
Orthopedic abnormalities	+	+	−	−	−
Behavioral concerns	−	+	−	+	+

[a] + = characteristic was present, − = characteristic was not present, ± = variability in appearance of the characteristic across repeated assessments.

Table 9. Physical Measure Results at Baseline 10 Weeks, and Discharge (27 Weeks)[a]

Measure	Baseline initial evaluation (10 days postsurgery)	At 10 weeks (after Standard Hand Rehabilitation protocol[b])	At 27 weeks (after Standard Hand Rehabilitation Protocol with ESM)
Active range of motion (pain-free) elbow flexion–extension	−15°–115°	−15°–135°	−10°–145° (functional range)
Sensory			
Size and type of protection at incision site[c]	8 cm x 8 cm gel pad 1/4" thick	3 cm x 4 cm gel pad 1/8" thick	2 cm x 4 cm foam pad 1/8" thick
Frequency of wearing pad[d]	Worn at all times	Intermittent	Intermittent
Hand Dowel Test[c]	Not tested secondary to postsurgical contraindications	Tolerated 3 out of 10 textures	Tolerated 7 out of 10 textures
Grip strength (in pounds) (right/left)	Not tested secondary to postsurgical contraindications	Right–25 Left–65	Right–46 Left–62.5
Quality of movement patterns during functional activities (right upper extremity only)	Not tested secondary to postsurgical contraindications	Robotlike (1 joint moves at a time)	Fluid, coordinated (joints move simultaneously)

[a] Reprinted with permission of the American Occupational Therapy Association from Toth-Fejel GE, Toth-Fejel GF, Hedricks CA. Occupation-centered practice in hand rehabilitation using the experience sampling method. *Am J Occup Ther.* 1998;52:381-385.

Note. ESM = experience sampling method.
[b] See Blackmore & Hotchkiss (1996).
[c] Test based on Downey Hand Center Hand Sensitivity Test (Barber, 1990).
[d] Worn as needed during functional tasks involving excessive tactile input near or on elbow incision site.

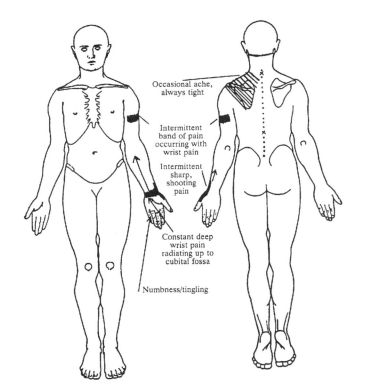

Occasional ache,
always tight

Intermittent
band of pain
occurring with
wrist pain

Intermittent
sharp,
shooting
pain

Constant deep
wrist pain
radiating up to
cubital fossa

Numbness/tingling

Figure 15. *Body chart illustrating where the patient reported pain when first examined.*[5]

Evaluation, Diagnosis, and Prognosis (Including Plan of Care)

Evaluations are clinical judgments that clinicians make for the purpose of establishing a diagnosis and prognosis. **Figure 12** defines these terms as they are used by the *Guide to Physical Therapist Practice.*[3]

Evaluations are based on a synthesis of all of the data that you reported in the systems review and tests and measures section. Now it's time to explain how you used each piece of data to establish a diagnosis, prognosis, and plan of care. Which test results helped rule out a diagnosis? Which results led you toward a diagnosis that you then confirmed with other data? Which pieces of information did you use to arrive at a hypothesis about the cause of the patient's problem? As with every other part of a case report, put your thought process in writing so that it is clear to readers (and to yourself).

Case report writers who clearly describe their evaluation, diagnosis, and prognosis processes make their decision making explicit and contribute valuable examples of these aspects of patient/client management. Few such examples currently exist in the literature. Similarly, few examples of the entire process of evaluation used in making decisions for clients receiving occupational therapy services (**Figure 13**) exist in the literature.

Diagnosis. In the best of all rehabilitation worlds, therapists would be able to identify a cluster (eg, of signs or symptoms, impairments, functional limitations, and disabilities), syndrome, or category as part of diagnostic classification for all patients, which then would lead to the most appropriate intervention. Unfortunately, this "best of all worlds" does not yet exist—with a few exceptions.

Table 10. Classification Categories, Key Examination Findings, and Treatment Approaches for Patients With Acute Low Back Symptoms According to the Treatment-Based Classification System Described by Delitto et al[a,17]

Classification	Key Signs and Symptoms	Treatment Approach
Extension	Flexion activities worsened symptoms (sitting, bending) Symptoms improved with extension movement testing Symptoms worsened with flexion movement testing	Extension exercises Restriction of flexion (education/bracing)
Flexion	Extension activities worsened symptoms (standing, walking) Symptoms improved with flexion movement testing Symptoms worsened with extension movement testing	Flexion exercises Restriction of extension (education/bracing) Partially unloaded walking
Mobilization (lumbar/sacroiliac)	Sacroiliac: positive sacroiliac tests Lumbar: opening or closing pattern with movement testing	Mobilization/manipulation
Immobilization	Frequent prior episodes due to minimal spinal perturbations Prolonged static postures worsened symptoms Symptoms worsened with sustained movement testing Symptoms improved with repeated movement testing	Avoidance of end-range or sustained postures (bracing/education) Trunk strengthening and stabilization exercises
Lateral shift	Visible lateral shift (lateral translation of the trunk relative to the pelvis) Asymmetrical side-bending range of motion Symptoms improved with pelvic translocation movement testing, worsened with opposite translocation	Pelvic translocation exercise in standing or prone position Pelvic translocation exercise combined with extension Autotraction
Traction	Radicular symptoms Symptoms did not improve with any movement tests Symptoms worsened with most movement tests	Mechanical traction Autotraction

[a]Delitto A, Erhard RE, Bowling RW. A treatment-based classification approach to low back syndrome: identifying and staging patients for conservative treatment. *Phys Ther.* 1995;75:470-485.

The *Guide to Physical Therapist Practice*[3] contains preferred practice patterns, into which patients are classified based on the physical therapist's evaluation of the examination data; however, the practice patterns provide only the "boundaries within which a physical therapist may design and implement plans of care."[3(p35)] Case report writers might specify the practice pattern into which they classify the patient, as delineated in the Guide, but they also might provide a more specific diagnosis, if one can be determined. A case report by Fritz[17] gives a good example of a diagnostic classification approach for patients with low back syndrome that is specific and guides intervention (**Table 10**).

Sometimes the evaluation and the diagnostic process reveal findings that are outside the scope of the therapist's knowledge, experience, or expertise and that therefore require the therapist to refer the patient to an appropriate practitioner.[3] Gray's case report[18] is an example of such a situation. His evaluation indicated that a patient with a diagnosis of sciatica might actually have intermittent vascular claudication. The therapist referred the patient back to the physician to rule out occlusive vascular disease, which a vascular specialist subsequently diagnosed and surgically repaired.

When the diagnostic process does not yield an identifiable cluster, syndrome, or category, therapists must develop hypotheses about the cause of the patient's problem and must design possible solutions.

When the diagnostic process does not yield an identifiable cluster, syndrome, or category, therapists must develop hypotheses about the cause of the patient's problem and must design possible solutions. The hypothesis may relate to the identification of a particular pathology that the clinician believes to be responsible for the problem, or it may relate to the determination of the impairments that appear to contribute to the the functional limitations or the disability reported by the patient. In either case, hypothesized causes are critical aspects of clinical decision making. Because the hypothesized causes of the problem link the evaluation to the prognosis and plan of care, authors of case reports are obligated to explain their hypotheses and how the data contributed to them.

In experimental studies, a hypothesis is a testable idea about cause. Because case reports lack the controls of experimental studies, hypotheses cannot be tested in the same way they are tested in research. But hypotheses *are* tested informally in case reports through the data collected and the logical arguments provided by the author.

Hypotheses *are* tested informally in case reports through the data collected and the logical arguments provided by the author.

Mueller and Diamond[19(p1918)] described a 69-year-old man with a diagnosis of diabetes mellitus, peripheral neuropathy, and a right plantar ulcer who was referred for intervention for the ulcer. After completing their examination, the authors hypothesized that

> The patient had a chronic plantar ulcer secondary to insensitivity and deformities at his foot. The insensitivity and deformities appeared to allow increased unnoticed pressure under the patient's metatarsal heads during weight bearing, which caused skin breakdown.

Mueller and Diamond informally tested their hypothesis by applying an intervention designed to address the factors identified in their hypothesis. They developed a procedure to normalize pressure under the metatarsals, and the ulcer healed. The outcome (healed ulcer) supported the credibility of their hypothesis—but lacking the controls of research, the case report could *not* prove that the intervention caused the ulcer to heal.

Moyers and Stoffel[20(p641)] proposed and tested a hypothesis regarding a patient scheduled for surgery for recurrent bilateral carpal tunnel syndrome, carpometacarpal arthritis of the right thumb, and an osteophyte on the left trapezoid. The examination interview with the patient and her husband suggested that the patient drank an excessive amount of alcohol.

> Obviously, continued drinking during treatment could limit the options for controlling postsurgical pain (eg, transcutaneous nerve stimulation in place of medication) (*Acute Pain Management Guideline*, 1992), could ultimately interfere with the client's progress toward the goals of rehabilitation, could prevent implementation of the second surgical procedure, and could potentially increase the time off from work.

The authors tested their hypothesis by using a motivational interviewing approach, which led to a diagnosis of substance dependence and ultimately to the patient's participation in a detoxification program.

A hypothesis was developed and informally tested by Riddle and Freeman[21(p1914)] with a patient with a diagnosis of bilateral plantar fasciitis and Achilles tendinitis. The patient had severe foot pain when taking the first few steps each morning and was unable to teach aerobic classes because of severe pain. The authors put forth the following hypothesis:

Table 11. Symptoms That Contribute to Initial Working Hypotheses After the Patient Interview[23]

Symptom	Working Hypothesis
Symptoms in the L-5 dermatome	L-5 chronic nerve root irritation
Symptoms were nonirritable and moderately severe	
Stage of the pathology was chronic and stationary	
Pain with getting in and out of car (neck flexion component)	Adverse neural tissue tension component
Worsening of symptoms with the use of his clutch (knee extension component)	
Pain on the initiation of ambulation that dissipated quickly and returned later	
Difficulty with extension activities (ie, walking and standing)	Extension dysfunction

The patient was unable to dance without pain and was unable to ambulate pain free in the morning because of inflammatory processes. We believed these inflammatory processes were located bilaterally in the area of the insertion of the plantar fascia and in the area of the triceps surae tendon.... We believed that these inflammatory processes were precipitated by the abnormal alignment of each rear foot and forefoot, which we had identified when taking measurements of forefoot and rear-foot positions during the examination. We believed that this abnormal alignment predisposed the patient to developing symptoms caused by forces that occurred repetitively during high-impact aerobic dancing. When foot malalignments are present during repetitive upright activities, excessive forces are thought to be applied to the soft tissues that support the longitudinal arch of the foot.[9] Soft tissues that are thought to assist in the support of the longitudinal arch are the plantar fascia and the triceps surae.[9]

Gill-Body and colleagues[13(p133)] reported on the cases of two patients with peripheral vestibular dysfunction, one of whom complained of a 3-month history of difficulty walking outdoors, ringing in the right ear, and an inability to return to work as a tour guide due to her inability to stand on a moving bus and walk in a straight line while maintaining balance. After the examination, the authors hypothesized the following:

1. The patient's decreased cervical range of motion could be related to her voluntarily holding her head still during gait and other functional activities; decreased cervical range of motion and alignment could impair postural responses[10] and were therefore worth addressing in intervention.

2. The patient's primary problem of impaired postural stability was related to her vestibular hypofunction on the right side, as supported by the posturography test results of difficulty with sensory conditions 5 and 6 [results obtained with an instrument designed to measure body sway under different conditions].

3. The patient clearly demonstrated some ability to utilize vestibular information for postural control in situations in which accurate visual and proprioceptive information were not as available (ie, sensory conditions 5 and 6 could be partially performed on some trials).

These three hypotheses were developed to guide intervention based on the examination findings. The authors devised an intervention program designed to address the impaired balance and range of motion that were identified in the hypotheses. Follow-up balance and range-of-motion measurements were reported after a course of intervention, as were other outcomes. (See **Chapter 8**, "Describing the Outcomes.") The authors provided data to support their hypotheses in the following way: They thoroughly described their intervention and how it was linked to their hypotheses, reported the preintervention and postintervention impairment measurements that were referred to in the hypotheses, and thoroughly described the changes that took place in the patient's functional ability.

Malouin and colleagues[22] took a different approach to informal hypothesis testing. They studied a series of patients with acute cerebrovascular accidents to determine whether a specific and aggressive intervention designed to restore gait patterns could be used safely and effectively. The authors also wanted to thoroughly describe the proposed intervention procedures. They referenced several studies that supported the hypothesis that intensive and early task-specific training was the rehabilitation approach of choice for patients with acute cerebrovascular accidents who had altered gait patterns. They reported a large amount of data to support their conclusion: "Early and intensive gait-related training is feasible and...can be very well tolerated by patients who are moderately to severely involved following a stroke."[22(p788)]

Because they were not conducting a research study, the authors did not test the hypothesis of whether their intervention approach was more effective than another approach. But their report *suggested* that a true experimental study would be an appropriate next step. This is an example of the role that case reports can play in providing data that can be used to justify larger, controlled experimental studies.

Case reports can play a role in providing data that can be used to justify larger, controlled experimental studies.

Tables and figures can be used to supplement the text describing hypotheses. Koury and Scarpelli[23] used a table (**Table 11**) to summarize what were thought to be the most important symptoms in a patient diagnosed with chronic lumbar nerve root irritation. The table links the symptoms reported by the patient to the causes hypothesized by the authors.

Case reports can be designed to informally test a variety of different forms of hypotheses. If you plan to informally test a hypothesis in your case report, ask yourself the following questions: Is the hypothesis stated clearly in the report? Is the theoretical basis for the hypothesis described? Is the hypothesis testable? If the hypothesis is testable, do the data provided in the report support or refute the hypothesis?

Prognosis. Determining a prognosis involves predicting the optimal level of function that a patient/client can achieve and a time line for reaching that level.

How did you decide, for example, that a child with cerebral palsy probably will not walk functionally and needs a power wheelchair? What did you consider before deciding, for the patient in your case report, that you could reduce the usual time that patients with low back pain receive workers' compensation? How did you decide that a patient with a stroke should be able to use his arm functionally within 2 months? What information made you think that 3 weeks of intervention would help a woman with hypermobility syndrome participate in her favorite recreational activities again?

Clinicians develop plans of care based on some implicit judgments about a patient's potential and the best way to attain it. In a case report, the decision-making process must be explicit.

Many clinicians, particularly students and new graduates, proclaim that they can't predict what a patient will ultimately be able to do or how long it will take to achieve goals. Clinicians still develop plans of care, however, based on some implicit judgments about a patient's potential and the best way to attain it. In a case report, the decision-making process must be explicit. You can determine and support prognoses in three primary ways: referencing published studies, making a presumptive argument, or considering your own clinical experience.

Referencing published studies often is the most accurate and credible way to determine a prognosis. In their evidence-based medicine text, Sackett et al[24(p95)] listed the elements of prognosis about which clinicians hope to find research evidence to help answer three questions: "a qualitative element (Which outcomes could happen?), a quantitative element (How likely are they to happen?) and a temporal element (Over what period of time?)." Unfortunately, relatively little research currently exists to help rehabilitation professionals answer these questions, but some studies are available, and you can find them by searching the literature. Some examples:

■ As with any literature search, a good place to start looking is in a database of systematic reviews of research articles. The Database of Abstracts of Reviews of Effectiveness, for example, includes a critical review of an article on treatment for soft tissue injuries of the ankle.[25] The reviewers concluded that "ankle injuries have a good prognosis, which is altered little by treatment." They went on to say, however, that early treatment might reduce acute symptoms. Both of these pieces of information could be important to consider in determining the prognosis and plan of care for a patient with soft tissue injury of the ankle.

■ Most of the time you will not find a systematic review to help you with your prognosis, but you might find one or more research articles that provide useful information. For instance, researchers have conducted studies of the prognosis for ambulation of children with cerebral palsy.[26-28] Researchers also have identified prognostic factors related to the length of time that patients with low back pain receive workers' compensation.[29] Other researchers have identified ways to predict upper-extremity function following stroke.[30,31] In their study of early shoulder and hand function as a predictor of recovery following stroke, Katrak et al,[30] for example, calculated and reported odds ratios, which are appearing more often in the literature and are useful for evidence-based decision making.[24] The need for more evidence-based decision making in this area was suggested by another study, in which the researchers found that occupational therapists and physical therapists tended to underestimate what patients would be able to do 6 months after a severe middle-cerebral artery stroke.[31]

If you cannot find research to help you determine a prognosis, you probably can *make a presumptive argument* for the prognosis. **Chapter 4** describes how to make a presumptive argument for the reliability and validity of measurements; a presumptive argument to support your prognosis is similar. The clinician develops theoretical arguments to support the decisions involved in determining a prognosis. Even if you cannot find research reports, perhaps your literature search will reveal clinical perspectives, case reports, and other peer-reviewed observations and opinions about the prognosis for patients who are similar to yours. Perhaps you can find related research that addresses certain aspects of the patient's problem, such as the healing time for soft tissue injuries, from which you can make a presumptive argument about the prognosis for a patient's specific type of injury.

Sometimes clinicians have no alternative other than to *base the prognosis on their own past experience or the experience of colleagues*. If you base the prognosis on experience, make sure that you clearly state whose experience it was. Too many authors use passive voice construction to avoid using the first person. An example: "It has been observed that most patients with these examination results are independent in ADL within 2 months." Who made this observation? Passive voice construction ("it has been observed") hides the actor. A clearer statement would be: "I have observed that most patients...."

Except in rare instances, avoid determining a prognosis based solely on your own experience. In a case report of a patient with hypermobility syndrome (HMS), Russek[33(p392)] used a combination of published opinion, a presumptive argument, and her own experience to determine a prognosis:

> Prognosis for HMS is mixed. On one hand, there is no cure for the disorder. The goal for treatment, therefore is not to return to "normal" (ie, not hypermobile) joint mobility but restoration of relatively pain-free function. That is, treatment does not eliminate the underlying impairment of excessive mobility. However, physicians specializing in HMS propose that treatment improves function and decreases disability.[6,35]

> Some authors[2,12,36-39] assert that HMS is not progressive and does not necessarily lead to progressive deformity or disability in the way that rheumatoid arthritis, for example, might. From this point of view, the prognosis is good. Individuals with HMS, however, have a greater incidence of many acute and chronic musculoskeletal disorders[5,11] and tend to develop more osteoarthritis than individuals without hypermobility.[3,40,41] Hypermobility syndrome also is associated with some other systemic disorders, such as mitral valve prolapse.[6] Overall, therefore, prognosis is fair to good. In the opinion of some physicians and my clinical experience, patients with HMS can function and their quality of life often can be improved with treatment but they will usually have chronic or recurrent problems.

Russek did not include a time line for improvement. Today, reviewers, editors, and most instructors expect to see that kind of time line in a case report.

Plan of care. According to the *Guide to Physical Therapist Practice*,[3(p46)] the plan of care includes "the anticipated goals and expected outcomes, predicted level of optimal improvement, specific interventions to be used, and proposed duration and frequency of the interventions that are required to reach the anticipated goals and expected outcomes." *The Guide to Occupational Therapy Practice*[4] describes similar elements for the intervention plan: long-term functional goals; short-term goals; intervention procedures; type, amount, frequency, and duration of intervention; and recommendations for need for occupational therapy services and referrals.

If you look at case reports published to date (**Appendix 4** provides a list of sample reports), you will find that the authors almost always described the elements of the plan of care or the intervention plan, but they rarely described the decision making that led to each element. In the future, reviewers, editors, and instructors will be looking for descriptions of how case report writers made these decisions. As you write your case report, be sure you answer the question "why" as it relates to each element of the plan. Why these goals? Why this intervention to achieve the goals? Why this amount, frequency, and duration of intervention? As with other parts of your case report, make your decision making explicit!

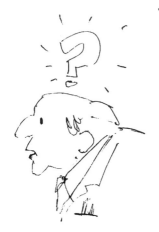

Next: What Did You Do, and Why and How Did You Do It?

Describing your patient or situation and the decision-making process leading to the intervention (if any) involves clarifying your clinical reasoning for the reader. Your rationale for the intervention that you used should be closely linked to the diagnosis or the hypothesized cause of the patient's problem and to the prognosis.

References

1   DeBakey L, DeBakey S. The case report, I: Guidelines for preparation. *Int J Cardiol.* 1983;4:357-364.

2   Depoy E, Gitlin LN. *Introduction to Research: Multiple Strategies for Health and Human Services.* St Louis, Mo: CV Mosby Co; 1994.

3   Guide to Physical Therapist Practice. 2nd ed. *Phys Ther.* 2001;81:9-744.

4   Moyers PA. *Guide to Occupational Therapy Practice.* Bethesda, Md: American Occupational Therapy Association; 1999.

5   Squires BP. Case reports: what editors want from authors and peer reviewers. *CMAJ.* 1989;141:379-380.

6   Anderson M, Tichenor CJ. A patient with de Quervain's tenosynovitis: a case report using an Australian approach to manual therapy. *Phys Ther.* 1994;74:314-326.

7   Watson CJ, Schenkman M. Physical therapy management of isolated serratus anterior muscle paralysis. *Phys Ther.* 1995;75:194-202.

8   Dunbar SB. A child's occupational performance: considerations of sensory processing and family context. *Am J Occup Ther.* 1999;53:231-235.

9   Gross MT, Schuch CP. Exercise programs for patients with post-polio syndrome: a case report. *Phys Ther.* 1989;69:72-76.

10 Beattie P. The use of an eclectic approach for the treatment of low back pain: a case study. *Phys Ther.* 1992;72:923-928.

11 Elstein AS, Shulman L, Sprafka S. Medical problem solving: a ten-year retrospective. *Evaluation and the Health Professions.* 1990;13(1):5-36.

12 Payton OD. Clinical reasoning process in physical therapy. *Phys Ther.* 1985;65:924-928.

13 Gill-Body KM, Krebs DE, Parker SW, Riley PO. Physical therapy management of peripheral vestibular dysfunction: two clinical case reports. *Phys Ther.* 1994;74:129-142.

14 Canélon MF. Job site analysis facilitates work reintegration. *Am J Occup Ther*. 1995;47:461-467.

15 Harris SR, Osborn JA, Weinberg J, et al. Effects of prenatal alcohol exposure on neuromotor and cognitive development during early childhood: a series of case reports. *Phys Ther*. 1993;73:608-617.

16 Toth-Fejel GE, Toth-Fejel GF, Hedricks CA. Occupation-centered practice in hand rehabilitation using the experience sampling method. *Am J Occup Ther*. 1998;52:381-385.

17 Fritz JM. Use of a classification approach to the treatment of 3 patients with low back syndrome. *Phys Ther*. 1998;78:766-777.

18 Gray JC. Diagnosis of intermittent vascular claudication in a patient with a diagnosis of sciatica. *Phys Ther*. 1999;79:582-590.

19 Mueller MJ, Diamond JE. Biomechanical treatment approach to diabetic plantar ulcers: a case report. *Phys Ther*. 1988;68:1917-1920.

20 Moyers PA, Stoffel VC. Alcohol dependence in a client with a work-related injury. *Am J Occup Ther*. 1999;53:640-645.

21 Riddle DL, Freeman DB. Management of a patient with a diagnosis of bilateral plantar fasciitis and Achilles tendinitis: a case report. *Phys Ther*. 1988;68:1913-1916.

22 Malouin F, Potvin M, Prévost J, et al. Use of an intensive task-oriented gait training program in a series of patients with acute cerebrovascular accidents. *Phys Ther*. 1992;72:781-793.

23 Koury MJ, Scarpelli E. A manual therapy approach to evaluation and treatment of a patient with a chronic lumbar nerve root irritation. *Phys Ther*. 1994;74:548-560.

24 Sackett DL, Straus SE, Richardson WS, et al. *Evidence-based Medicine: How to Practice and Teach EBM*. 2nd ed. New York, NY: Churchill Livingstone: 2000.

25 Abstract and commentary of: Ogilvie-Harris DJ, Gilbart M. Treatment modalities for soft tissue injuries of the ankle: a critical review. *Clin J Sport Med*. 1995:5(3);175-186. In: Database of Abstracts of Reviews of Effectiveness. 2001;1. Available at: http://nhscrd.york.ac.uk/darehp.htm. Accessed April 23, 2001.

26 Bleck EE. Locomotor prognosis in cerebral palsy. *Dev Med Child Neurol*. 1975;17:18-25.

27 da Paz AC Jr, Burnett SM, Braga LW. Walking prognosis in cerebral palsy: a 22-year retrospective analysis. *Dev Med Child Neurol*. 1994;36:130-134.

28 Watt JM, Robertson CM, Grace MG. Early prognosis for ambulation of neonatal intensive care survivors with cerebral palsy. *Dev Med Child Neurol*. 1989;31:766-773.

29 McIntosh G, Frank J, Hogg-Johnson S, et al. Prognostic factors for time receiving workers' compensation benefits in a cohort of patients with low back pain. *Spine*. 2000;25:147-157.

30 Katrak P, Bowring G, Conroy P, et al. Predicting upper limb recovery after stroke: the place of early shoulder and hand movement. *Arch Phys Med Rehabil*. 1998;79:758-761.

31 Olsen TS. Arm and leg paresis as outcome predictors in stroke rehabilitation. *Stroke*. 1990;21:247-251.

32 Kwakkel G, van Dijk GM, Wagenaar RC. Accuracy of physical and occupational therapists' early predictions of recovery after severe middle cerebral artery stroke. *Clin Rehabil*. 2000;14:28-41.

33 Russek LN. Examination and treatment of a patient with hypermobility syndrome. *Phys Ther*. 2000:80:386-389.

Chapter 7

Describing the Intervention

After describing the patient (or other entity), the examination, and the evaluation, the next step is to describe what was done to reach the identified goals and outcomes—that is, the next step is to describe the intervention. When the focus of the case report is an entity other than a patient, the "intervention" can take many forms. Both the decision-making process that led to the intervention decisions and the components of the intervention should be clearly described.

If case reports are to be useful to clinicians and are to serve as a basis for experimental studies, descriptions of the intervention rationale must be complete and understandable.

Intervention Rationale

Unfortunately, many case reports published in the rehabilitation literature do not adequately describe the rationale that the author used in deciding what interventions to use and how to apply them. The rationale for intervention is part of the decision-making process described in **Chapter 6**. Depending on the flow of the case report, the plan of care and its rationale could be addressed under the subhead of "prognosis," "plan of care,"[1] "intervention plan,"[2] or "intervention." In either case, the rationale must be addressed. Today, editors and reviewers make certain that it is!

Clinical decisions related to interventions can be classified into two types: those that relate to the type and amount of intervention initially chosen, and those that relate to why an intervention approach should be modified. The information reported in a case report to support these two types of decisions can come from a variety of sources, including published research reports, arguments for biological plausibility, and theoretical arguments that have been published in books or journals. You do not always have to reference the work of others when explaining why you made your intervention decisions; however, citing previously published work greatly strengthens the basis of many intervention decisions. Other intervention decisions may be based on the clinical environment or on the patient's environment. "Logic" and "common sense" may serve as a basis for intervention decisions, but the rationale must be consistent with existing evidence about the effectiveness or ineffectiveness of the intervention approach.

Selection of the initial interventions. One example of explaining rationale is found in the case report of Koury and Scarpelli,[3(p553-554)] who described why the initial intervention was chosen for a patient with low back pain:

> Initial treatment consisted of three 45-second bouts of left L-5 unilateral PA mobilizations, as described by Maitland.[2] We chose this treatment approach because we believe (1) the patient had a local joint dysfunction to which a left L-5 unilateral PA pressure was most comparable, (2) the problem was one of resistance greater than pain because on passive testing the examiner encountered resistance prior to any complaints of symptoms, (3) there were no contraindications to compressing the involved joint surfaces or structures, (4) PA mobilization helps to restore extension, and (5) unilateral problems respond to unilateral techniques.[2,32]

In a case report involving a patient diagnosed with lower-extremity hypertonia associated with static encephalopathy, Selby[4(p1922)] described why she chose to position her patient's feet in a specific way when using serial casting:

> The serial application of bivalved casts set in the subtalar neutral (STN) position...was used to gradually lengthen the child's tight tendons while allowing him to practice a heel-toe gait pattern. The STN position was chosen for the following reasons: 1) It reportedly provides maximum congruency of the foot and ankle joints, thereby providing an optimally stable position for weight-bearing; 2) the STN position has been described as a midposition for the foot around which the motions of supination and pronation occur[3]; and 3) I have found that the STN position produces the fewest problems with skin condition during use of casts and orthoses.

Many intervention regimens are designed to increase the force-generating capacity of a muscle or a group of muscles. Watson and Schenkman[5(p200)] described their rationale for the strengthening exercise program that they designed for a patient with paralysis of the serratus anterior muscle:

> Strengthening exercises for the lower trapezius muscle, the serratus anterior muscle, and the rotator cuff were to be performed every other day (30 repetitions each). Strengthening of the lower trapezius muscle has been described as one of the major aims of therapy in the case of serratus anterior muscle paralysis secondary to the ability of the lower trapezius muscle to protect serratus anterior muscle from elongation.[3] The patient performed the lower trapezius muscle exercise in the prone-lying posi-

tion with the affected upper extremity over the side of the table.... In this position, the patient was instructed to laterally rotate the shoulder and then flex through the full pain-free ROM. The prone position was selected to reduce the effects of gravity and to allow scapular mobility, which could be hindered in the supine position. Although contraction of the lower trapezius muscle does produce some scapular adduction, this is not its primary action. This patient was initially thought to have hypertrophy of the upper trapezius muscle, probably secondary to increased functional demands placed on the muscle; strengthening exercises were therefore not specifically addressed.

In this example, the rationale for several clinical decisions was described, including 1) why it was important to strengthen the lower trapezius muscle, with a reference to a published paper to support the authors' decision, 2) why the patient was positioned in a particular way, and 3) why the upper-trapezius muscle was not exercised. All of these decisions clarify for the reader why the authors did what they did.

Modification of the interventions. Gill-Body and colleagues[6(p133)] defined the criteria they used to determine when the rehabilitation program of a patient with peripheral vestibular dysfunction should be progressed. The program was divided into three phases:

> The patient progressed to each new phase during weekly visits to the physical therapy clinic as her performance on the previous phase improved to the point at which the individual exercises could be performed easily and without an increase in the perception of disequilibrium.

Flowers et al[7(p65)] devoted a major portion of their case report about a patient with finger extensor tendon lacerations to a description of the progression of intervention based on the reexamination and reevaluation. A small sample of their decision making:

> The patient was unable to return to the clinic for 5 days (February 14), at which time a 5-degree improvement in the extension lag (25°) was noted along with no change in flexion (90°). We were encouraged, but reluctant to place too much emphasis on only a 5-degree change in measurement. No change was made in the program.... On February 21, the extension lag had improved to 20 degrees and the flexion increased back to 90 degrees. The improving extension was interpreted as evidence of desirable remodeling at the attenuated repair site. The persistent 20-degree extension lag, however, also suggested a potential tendon adhesion. It was now approximately 8 weeks postsurgery. A decision was made to institute gentle resistive extension exercise based on our hypothesis that the extension lag was due to a restricting adhesion. Because it was now about 8 weeks postsurgery, we felt that maturation of the scar at the repair site provided sufficient tensile strength to allow resistive extension.

The authors' explanation for why intervention was changed is an important part of case reports. Without an adequate explanation, the reader can only speculate as to why intervention might have been altered.

How Was the Intervention Applied?

In addition to explaining why the intervention was selected and why it changed over time, authors must describe how the intervention was applied—so clearly and completely that another therapist could replicate the intervention with a similar patient. Interventions described in case reports appear primarily in text format, tables or figures, or both. The challenge is to determine which formats will do the best job of operationally defining your interventions.

Malouin et al[8(p782)] wrote a clear operational definition of the intervention applied to a group of patients diagnosed with an acute cerebrovascular accident. This is only an excerpt, but the authors' use of operational definitions still is clear:

> Two daily physical therapy sessions, each of 60 minutes' duration, were planned for each patient from about the eighth day after stroke, 5 days a week, for a 5-week period.... The main objective of the program was to promote gait relearning by means of intensive SGT [special gait-related training] activities introduced early in the rehabilitation process. It was thus important to practice different activities preparatory to independent standing and walking.... As soon as a patient was able to stand and take a few steps, walking was started on the treadmill. Treadmill training was initiated at two velocities: 0.045 and 0.09 m/s. The velocity was progressively increased according to individual capacity. A safety harness consisting of a climber's belt and a pulley system...was used to guard against falls. Other safety modifications, such as padding of the front panel and the treadmill rails, were made. The training was carried out by two physical therapists from the hospital at which the study was carried out. Generally, a patient was treated by the same therapist over the 5-week program.

The authors defined the intervention programs more thoroughly later in the manuscript and specifically defined the criteria for progression of the interventions. They also provided data that described the extent of the patient's participation in the intervention.

Some clinical decisions can relate to very specific parts of an intervention, so the intervention description must be just as specific. Olney and colleagues[9(p866)] described use of biofeedback and a gait analysis system with a patient who had a gait disturbance:

> We instructed the patient that a sound would be heard each time she reached the target value within the prescribed phase of the gait cycle and that the feedback coach would give her a score after each six-stride walk.

Table 12. Individual Compliance with Treatment Protocol Over the 5-Week Training Program[8]

Patient No.	No. of Physical Therapy Sessions	Mean Duration of Treatment (min)	Total Treatment Time (h)	% SGT[a]
101	43	56.4	40.42	25.0
106	48	50.9	40.72	27.2
108	50	47.6	39.67	35.5
113	50	52.4	43.67	40.5
201	41	55.8	38.13	28.0
205	39	49.3	32.05	15.7
208	50	55.3	46.10	25.1
211	47	44.5	34.86	40.4
212	50	57.5	47.92	32.5
$\bar{X}$	46.8	52.2	40.39	30.0
SD	4.5	4.5	5.1	8.1
Range	39–50	44.5–57.5	32.1–47.9	15.7–40.5
Maximum value possible	50	60	50	100
% of maximum value	93.6	87	80	30

[a]Percentage of treatment time devoted to special gait training activities.

After a few trials, Mrs P was able to obtain the beep with each stride, but she accomplished it by using an exaggerated flexion synergy, elevating her pelvis, and flexing her hip to accomplish the knee flexion. The physical therapist instructed her to allow her pelvis to drop rather than to elevate it and to lift her heel and allow her knee to bend before her forefoot left the ground. She was told that the beep should occur soon after this movement. The target value was decreased from 5 degrees to 3 degrees over the average maximum degrees of flexion to make the task easier. She did not use the abnormal pattern after this instruction.

Patient participation. Patient participation is an important issue to address in all case reports that describe the implementation of interventions. ("Participation" is preferred to "adherence" or "compliance" because it better reflects the partnership that should exist between patient and therapist.) Malouin et al[8] devoted an entire section in their report to this issue, summarizing in a table the data that described the frequency and duration of intervention (**Table 12**). Sometimes a brief description of a patient's report is all that is needed. The patient could be asked, for example, to keep a daily log of the number of times an exercise program was done. The log should then be used to describe how frequently a patient reported exercising.

An issue related to patient participation is whether the planned intervention was actually carried out. A patient may carry out a home exercise program but may be doing the exercises incorrectly. Descriptions that address both the extent of participation and the correctness of application strengthen a case report.

<u>Posterior Thigh Pain in a Patient With Low Back Pain</u>

<u>Description of Intervention</u>

Some key elements are required, as this abbreviated example shows. An initial dosage is reported with justification for using this dosage; the exercise is described in detail, including patient positioning, use of the home environment, and duration and frequency; and progression of intervention and the rationale for progression are reported. The change in patient status is also reported with progression:

Plan of Care

The patient was seen in the clinic twice the first week and once a week the following 3 weeks. We believed that because the patient's symptoms were intermittent in nature and there was no evidence of neurological involvement, we could most efficiently manage the patient by seeing him twice the first week. We believed that we could establish an appropriate regimen at the first visit and that the second visit could be used to ensure that the patient was performing the exercise safely and correctly. We only needed to see him one time per week after the first week to conduct a reexamination and to make modifications in the program, if necessary. The intervention consisted of exercise.

Exercise

Hamstring stretching: The patient was instructed to perform a hamstring stretching exercise in the following way. While lying supine on the floor in a doorway, the patient placed his left foot on the adjoining wall while maintaining the knee in full extension. The leg was placed at a height that initially provoked the pain symptoms in the left thigh. Based on the premise of total end-range time described by McClure and Flowers,[1] we believed this dosage of intervention would allow for improvements in the impaired straight leg raise (SLR) without worsening the pain.

Progression of intervention was determined by the patient's reported pain intensity during the exercise. As the intensity of the pain decreased, the patient's foot was positioned higher on the wall (the angle of the SLR was increased). During the first week the patient simulated a 45-degree SLR during the physical therapy session. The patient was instructed to hold the position for 30 seconds. Instructions were given to repeat the exercise once an hour for each hour the patient was awake.

By the second week, the patient had progressed to a position of approximately 55 degrees for the SLR. He was instructed to hold this position for a period of 1 minute per every waking hour. Because he improved his angle of SLR, we instructed him to increase the duration of the exercise. We believed a longer duration would increase total end-range time and facilitate further improvements. By the third week, the patient had progressed to a 65-degree SLR that was held for a period of 3 minutes, five times per day. We reduced the frequency of daily exercise because the patient was able to tolerate a longer duration of exercise per session. We kept the total end-range time constant (approximately 15 minutes) because this amount of time seemed to be resulting in improved SLR performance.

By the fourth week, the patient had progressed to a 75-degree SLR during the exercise. The frequency and duration were not changed.

Compare the above description with the following:

Plan of care: The patient was seen in the clinic twice the first week and once a week during the following 3 weeks. The intervention consisted of exercise.

Exercise

Hamstring stretching: The patient performed hamstring stretching for 30 seconds several times a day. The intervention was progressed every week based on patient tolerance. The treatment lasted a total of 4 weeks.

What's missing? Although there is some description of intervention dosage, no justification for this dosage is given. The exercise is named but not described. Because there are many ways to perform hamstring muscle stretching, it would be important to describe how it was done in this case. There is very little explanation of progression and no explanation of the rationale for progression.

References

1 McClure PW, Flowers KJ. Treatment of limited shoulder motion using an elevation splint. *Phys Ther*. 1992;72:57-62.

The case report of Mitchell and Versluis[10(p392)] illustrates how a patient's home exercise program can be operationally defined. The patient had an above-knee amputation and had recently received a heart transplant:

> A home exercise program was prescribed to increase the patient's muscle strength and she was instructed in proper positioning of the residual limb to prevent contractures. The home exercise program consisted of bilateral lower extremity hip flexion, extension, and abduction and right knee extension. Upper extremity exercises consisted of shoulder flexion and abduction and elbow flexion and extension. The exercises were to be performed twice daily for 10 repetitions initially. The patient was progressed from performing active ROM [range of motion] on the lower extremities to resistive exercise, and the number of repetitions was increased to 20. The patient was instructed to lie prone for 20 minutes daily to prevent hip flexion contractures. In addition, the patient was instructed to use a perceived exertion scale (ie, shortness of breath, sweating), rather than monitoring her heart rate and blood pressure, as is common in cardiac patients without heart transplant, because the transplanted denervated heart does not respond with typical parasympathetic and sympathetic changes to exercise.

Home exercise programs commonly are described in case reports. The home exercise program described above illustrates one way of operationalizing a home program. Mitchell and Versluis defined the type of exercises that were done, the number of repetitions for each exercise, and the criterion used to stop exercise. Authors can enhance an operational definition of a home program by describing the patient position during exercise and the amount and type of resistance used. Editors and reviewers ask for those details.

Dunbar[11(p233)] also operationally defined a home program that was carried out by the mother of a child with sensory processing problems: "While discussing the type of involvement that she was able to provide, while taking her other obligations into consideration, the mother agreed to take Sara to the park at least once daily for 1 hr, and she agreed to integrate other sensory activities into her daily caregiving routine. Several types of vestibular and proprioceptive activities that Sara appeared to need were available at the park: monkey bar climbing, slide play, and games incorporating running and jumping." Dunbar then went on to describe other types of activities that were incorporated into daily activities.

Using Tables and Figures to Summarize

The use of a table to summarize interventions is advantageous for two reasons. First, the reader can see the "big picture" when interventions are summarized in a table. Descriptions of interventions in a text format sometimes are difficult to follow, especially when the descriptions are lengthy. Second, the use of a table allows the reader to easily follow the chronology of intervention. For some examples of how tables and figures have been used in published case reports, see the following pages.

Table 13. Summary of Treatments[3]

Findings	Treatment	Reassessment	Working Hypothesis
Initial evaluation (day 1)			
Extension with over-pressure increased buttocks pain	Left L-5 unilateral posteroanterior (PA) mobilizations (three bouts)	Extension with over-pressure normal	Extension dysfunction
Left lumbar quadrant test increased thigh pain		Left lumbar quadrant test increased ROM	L-5 chronic nerve root irritation
Right side bending with over-pressure reproduced thigh burning			
Flexion −15 cm (−6 in) from fingertips to floor reproduced leg pain		Flexion, right side bending, SLR, and slump unchanged	Adverse neural tissue tension test (ANTT) component
Straight leg raising (SLR) to 65° reproduced burning pain			
Slump test at −15° of knee extension reproduced numbness and tingling			
Day 2			
Flexion −15 cm from fingertips to floor increased leg pain	Left L-5 unilateral PA mobilizations (three bouts) with increased vigor	No change in remaining comparable signs	L-5 chronic nerve root irritation
SLR to 65° reproduced burning pain	Exercise program for abdominal, gluteal, and quadriceps femoris muscles		ANTT component
Slump test at −15° of knee extension reproduced numbness and tingling			
Extension and quadrant tests were full range of motion (ROM) and painless to over-pressure			
Day 3			
Flexion −15 cm from fingertips to floor increased leg pain	Left L-5 unilateral PA mobilizations (three bouts)	7.6-cm (3-in) increase in flexion	L-5 chronic nerve root irritation
SLR to 65° reproduced burning pain	Three general lumbar rotations to the left	No change noted in right side bending, SLR, or slump	ANTT component
Slump test of −15° of knee extension reproduced numbness and tingling			
Right side bending with over-pressure reproduced thigh burning			
Day 4			
Flexion −7.6 cm from fingertips to floor increased leg pain	Left L-5 unilateral PA mobilizations (three bouts)	Fingertips to floor increased leg pain	L-5 chronic nerve root irritation
SLR to 65° reproduced burning pain	Three general lumbar rotations to the left	SLR to 75° increased leg symptoms	ANTT component
Slump test at −15° of knee extension reproduced numbness and tingling	Hold-relax SLR	Slump test increased numbness and tingling at −10° of knee extension	
Day 5			
Flexion full, but with over-pressure increased leg symptoms	Three bouts of left L-5 unilateral PA mobilizations	All active movements and SLR were full ROM and painless to over-pressure	ANTT component

(continued)

Table 13. Continued

Findings	Treatment	Reassessment	Working Hypothesis
Day 5			
SLR to 75° with neck flexion (NF) and dorsiflexion (DF) components increased burning sensation	Three general lumbar rotations to the left	Slump test at −5° of knee extension reproduced numbness and tingling	L-5 chronic nerve root irritation
Slump test at −10° of knee extension reproduced numbness and tingling	Three bouts (45 s) of SLR at 75°		
Right side bending was full ROM and painless to over-pressure			
Day 6			
Slump test at −5° of knee extension reproduced numbness and tingling	Slump test with the components of NF and DF at −5° of knee extension	Slump reproduced numbness and tingling with the components of NF and DF	ANTT component
All other tests negative			L-5 chronic nerve root irritation
Day 7			
Slump test with components of NF, DF, and hip flexion reproduced numbness and tingling	Slump test with the components of NF, DF, and hip flexion	Slump test normal stretch	Resolving nerve root
			Minimal ANTT component
Day 8			
No objective signs noted	Reviewed home exercise	No physical signs	Discharged to home exercise program, no longer experienced any symptoms or physical signs and was not limited functionally

■ **Table 13** contains an intervention summary from Koury and Scarpelli's[3] case report on a patient with low back pain. At a glance, the reader can determine how many types of interventions were used, what the interventions were, and why those interventions were selected. One problem with describing interventions in tabular format is that the descriptions are too brief. Koury and Scarpelli solved that problem by supplementing the table with complete operational definitions in the text.

■ Gill-Body and colleagues[6] created a different type of table to report an intervention approach used for a patient with unilateral vestibular dysfunction (**Table 14**). The table lists the intervention activities and describes the rationale for the different phases of intervention. Again, the authors supplemented the information in the table with descriptions in the text.

Table 14. Vestibular Rehabilitation Treatment Program and Its Rationale for Patients With Unilateral Vestibular Dysfunction[6]

Rationale	Treatment Activity[a]
Phase 1	
1. Encourage active extraocular movements	Extraocular movements, self-selected speed
2. Enhance vestibular adaptation	Visual fixation, EO, stationary target, slow head movements, near targets
3. Encourage resetting of VOR gain	Imaginary visual fixation, EC, small head movements, self-selected speed
4. Promote utilization of somatosensory and vestibular inputs for postural control	Static stance, EO and EC, feet together, arms outstretched, book on head
5. Improve dynamic postural control utilizing all sensory inputs	Gait with narrowed base of support, EO
6. Improve dynamic postural control utilizing all sensory inputs	March in place slowly, EO
7. Decrease cervical musculature tightness	Active neck range of motion, all directions, slow movements
Phase 2	
1. Promote use of VOR at various speed head movements	Visual fixation, EO, stationary target, fast and slow movements, near targets
2. Enhance vestibular adaptation by inducing retinal slip	Visual fixation, EO, moving target in opposite direction, slow head movements
3. Promote utilization of somatosensory and vestibular inputs for postural control	Static stance, semitandem, EO and EC, arms close to body, book on head
4. Promote use of somatosensory inputs for postural control	Static stance on foam surface, EO, book on head
5. Improve dynamic postural control utilizing somatosensory inputs	Gait with narrowed base of support, EO, book on head
6. Improve dynamic postural control utilizing somatosensory inputs	Gait with normal base of support, EO, book on head
7. Decrease cervical muscle tightness	Active neck range of motion, all directions, slow movements
Phase 3	
1. Enhance vestibular adaptation	Visual fixation, EO, stationary target, fast and slow head movements, near and far targets
2. Enhance vestibular adaptation	Visual fixation, EO, moving target, slow and fast head movements
3. Promote use of somatosensory and vestibular inputs for postural control	Static stance on foam surface, EC, with and without book on head
4. Improve dynamic postural trol utilizing vestibular and somatosensory inputs	Gait with narrowed base of support, EC, with and without book on head
5. Improve dynamic postural control when head is moving utilizing all sensory inputs	Gait with normal base of support, fast head movements
6. Improve dynamic postural control utilizing somatosensory and vestibular inputs	March in place slowly, EO and EC, with and without book on head
7. Decrease cervical muscle tightness	Active neck range of motion, all directions, slow movements

[a]EO=eyes open; EC=eyes closed; VOR=vestibular ocular reflex.

Table 15. Biofeedback-Monitored Protocol[a]

Visit	Motion	Time (Minutes)	Repetitions/Threshold
1	Humeral flexion to 90° with external rotation	15	To fatigue
	Abduction to 90° with external rotation	15	To fatigue
2	Humeral flexion with external rotation	15	Increase repetitions Increase threshold
	Abduction with external rotation	15	Increase repetitions Increase threshold
	Horizonal abduction from 90° of flexion	15	To fatigue
3	Humeral flexion with external rotation	5	50 repetitions
	Humeral flexion at neutral	5	50 repetitions
	Humeral flexion with internal rotation	5	50 repetitions
	Abduction with external rotation	5	50 repetitions
	Abduction at neutral	5	50 repetitions
	Abduction with internal rotation	5	50 repetitions
4	Same as Visit 3	5	Increase repetitions Increase threshold
	Reaching behind back	5	
	Functional activities	5	
5	Visit 4 motions with light weight (1.36 kg)*		Three sets of 10 for each motion
Week 3	Same motions with increasing weights, rotator cuff strengthening, plyometrics, PNF, scapular stabilization		

*3 lbs.

PNF = Proprioceptive neuromuscular facilitation.

[a]Reprinted with permission of Williams & Wilkins, Baltimore, Md from Young MS. Electromyographic biofeedback use in the treatment of voluntary posterior dislocation of the shoulder: a case study. *J Orthop Sports Phys Ther*. 1994;20:171-175.

■ In a case report written by Young,[12] a table was created to summarize the types of exercises used by a patient who had repeated posterior dislocations of the glenohumeral joint (**Table 15**). The table concisely describes the temporal sequence of the program, the type of exercise used, the duration of the exercise, and the number of repetitions used for each exercise. Young also supplemented the table with text to operationally define the intervention.

Table 16. Chronological Description of Treatment and Passive Range of Motion (PROM).[13]

Weeks Postinjury	Treatment	PROM (°)		
		Flexion	Abduction[a]	Lateral Rotation[b]
0	Fracture/dislocation			
6	Moist heat, ultrasound, pendulum, low-grade manual therapy, ice post-exercise (visits three times per week)	80	60	5
6+day	Increase to high-grade manual therapy, continuous passive motion, home program (three times per day): pendulum, wand, ice	80	60	5
8	Allow gentle activities of daily living	100	75	15
10	Reduce visits to twice per week, discontinue ultrasound, add elevation splint 1 hour four times per day	105	85	20
12	Discontinue all treatment in clinic, continue to monitor outcome of home program, add strengthening, increase splint time to 2 hours four times per day	130	105	40
13	No change	140	120	50
14	No change	155	145	65
15	No change	165	160	65
16	No change	165	165	70
25	Patient discharged	175	170	80

[a]Abduction measured with the arm 40° to the coronal plane.

[b]Lateral rotation measured with the arm by the side.

■ McClure and Flowers[13] used a table to summarize the chronological progression of the intervention and the changes in status in a patient with limited glenohumeral range of motion following a fracture and dislocation of the humeral head (**Table 16**).

■ Twist[14] used a figure to illustrate the electrode placements used in the intervention for a patient with a spinal cord injury (**Figure 16**).

■ Cibulka[15] used figures to illustrate the method for applying a joint mobilization procedure to the first metatarsophalangeal joint of a patient who had forefoot pain (**Figure 17**).

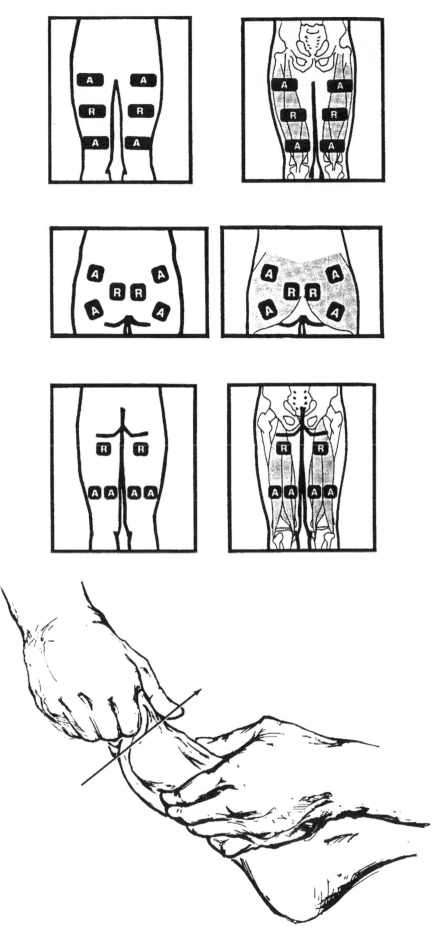

Figure 16. *Electrode placement: quadriceps femoris muscles (top diagrams); gluteus maximus muscles (center diagrams); hamstring muscles (bottom diagrams). (A = active electrodes; R = reference electrodes.)[14]*

Figure 17. *Method for stabilizing and evaluating metatarsophalangeal (MTP) joint dorsiflexion and mobilizing MTP joint by translating (in direction of arrow) proximal phalanx dorsally with metatarsal bone stabilized.[16]*

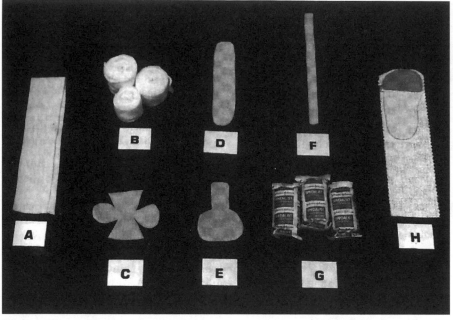

Figure 18. *Equipment: (a) stockinette, (b) cast pad, (c) bimalleolar pad, (d) tibial pad, (e) heel pad, (f) strip for cast cutter protection, (g) plaster, (h) footplate.*[16]

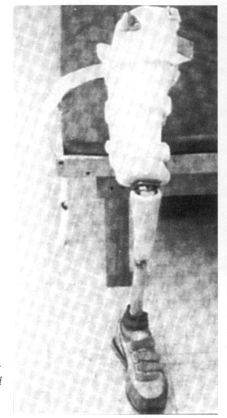

Figure 19. *Temporary contoured adducted trochanteric-controlled alignment method (CAT-CAM) prosthesis with removable lateral wall.*[9]

Figure 20. *(right) A) Internal/external rotation with 45° of abduction. This exercise shows internal rotation and was a progression of the treatment. The rope from the pulley apparatus was perpendicular to the patient's lower arm. This allowed for maximum resistance in the middle range and decreasing resistance at the end range and allowed the optimal stimulus for the muscle to occur. At the start of the treatment, the patient performed three sets of 40 repetitions against a graded weight resistance of 0.5 kg, and after 2 ½ months of treatment, the weight resistance had been increased to 1 kg. (left) B) Internal/external rotation with 70° of abduction. The figure shows external rotation and was a further progression of the treatment. As the patient recovered, he was working through an increasingly greater range of motion. At this point, the patient performed three sets of 40 repetitions with a weight resistance of only 0.5 kg. Reprinted with permission of Williams & Wilkins, Baltimore, Md, from Torstensen TA, Meen HD, Stiris M. The effect of medical exercise therapy on a patient with chronic supraspinatus tendinitis: diagnostic ultrasound—tissue regeneration: a case study. J Orthop Sports Phys Ther. 1994;6:319-327.*

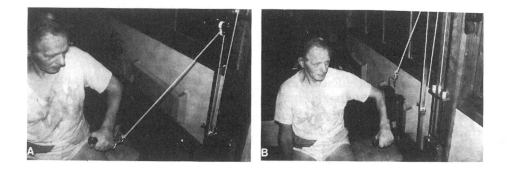

■ To enhance their operational definition of a serial casting intervention for correcting contractures following an acute burn injury, Johnson and Silverberg[16] used a figure that illustrated the equipment used to make serial casts (**Figure 18**).

■ Mitchell and Versluis[10] included a photograph of a temporary prosthesis used in the management of a patient with an above-knee amputation (**Figure 19**).

■ Torstensen and colleagues[17] included several photographs in their case report to clarify the operational definitions of the exercises that were used for a patient with a diagnosis of supraspinatus tendinitis (**Figure 20**).

■ Watson and Schenkman[5] used diagrams to operationalize exercises (**Figure 21**).

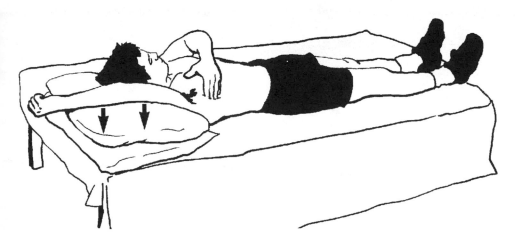

Figure 21. *Diagram illustrating serratus anterior muscle strengthening by upwardly rotating the scapula while simultaneously flexing the humerus; the patient is palpating to determine whether the serratus anterior muscle is contracting.*[5]

Appendix
Audiotape Script for Dressing Training

Time	Cue	Instruction
	1	"Ethel, listen to the tape. It is time to dress."
	2	"Look at your bed. Do not touch your clothes until told to do so by the tape."
12 sec	3	"Take off your nightgown."
5 sec	4	"Put your nightgown on your bed BEHIND your pile of clothes."
1 min 30 sec	5	"Pick up your bra. Put it on."
1 min 50 sec	6	"Put on your blouse [slight pause] and button it."
45 sec	7	"Put on your underpants."
1 min 40 sec	8	"Put on your pants."
50 sec	9	"Take ONE sock and put it on."
50 sec	10	"Take the other sock and put it on."
60 sec	11	"Take ONE shoe. Put it on and tie it."
60 sec	12	"Take the other shoe. Put it on and tie it."
	13	"STOP. Make sure you have put on all of your clothes. Check your bra. Check your blouse. Check your underpants. Check your pants. Check your left sock. Check your right sock. Check your left shoe. Check your right shoe."
	14	"You are finished dressing. STOP."

Figure 22. *An appendix used to provide information about a specific component of an intervention. Reprinted with permission of the American Occupational Therapy Association from Cook EA, Luschen L, Sikes S. Dressing training for an elderly woman with cognitive and perceptual impairments. Am J Occup Ther. 1991;45:652-654.*

Using Appendixes to Provide Specific Information

Appendixes also can be used to provide information about interventions. Cook et al[18] used an appendix to describe one of the components of dressing training for elderly patients with cognitive and perceptual impairments (**Figure 22**).

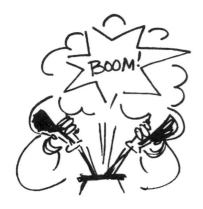

Next: What Happened?

"Outcomes" are more than changes in the patient's impairments, such as range of motion. Case reports should include changes in the patient's ability to do those things that are important to that patient—getting dishes out of a cabinet, walking to the bathroom. There are many ways to depict outcomes. Be creative!

References

1   Guide to Physical Therapist Practice. 2nd ed. *Phys Ther*. 2001;81:9-744.

2   Moyers PA. *The Guide to Occupational Therapy Practice*. Bethesda, Md: American Occupational Therapy Association; 1999.

3   Koury MJ, Scarpelli E. A manual therapy approach to evaluation and treatment of a patient with a chronic lumbar nerve root irritation. *Phys Ther*. 1994;74:548-560.

4   Selby L. Remediation of toe-walking behavior with neutral-position, serial-inhibitory casts: a case report. *Phys Ther*. 1988;68:1921-1923.

5   Watson CJ, Schenkman M. Physical therapy management of isolated serratus anterior muscle paralysis. *Phys Ther*. 1995;75:194-202.

6   Gill-Body KM, Krebs DE, Parker SW, Riley PO. Physical therapy management of peripheral vestibular dysfunction: two clinical case reports. *Phys Ther*. 1994;74:129-142.

7   Flowers KR, McClure PW, McFadden C. Management of a patient with lacerations of the tendons of the extensor digitorum and extensor indicis muscles to the index finger. *Phys Ther*. 1996;76:61-66.

8   Malouin F, Potvin M, Prévost J, et al. Use of an intensive task-oriented gait training program in a series of patients with acute cerebrovascular accidents. *Phys Ther*. 1992;72:781-793.

9   Olney SJ, Colborne GR, Martin CS. Joint angle biofeedback and biomechanical gait analysis in stroke patients: a case report. *Phys Ther*. 1989;69:863-870.

10 Mitchell CA, Versluis TL. Management of an above-knee amputee with complex medical problems using the CAT-CAM prosthesis. *Phys Ther*. 1990;70:389-393.

11 Dunbar SB. A child's occupational performance: considerations of sensory processing and family context. *Am J Occup Ther*. 1999;53:231-235.

12 Young MS. Electromyographic biofeedback use in the treatment of voluntary posterior dislocation of the shoulder: a case study. *J Orthop Sports Phys Ther*. 1994;20:171-175.

13 McClure PW, Flowers KR. Treatment of limited shoulder motion: a case study based on biomechanical considerations. *Phys Ther*. 1992;72:929-936.

14 Twist DJ. Acrocyanosis in a spinal cord injured patient—effects of computer-controlled neuromuscular electrical stimulation: a case report. *Phys Ther*. 1990;70:45-49.

15 Cibulka MT. Management of a patient with forefoot pain: a case report. *Phys Ther*. 1990;70:41-44.

16 Johnson J, Silverberg R. Serial casting of the lower extremity to correct contractures during the acute phase of burn care. *Phys Ther*. 1995;75:262-266.

17 Torstensen TA, Meen HD, Stiris M. The effect of medical exercise therapy on a patient with chronic supraspinatus tendinitis: diagnostic ultrasound—tissue regeneration, a case study. *J Orthop Sports Phys Ther*. 1994;6:319-327.

18 Cook EA, Luschen L, Sikes S. Dressing training for an elderly woman with cognitive and perceptual impairments. *Am J Occup Ther*. 1991;45:652-654.

Chapter 8

Describing the Outcomes

For the purpose of a case report, "outcome" is defined as the status of the patient, other entity, or situation following intervention. When the case report describes nonpatients (eg, students), the outcome usually relates to how those nonpatients function in the environment described in the report. When the case report describes patients, the outcome usually relates to the patient's ability to complete physical actions, tasks, or activities (functional limitations and disabilities). Outcomes also can relate to risk reduction/prevention; health, wellness, and fitness; societal resources; and patient/client satisfaction.[1] Remember: Case reports can only describe outcomes; they can't prove that interventions *cause* outcomes.

Some case reports describe changes in impairments, such as range of motion or pain, as an outcome—but that's not enough. At a minimum, case reports should describe changes that occur in the functional limitations and disabilities. After all, improvement in impairments may not always relate to the aim of intervention, which is to improve a patient's ability to perform real-life activities.

Outcomes can be measured using one or more of the tests and measures designed to assess the patient's ability to function. (**Appendix 2** contains a list of references to some published studies on the reliability and validity of measurements obtained with some commonly used tests and measures.) It is not necessary to use a published test or measure, however, if the outcome can be better described through the *patient's report* of changes in functional limitations and disabilities. Some published tests and measures are not responsive enough to detect changes that are meaningful for individual patients; others may not contain items that measure the patient's desired outcomes. Case reports are strengthened if the patient's reports of progress are obtained during the course of intervention as well as at the end of

What is an outcome? It can be how a group of people function in a given environment, or it can be the status of patients after an intervention.

intervention and if long-term follow-up information is obtained, even from a simple telephone call. Outcomes can be depicted in text, tables, or a variety of figures.

Outcomes in Text

Anderson and Tichenor[2(p323)] reported the following outcome after an intervention program for a patient with a diagnosis of de Quervain tenosynovitis:

> When discharged, she reported having no pain at night, no wrist and hand pain, no numbness, and no sharp pain in the thumb or radiating pain up the lateral aspect of the radius. The pain in the deltoid muscle remained the most resistant to change, with exacerbations occurring for no identifiable reason. The patient reported she was still unable to vacuum or lift heavy pots because of weakness.

The outcome described by Anderson and Tichenor illustrates the importance of reporting on the patient's ability to perform functional activities. Despite the resolved pain and numbness (impairments), the patient still was unable to use the vacuum cleaner or lift heavy objects (functional limitation), and her ability to perform the role of homemaker was still limited (disability).

In her case report of a child with sensory processing problems, Dunbar[3(p233-234)] first described improvement in impairment, as measured by a standardized test, and then improvement in functional limitations and disabilities that were important to the child's family:

> Sara had made tremendous gains evidenced by an increase in scores on the DeGangi-Berk Test of Sensory Integration. Her retest score increased by 8 points (from 7 to 15) for postural control, by 17 points (from 4 to 21) for bilateral motor integration, and by 14 points (from 0 to 14) for reflex integration. Specific improvements in Sara's behavior and occupational performance that had meaning for this particular family were an ability to quietly color and engage in other tabletop play for a 2-hour airplane trip, cessation of head banging, diminishment of tantrums, and sleeping though the night.

Another outcome that Dunbar described was Sara's mother's statement that she had increased awareness of ways in which she could help her daughter.

The case report of McClure and Flowers[4(p934)] reports the outcome both at the time of termination of physical therapy services and at follow-up. The authors developed and applied an intervention for a patient whose shoulder was immobilized following a dislocation and fracture of the head of the humerus:

> Twenty-five weeks after her injury, the patient had achieved almost full pain-free PROM [passive range of motion].... She was independent in activities of daily living including dressing, bathing, cooking, typing, and lifting the types of objects she was able to lift prior to her injury. At

1-year and 5-year follow-ups, she had no complaints of pain and she had full function and ROM.

The case report of a patient with peripheral vestibular dysfunction, written by Gill-Body and colleagues,[5(p133)] shows how impairment, functional limitation, and disability measurements can be used to describe the outcome of intervention. They used a self-report measure to describe the change in disability, the Dizziness Handicap Inventory (DHI):

At the conclusion of the 8-week period of intervention, the patient reported a slight decrease in the intensity of her sensation of disequilibrium (3/10) and improvements in four physical and two functional activities previously reported to be problematic on the DHI. No items on the DHI were reported to be worse. Clinical balance assessment revealed no change in ability to perform unilateral stance with eyes open or eyes closed. Tandem stance with eyes closed could be performed for 20 seconds (improved from 5 seconds). Stance with eyes closed and with feet together on the floor and on foam could be performed without any observable increase in sway for 60 seconds. Tandem gait with eyes open could be performed for seven steps (improved from five steps). The patient's active cervical range of motion was full, and she no longer reported any feelings of muscular pulling during active cervical movements. Posture was improved, as noted by a more erect stance and only a minimally displaced forward head. During observation of gait, her base of support appeared normal and she demonstrated some arm swing and trunk rotation. She was able to walk in a straight line without difficulty but continued to stagger to the side if she attempted to turn quickly. She was able to ambulate in a straight path without slowing her speed of gait while rotating her head from side to side with only occasional cross steps.

Note how the authors linked measurement of impairment and functional limitation to measurement of the patient's self-perceived disability. Linking measurements of impairment, functional limitation, and disability gives the reader insights into what impairment measurements may be the most relevant to the patient's function. Because therapists frequently base their intervention decisions on the types of impairments that exist, this approach is strongly recommended.

Linking measurements of impairment, functional limitation, and disability gives the reader insights into what impairments may be the most relevant.

Young[6(p173)] concisely described the outcome for a patient with a recurring dislocation of the shoulder: "One year postdischarge from physical therapy, her shoulder had not dislocated and she was throwing the shot put for her high school track team." In contrast, Watson and Schenkman[7(p201)] gave a detailed description of the outcome for a patient with paralysis of the serratus anterior muscle:

After 5 months of physical therapy, and 10 months after the onset of right shoulder pain, the patient had retained full shoulder PROM [passive range of motion]. The patient's serratus anterior muscle strength improved to Poor plus, but his muscle strength was otherwise unchanged throughout the upper extremity. The increase in serratus anterior muscle strength resulted in increased scapular abduction and

Posterior Thigh Pain in a Patient With Low Back Pain

Outcomes

Consider the following statement:

> Straight leg raise (SLR) was improved to 100% of full range of motion without pain in 4 weeks. The patient returned to work and was able to do all of his recreational activities. The patient accomplished all of his goals.

This statement reports impairment and disability status for the end of the episode of care, but there is no description of how these elements changed throughout the course of intervention. There is no mention of home exercise programs or follow-up reexaminations. In some cases, the author may decide that home exercises and follow-up are not necessary; if so, the author should explain why they were not needed.

> Reexamination during the second week of intervention indicated that the SLR range of motion increased to 55 degrees on the left leg. No change in functional limitation or disability status was observed. At week 3, left SLR range of motion was 65 degrees. The patient was now able to walk rapidly without a decreased step length on the left side. He was able to drive for 2 hours before noticing posterior thigh pain. Thigh pain when getting in and out of his truck was reduced to a level 4 on the visual analogue scale (VAS), compared with a level 7 on the scale 2 weeks before.
>
> The left SLR range of motion was 75 degrees by week 4 of the program. The patient reported being able to drive his truck for 6 hours before noticing thigh pain and being able to get in and out of his truck without pain. At the beginning of week 5, the left SLR range of motion was 80 degrees and was comparable to that of the uninvolved side. The patient was able to work without discomfort. He was participating in "light" soccer, but was not playing any games. Physical therapy was discontinued. The patient was instructed to continue with the hamstring muscle exercise 3 times per week as a maintenance program. In our experience, this program is sufficient to maintain soft tissue flexibility.
>
> At 1 month and 6 months postdischarge, we made follow-up telephone calls. The patient reported that he was playing soccer at the level he was playing prior to the onset of his problem. He was able to do his full-time job without discomfort at both 1 month and 6 months.

Note that changes are reported in both impairments and disability at periodic intervals throughout the course of intervention. Descriptions of discharge planning (maintenance exercise program) and follow-up reports also are included.

upward rotation during humeral elevation. As a result, he had increased shoulder AROM [active range of motion] to 145 degrees of abduction and 155 degrees of flexion.... At that time, the patient moved out of state....

The patient reported that after moving he followed up with physical therapy but was limited to only three monthly visits secondary to restrictions from his health maintenance organization. He reported that his shoulder started to dramatically improve approximately 1 year after the onset of pain. The patient's medical records were obtained from the treating physical therapist. At the time of the patient's last visit, 13 months after the onset of pain, his serratus anterior muscle strength had increased to Good plus. He had scapular winging, but full right shoulder AROM.

At the writing of this case report, it had been approximately 17 months since the onset of pain and the patient stated that he felt "90% improvement" in the use of his right shoulder. He reported pain-free use of his affected upper extremity, but noticed that the right upper extremity fatigued more easily than the left upper extremity. He stated that he was able to lift light weights, including his child, over his head and no longer had the sensation of the shoulder sliding out of place.

First, this description summarizes the chronology of the patient's recovery and consistently frames the outcome relative to the time that passed since the onset of symptoms. Second, the description is thorough and addresses external factors judged to be important in this patient's care (eg, the restrictions in insurance coverage). Third, the authors included descriptions of all the factors that were assessed by the therapists, that is, changes in impairment and functional limitations.

The outcome reported by Mitchell and Versluis[8(p393)] for a patient with an above-knee amputation illustrates another point about descriptions of outcome in particular and descriptions of outcome in case reports in general. Not every outcome in a case report will suggest that the intervention succeeded in guiding the patient toward achieving all goals. Sometimes goals just aren't reached! Unattained goals, however, do not preclude the usefulness (and potential publication) of a case report. Mitchell and Versluis wrote:

A follow-up telephone call at six months postintervention revealed the patient still ambulating with a temporary prosthesis and two straight canes for an unlimited distance. The patient reported that she was riding a stationary bike up to 15 miles a day and continuing with her home exercise program. When asked about future plans for a definitive prosthesis, the patient reported that weight fluctuations prohibited a permanent prosthesis at this time.

The case report by Phillips and Audet[9(p523)] also illustrates the point that the patient does not have to meet all goals for a case report to be publishable. The authors used serial casting to treat the knee joints of a patient with cerebral palsy:

> When [the patient] was seen at the clinic 4 weeks after discharge, he was ambulating independently without his braces using two straight canes and without excessive hip flexion, knee flexion, or hip internal rotation; his heels were flat during the stance phase of gait. Active dorsiflexion at heel-strike was not achieved.

Outcomes in Tables

In a table that is unusual, Schindler et al[10] described bilateral tendon transfer outcomes for a patient with C-5 quadriplegia, both in terms of what happens in "real" life (usual routine postsurgery) and what would be "ideal" (if time allows postsurgery) (**Table 17**). Tables can be particularly useful for summarizing chronological changes in impairments, functional limitations, or disabilities. Gill-Body and colleagues[5] summarized the changes in a patient's self-perceived level of disability as measured with the Dizziness Handicap Inventory (DHI). The patient was diagnosed with bilateral vestibular hypofunction, and the table illustrates the changes that took place in the DHI over two time intervals (**Table 18**). Head and Patterson[11] created a table that concisely summarized their client's problems, the adaptive equipment intervention selected to address each problem, the outcome, and the cost (**Table 19**).

Table 17. Functional Assessment Scale Scores Before and After Surgery[a]

	Pre-surgery	Usual Routine Post-surgery	If time allows Post-surgery
Dressing			
Upper extremities	1	3	4
Lower extremities	1	1	1
Communications			
Typewriter/computer	1	1	7
Write	1	7	7
Telephone	1	7	7
Turn pages	1	7	7
Homemaking			
Cold food	1	4	6
Stove top			
or electric skillet	1	1	1
Oven or microwave	1	1	4
Marketing	1	1	1
Light cleaning	1	1	1
Heavy cleaning	1	1	1
Laundry	1	1	1
Bladder Management			
Empty leg bag	1	6	6
Put on leg bag	1	1	1
Leg bag connections	1	1	1
Clothing/clean-up	1	1	1
Feeding			
Feeding	4	7	7
Spoon/fork	4	7	7
Cup/glass	1	7	7
Cut food	1	1	1
Light Hygiene			
Grooming	1	4	7
Brush/comb hair	1	7	7
Brush teeth	4	5	7
Shave	1	3	7
Wash face & hands	1	7	7
Bathing			
Bathing/showering	1	4	4

Key

Levels		
7 Complete Independence (Timely, Safely)	No	
6 Modified Independence	Helper	
Modified Dependence		
5 Supervision		
4 Minimal Assist (Subject = 75%+)		
3 Moderate Assist (Subject = 50%+)	Helper	
Complete Dependence		
2 Maximum Assist (Subject = 25%+)		
1 Total Assist (Subject = 0%+)		

[a]Reprinted with permission of the American Occupational Therapy Association from Schindler L, Robbins G, Hamlin C. Functional effect of bilateral tendon transfers on a person with C-5 quadriplegia. *Am J Occup Ther*. 1994;48:750-757.

Table 18. Self-Reported Changes on Dizziness Handicap Inventory for Patient With Bilateral Vestibular Hypofunction.[a,5]

Physical/Functional Factors

0- to 8-Week Changes	9- to 16-Week Changes	Emotional Factors
+ Ability to look up	+ Ability to look up	+ Less feeling of embarrassment in front of others
+ Ability to move head quickly	+ Ability to move head quickly	+ Less fear that others think individual is intoxicated
++ Ability to walk down aisle of supermarket	+ Ability to walk down aisle of supermarket	− Ability to participate in social activities
++ Ability to do job	+ Ability to walk down a sidewalk	− Feelings of depression

[a]+=item rated as "a little improved"; ++=item rated as "much improved"; −item rated as "a little worse."

Table 19. Summary of Interventions[a]

Summary of Interventions

Problem	Intervention	Outcome	Cost
Unsafe, limited mobility	Powered wheelchair	Trial use—not accepted by client because he did not feel safe	Loaner from stock
	Lightweight manual wheelchair	Independent in indoor mobility	$360
Limited bed mobility	Electric hospital bed	Independent	$650
Inaccessible home entrance	Wheelchair ramp	Able to enter and exit home with assistance	$1200
Unable to open containers	Loop scissors, tab gripper, jar lid opener	Used infrequently	$20
Difficulty with feeding and drinking	Long straw, lightweight cup with handle, nonskid mat	Able to perform activities with greater ease	$40
Unable to wear shoes	Special booties	Increased warmth and protection from trauma	$50
Difficulty holding toothbrush	Tubing to build up handle	Independent	$3
Unable to pick up objects from floor	Dressing stick	Used to pick up some items (e.g., clothing) and to extend reach	$10

[a]Reprinted with permission of the American Occupational Therapy Association from Head J, Patterson V. Performance context and its role in treatment planning. *Am J Occup Ther*. 1997;51:453-457.

Outcomes in Histograms

Balogun and Okonofua[12] used a histogram to illustrate changes in the perception of pain intensity over time for a patient with a diagnosis of pelvic inflammatory disease (**Figure 23**).

Outcomes in Line Graphs

Crum[13] used a series of line graphs to summarize the changes that took place in temporomandibular joint range of motion in a group of patients with spinal cord injury (**Figure 24**).

McClure and Flowers[4] used a different type of line graph to illustrate the changes in range of motion that took place over time in a patient with limited motion of the shoulder (**Figure 25**).

Morrison[14] used a line graph to demonstrate the changes that occurred in a patient's vital capacity over several intervention sessions (**Figure 26**). The patient was diagnosed with quadriplegia and was treated with electromyographic biofeedback. The goal of biofeedback training was to improve his accessory breathing muscle activity and therefore his vital capacity. **Figure 27** shows the amount of time the patient was taken off the ventilator during each intervention session.

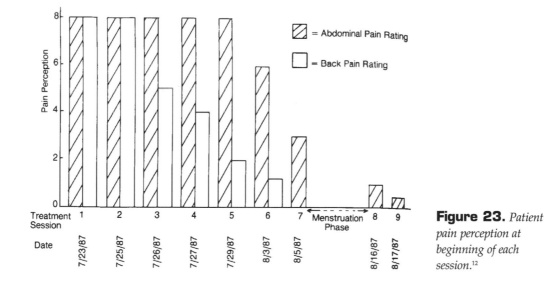

Figure 23. *Patient pain perception at beginning of each session.*[12]

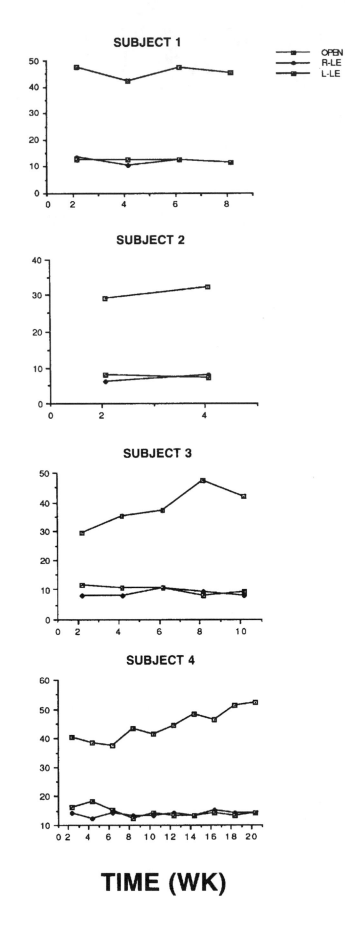

Figure 24. *Active range-of-motion measurements (in millimeters) of temporomandibular joint. (R-LE = right lateral excursion; L-LE = left lateral excursion.)*[13]

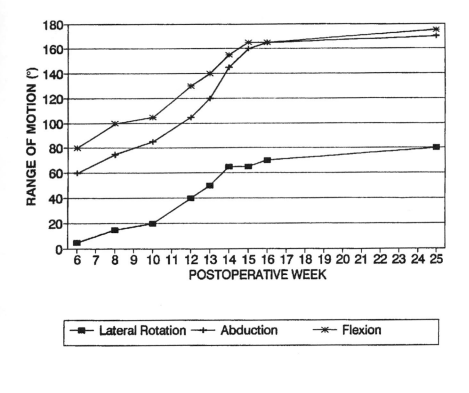

Figure 25. (left) Range-of-motion data for shoulder movements of lateral rotation, abduction, and flexion in 57-year-old female patient following fracture and dislocation of right humeral head.[4]

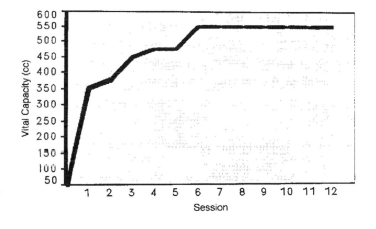

Figure 26. Vital capacity of patient with high-level quadriplegia during (sessions 1-6) and after (sessions 7-12) electromyographic biofeedback training.[14]

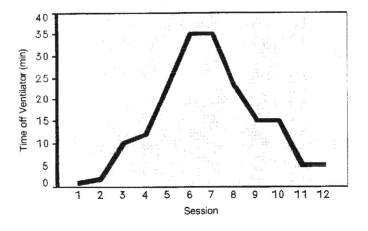

Figure 27. Amount of time off mechanical ventilator achieved by patient with high-level quadriplegia during (sessions 1-6) and after (sessions 7-12) electromyographic feedback training.[14]

Outcomes in Scans and Photographs

Cibulka et al[15] hypothesized that a patient's symptoms of left-leg pain were due to the excessive forces under the forefoot resulting from a forefoot-contact running style. They used two F-scans to illustrate the plantar pressure distribution of the patient before and after training in a heel-toe running style (**Figures 28, 29**).

Mueller and Diamond[16] used photos of a patient's foot to illustrate the changes that took place in a plantar ulcer (active pathology) that was treated using a total contact cast (**Figures 30, 31**).

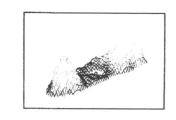
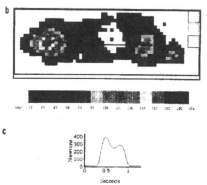

Figure 28. *(top left) An F-scan of the left foot during the stance phase of the forefoot contact running style. The patient was running at 5.2 mph (8.3 km/h) in running shoes. A) The composite peak vertical pressures on the plantar surface of the foot showing larger vertical pressures in the forefoot. B) The vertical pressures on the plantar surface of the foot demonstrating the path of center of pressure beginning and ending in the forefoot. C) A graph of the peak vertical pressure-time curve during the stance phase of the running cycle. Key is shaded in kiloPascal (kPa); 1 kPa = 0.145 lb/inch².*

Figure 29. *(top right) An F-scan of the left foot during the stance phase of the heel contact running style. The same patient was again running at 5.2 mph (8.3 km/h) in running shoes. A) The composite peak vertical pressures on the plantar surface of the foot showing larger vertical pressures in the heel and more distribution of pressure throughout the forefoot. B) The vertical pressures on the plantar surface of the foot demonstrating the path of center of pressure extending throughout the entire foot. C) A graph of the peak vertical pressure-time curve during the stance phase of the running cycle. Key is shaded in kiloPascal (kPa); 1 kPa = 0.145 lb/inch².*

Reprinted with permission of Williams & Wilkins, Co, Baltimore, Md, from Cibulka MT, Sinacore DR, Mueller MJ. Shin splints and forefoot contact running: a case report. J Orthop Sports Phys Ther. 1994;20:98-102.

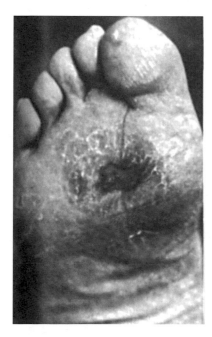
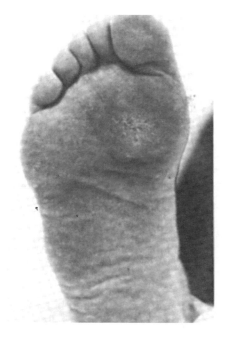

Figure 30. *(bottom left) Plantar ulcer after treatment with total contact casting for 85 days.*

Figure 31. *(bottom right) Plantar surface of patient's foot at 6-month follow-up visit.[16]*

Outcomes in Radiographs

In Wieder's description of the intervention of a patient with a diagnosis of traumatic myositis ossificans,[17] radiographs were used to illustrate the changes that took place in the pathology following a course of intervention (**Figures 32, 33**).

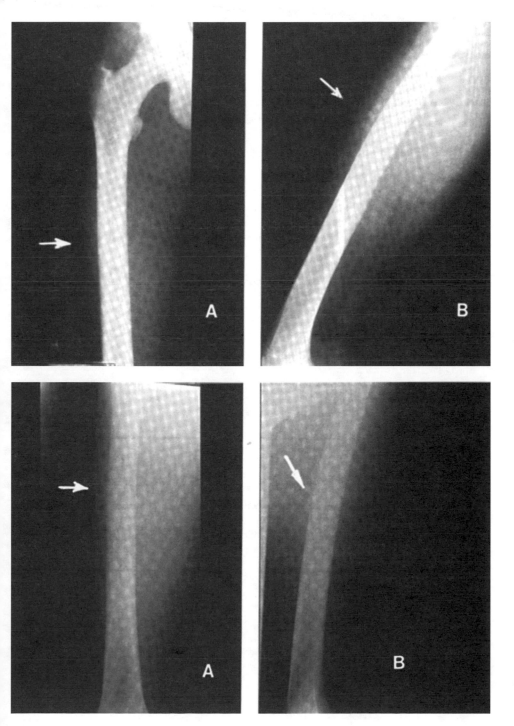

Figure 32. *Pretreatment radiographic films of right femur of patient with myositis ossificans: (A) anterior-posterior view; (B) lateral view.*[17]

Figure 33. *Posttreatment radiographic films of right femur of patient with myositis ossificans: (A) anterior-posterior view; (B) lateral view.*[17]

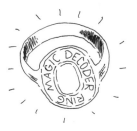

Next: What Does Your Case Report Mean?

Changes in impairments can be important to report, but impairment measurements must be linked to changes in functional limitations and disabilities. Changes in radiographs, vital capacity, range of motion, developmental test results for children, or foot pressure are not enough. Changes in ability to lift boxes, shop for groceries, take care of children, work at a computer, play sports, or do other activities that are important to patients also must be reported. Once you've done that, it's time to offer possible explanations for what happened in the case.

References

1 *Guide to Physical Therapist Practice.* 2nd ed. Phys Ther. 2001;81:9-744.

2 Anderson M, Tichenor CJ. A patient with de Quervain's tenosynovitis: a case report using an Australian approach to manual therapy. *Phys Ther.* 1994;74:314-326.

3 Dunbar SB. A child's occupational performance: considerations of sensory processing and family context. *Am J Occup Ther.* 1999;53:231-235.

4 McClure PW, Flowers KR. Treatment of limited shoulder motion: a case study based on biomechanical considerations. *Phys Ther.* 1992;72:929-936.

5 Gill-Body KM, Krebs DE, Parker SW, Riley PO. Physical therapy management of peripheral vestibular dysfunction: two clinical case reports. *Phys Ther.* 1994;74:129-142.

6 Young MS. Electromyographic biofeedback use in the treatment of voluntary posterior dislocation of the shoulder: a case study. *J Orthop Sports Phys Ther.* 1994;20:171-175.

7 Watson CJ, Schenkman M. Physical therapy management of isolated serratus anterior muscle paralysis. *Phys Ther.* 1995;75:194-202.

8 Mitchell CA, Versluis TL. Management of an above-knee amputee with complex medical problems using the CAT-CAM prosthesis. *Phys Ther.* 1990;70:389-393.

9 Phillips WE, Audet M. Use of serial casting in the management of knee joint contractures in an adolescent with cerebral palsy. *Phys Ther.* 1990;70:521-523.

10 Schindler L, Robbins G, Hamlin C. Functional effect of bilateral tendon transfers on a person with C-5 quadriplegia. *Am J Occup Ther.* 1994;48:750-757.

11 Head J, Patterson V. Performance context and its role in treatment planning. *Am J Occup Ther.* 1997; 51:453-457.

12 Balogun JA, Okonofua FE. Management of chronic pelvic inflammatory disease with shortwave diathermy: a case report. *Phys Ther.* 1988;68:1541-1545.

13 Crum NA. Signs of temporomandibular joint dysfunction in spinal cord injured patients wearing halo braces: a clinical report. *Phys Ther.* 1990;70:132-137.

14 Morrison SA. Biofeedback to facilitate unassisted ventilation in individuals with high-level quadriplegia: a case report. *Phys Ther.* 1988;68:1378-1380.

15 Cibulka MT, Sinacore DR, Mueller MJ. Shin splints and forefoot contact running: a case report. *J Orthop Sports Phys Ther.* 1994;20:98-102.

16 Mueller MJ, Diamond JE. Biomechanical treatment approach to diabetic plantar ulcers: a case report *Phys Ther.* 1988;68:1917-1920.

17 Wieder DL. Treatment of traumatic myositis ossificans with acetic acid iontophoresis. *Phys Ther.* 1992;72:133-137.

Chapter 9

"The Discussion": Time for Reflection

Based on your process of analysis or inquiry, the discussion section suggests possible explanations for what happened in your case. It cannot offer bold statements of "conclusion," however. A case report provides insight into clinical practice through description and analysis; it does not provide proof of effectiveness.

Although the discussion is less structured than the case description, it should cover several topics. The discussion should provide the link to the purpose of the case report and to the literature, reflect on the case management and outcomes, suggest possible alternative explanations for what happened, and pose research questions. It may be tempting to merely summarize the case management and outcomes. Instead, invest the time and energy to thoughtfully reflect on what your case report *means*.

You know more about the case than anyone else does. Your well-reasoned alternative explanations for what happened can contribute to the body of professional knowledge.

Link the Case to Its Purpose

A good way to begin the discussion is to use the first paragraph to remind the reader of the overall theme of the case and how your case is directly tied to that theme. In a case report involving a patient, the discussion usually begins with a general statement about the major clinical problem that the case illustrates.

In their case report about a female runner with a stress fracture and a negative bone scan, Sterling et al[1] introduced the discussion in this way: "Stress fractures of the hip can be an enigma to the practicing clinician and may be misdiagnosed due to minimal physical findings on examination.[23] The patient in this case [had] pain during periods of weight bearing, tenderness.... These symptoms are common in stress fractures of the proximal femur.[17,19,23,39,42]" Anderson and Tichenor[2] began their discussion by restating the problem and the specific focus of their case: "Physical therapists frequently treat patients who have a diagnosis of deQuervain's tenosynovitis or CTS [cumulative trauma syndrome]. The importance of this case study lies in the therapists' analysis of signs and symptoms to implement treatment and to obtain a response that dictated the direction of future treatments."

Relate the Case to the Literature

As the discussion continues, it should provide evidence of how the case fits within the context of the literature. In the introduction section, you used the literature to identify what had already been done in your topic area and to identify the boundaries for your case; in the discussion, you focus on how your case and findings compare with what is cited in the literature.

In their introduction, Sterling et al[1] cited literature that explained stress fractures, their causes, and their relationship to sports. That introduction set the stage for the purpose of the case, which was to describe an example of when the clinical algorithm does not fit with the patient's symptoms. The case description showed the misfit between the clinical data and the negative test results; the discussion used the literature to highlight what is known about early diagnosis of stress fracture. Although bone scintigraphy is considered to be the most sensitive test, the scan was negative in this case. Other literature was discussed.

Not all patient/client management proceeds as planned. Moyers and Stoffel[3] started their discussion by commenting on their patient's unexpected substance abuse problem and then linked the problem to the literature to heighten readers' awareness of the extent of substance abuse on the job:

> This case required a pragmatic approach for working holistically to resolve an unanticipated problem of substance abuse that threatened the success of the client's rehabilitation plan and the outcome of returning her to work. Given that the incidence of dangerous substance use on the job ranges from 10% to 20% in the United States despite the existence of Employee Assistance Programs since the 1940s (Backer, 1987; Miller, 1995), the emergence of complications in rehabilitation related to a substance use disorder should not be surprising.

As you prepare to write your discussion, it is likely that you will go back to the literature to reread what you cited in the introduction and to seek other literature that may be helpful in explaining what happened in your case. Note how Malouin et al[4] placed their cases in the context of the literature:

The practice of initiating rehabilitation as early as possible is not new. Early rehabilitation has been associated with reduced patient fatality and improved quality of survivorship following stroke.[13,23,24] Moreover it has been found that the time between stroke onset and initiation of intensive rehabilitation specifically affected transfers and ambulation training.[22] Our [report] demonstrates that patients can successfully cope with task-oriented (balance and gait) activities during the first week after stroke.

You also may restate and summarize key points from the literature that are directly tied to your case, as Denislic et al[5] did in a case report on a patient who had neuropathy associated with Sjögren syndrome. They noted, for instance, that different types of polyneuropathy—predominantly sensory forms—had been described in patients with primary Sjögren syndrome and that there was an emphasis on accurate assessment of sensory and autonomic nervous system in primary Sjögren syndrome caused by peripheral nervous system involvement.

When relating your case to the literature, a "funnel" approach may help. First, think about the broadest dimension of your case, such as "manual therapy," "vestibular dysfunction," or "professional socialization." Even though you may have focused on a specific application of a specific intervention, your case report is likely to relate to a much broader knowledge base in the profession. Consider how your specific case relates to this knowledge to help the profession bridge the gap between theory and practice. If your concrete example illustrates application of an abstract concept, make the connection explicit in the discussion. In a case report describing the use of an eclectic approach with an athlete who had low back pain, Beattie[6] showed how theoretical models of impairment and disability can apply to real patient data. The discussion said in part:

> In many manual therapy evaluative approaches, a great emphasis is placed on identifying and treating impairments such as abnormal joint mobility.[10,16,17] Few authors, however, discuss the importance of relating these impairments to the patient's disability. I believe that it is critical to evaluate all of the predisposing factors to the patient's disability, using a logical process. For example, "normal joint mobility" is a meaningless statement unless it is referenced to some activity, in this case normal joint mobility for the take-off phase of pole vaulting.[31]

In the discussion section of her case report of a child diagnosed with a sensory processing disorder, Dunbar[7] related the case back to Ayres' sensory integration theory. The information also could have been in the introduction to provide rationale for the testing and intervention. The discussion said in part:

> A vestibular-bilateral and sequencing disorder is one example of the type of sensory integrative dysfunction a young child can experience. This disorder is characterized by poor postural mechanisms, inadequate bilateral integration, and underresponsive vestibular systems. Tests and clinical observations of Sara's difficulty with coordinating both sides of her body and her continuous movement in play indicated concerns in this area. It is believed that children with this type of disorder usually need more intense

Consider how your case relates to a much broader knowledge base to help the profession bridge the gap between theory and practice.

Posterior Thigh Pain in a Patient With Low Back Pain

Discussion

In the grossly overstated discussion below, the authors conclude that their report proves effectiveness, which is inappropriate for case reports. They also make a generalization that all patients with back and leg pain should receive the intervention. This notion also is inappropriate, because they observed only one type of patient:

This case report proves that stretching exercises are a vital element in managing patients with leg pain associated with low back pain. We recommend that when patients with leg pain have a history of low back pathology, they should be started on an aggressive stretching program to alleviate the pain and restore function.

What would be a reasonable conclusion statement? Consider the following:

This case demonstrates the use of stretching exercises to manage a patient with leg pain that was associated with low back injury. The selection of intervention was based on the patient's response to stretching of soft tissues in the lower extremities and spine. We do not believe that all patients with low back pathology and associated leg pain should be managed using stretching exercises. However, in cases in which the condition is not acute and pain is reproduced with tests that attempt to lengthen the involved tissues, the use of stretching exercises to improve the flexibility of these tissues may be helpful in alleviating the pain and restoring function.

In the example above, the authors restrict their claims to the limits of the case report. They emphasize that the case only demonstrates, and does not necessarily prove, that this intervention can be effective. They are also careful to note that their findings apply only to a specific type of patient with leg pain associated with back pain and not to all patients with back and leg pain.

sensory input to perceive the same type of sensation as children without this disorder (Mailloux and Burke, 1997).

Whether your case lends support to or departs from the existing literature, you should continually monitor your language so that you do not slip into statements of cause and effect, such as "In contrast to previous reports, I found that microcurrent electrical stimulation was very effective in reducing pain from peripheral neuropathy in patients with AIDS." You should state only what happened in your specific case, without making a claim that the intervention *caused* the outcome: "Although inconsistent with previous reports, the patient's lower extremity pain was reduced following microcurrent electrical stimulation."

Santiesteban[8] wrote carefully about the possible clinical application of an intervention approach for temporomandibular joint (TMJ) dysfunction. He did not imply any cause and effect:

> The appliance described in this case report may be useful for physical therapists treating certain types of TMJ dysfunction. I am not suggesting that this appliance should substitute for a more carefully made and professionally fitted appliance, but it may be useful for those patients who cannot afford a professionally made appliance. It may also be useful for screening patients for the professionally made appliance.

Explain Your Hunches

McClure and Flowers[9] used their case to question the concave-convex arthrokinematic theory of joint movements as applied to a stiff shoulder joint. They posed another theoretical explanation, careful to explain their hunches in the context of the case report:

> In our opinion, any form of stretching dependent on therapist technique, such as high-grade mobilization, has limited application because, as Brand has noted, "any elongation of tissue accomplished by stretch will shorten again once the force is relaxed."[31(849)] Therefore, in our view, the increase in tissue length produced by a brief session of high-grade mobilization serves only to temporarily deform the tissue rather than to produce a permanent length change.... Although this temporary elongation may be very useful for facilitating further exercise and function, permanent elongation of a tissue is probably accomplished through another mechanism—remodeling.

Beattie[6] used broad theoretical concepts from a disability model to frame a patient case. In the introduction of his report, he used the concepts of impairment and disability; in the discussion section, he returned to these two concepts as a central organizing framework for the discussion. The patient's impairment was "painful stiffness of spinal motion," whereas the patient's disability was the inability to compete as a pole vaulter. Within the disablement framework, Beattie explained his hunches about how a clinician can relate impairment information to a patient's disability. He used a combined spinal movement (trunk extension, rotation, and side bending) for an intervention that seemed to be functionally related to the trunk motion that takes place during pole vaulting.

Alternative Explanations

Because it is not the intent of a case report to prove effectiveness, you must think about other possible factors related to the outcome. You know more about the case than anyone else does, and your well-reasoned alternative explanations can be important contributions to the professional literature.

Beattie[6] considered several possible explanations for his patient's improvement. Note that he used the discussion as an opportunity to "engage in a dialogue about the intervention"—not to demonstrate cause and effect.

> I believe that although the joint mobilization procedures may have been useful for reducing pain and restoring motion, the critical factor in the favorable outcome reported by this patient was his behavioral changes.[30] The patient's behavioral changes included the frequent performance of extension exercises and the "correction" of his habitual sitting posture.

In the discussion section of their case reports about patients with vestibular dysfunction, Gill-Body and colleagues[10] posed several questions about the reasons for their patients' outcomes. They suggested two possible answers:

> If the treatment program for the patient with UVD [unilateral vestibular dysfunction] were related to the improvements that were made, why might they have occurred? One possibility is that the patient was able to "train" her central nervous system, through the repetition of the various activities.... Another possibility is that the patient's increased range of cervical mobility, combined with the experience of performing activities and movements that she had been avoiding since her initial onset, allowed her central nervous system to "realize" that she indeed had some postural control that was present and available for use on a daily basis.[11]

Sometimes the alternative explanation is not about possible causes of the outcome, but about alternative case management, based on lessons learned. The discussion can be a time to admit "mistakes" and describe what effect the mistake may have had, with suggestions for the future, such as "I did not stabilize the metatarsal head with my hand. Consequently, the range of passive MTP [metatarsophalangeal] joint dorsiflexion appeared limited."[11]

Authors also have an opportunity to mention any missing or weak data. Beattie[6] used a combined spinal movement in the "quadrant position" as a test; however, this is a movement for which there currently is no reliable measurement. This was a limitation of the case, but it also made an excellent point about the kind of measure that is ultimately needed:

Because of the lack of available measures, I had to rely on the patient's perception of pain and stiffness in response to various active and passive trunk motions. This reliance on the patient's perceptions represents a limitation to this case [report]. The lack of measures that relate to patients who are potential candidates for manual therapy remains as an enormous barrier to the establishment of the efficacy of these treatments.

"Where Do We Go From Here?"

The end of the discussion is a place to write about the direction that research should take. The case report provides an in-depth look at clinical practice, but it does not give definitive answers about what should be done with similar cases in the future. Statements from previous case reports ("The application of this type of [gait] program to a larger population of patients who have had strokes, however, should be made with caution,"[3] "The effectiveness of mobilization in patients with osteophytes or intense arthrosis has not been demonstrated"[9]) indicate something about the nature of case reports: They should generate far more questions than answers.

In the discussion of her case report on the use of neuromuscular electrical stimulation for upper-extremity intervention with children with cerebral palsy, Carmick[12] made a comment that could be turned into more than one research question:

> It would be of interest to learn whether electrical stimulation could enhance motor learning and control enough to increase function so that the biomechanical changes that occur with growth deficiencies would not occur.

Flowers et al[13] identified a need for research based on their case of a patient with a finger extensor tendon laceration: "More research is needed to clarify the optimal timing and intensity of stress to extensor tendon repairs postoperatively."

Because a major purpose of case reports is to generate hypotheses for future research to help answer important questions that clinicians are asking, editors and reviewers expect authors to include research suggestions in the discussion sections of their case reports. This is a relatively recent development, however, so published case reports may not be the best source of examples. The conventional format of a research report, meanwhile, has long required suggestions for future research, so research reports may provide better models for this part of the discussion section. Fetters and Kluzik[14] made a number of suggestions for future research in their report of a study that compared the effects of two interventions on reaching by children with cerebral palsy:

> A new research strategy would be to analyze movement components such as speed, smoothness, cardiorespiratory effort, ability to isolate movement, and so forth prior to treatment and then assign groups for

intervention based on these common features of movement.... In future research, additional variables should be assessed following treatment. We had two examples of subjects reporting "tightness" of muscles following their experimental treatment regime.

Avoid simply recommending that future research be conducted with a larger number of subjects—that's so obvious that it's not helpful! You have learned something from the inquiry process that is part of writing a case report. How does what you learned contribute to new questions about practice and potential questions for research?

The Value of Intense Local Observation

Clinicians as "scholarly practitioners" are in the position to do intensive local observation and contemplation. Because you are in the trenches of practice, you are in the best position to observe and systematically collect data on specific patients. In trying to describe and account for what happened with patients, you are identifying the factors or variables that are important. You are describing the uncontrolled conditions and the personal characteristics and events that occurred during measurement and intervention. You, better than anyone else, know the "story of the person." You also are developing a data bank of clinical experience based on your continued analysis of cases. Your task is to observe, think, analyze, document, take action—and share what you've learned. The case report has provided a structure for you to do just that.

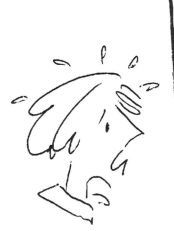

Next: Who's Afraid of Peer Review?

The hardest work is done. Now you need to "tie up the loose ends." You're about to take part in the peer-review process, something that may fill you with dread. But peer review is like anything else: The more you find out about it, the less daunting it becomes.

References

1   Sterling JC, Webb RFC, Meyers MC, Calvo RD. False negative bone scan in a female runner. *Med Sci Sports Exerc*. 1993;25:179-185.

2   Anderson M, Tichenor CJ. A patient with de Quervain's tenosynovitis: a case report using an Australian approach to manual therapy. *Phys Ther*. 1994;74:314-326.

3   Moyers PA, Stoffel VC. Alcohol dependence in a client with a work-related injury. *Am J Occup Ther*. 1999;53:640-645.

4   Malouin F, Potvin M, Prévost J, et al. Use of an intensive task-oriented gait training program in a series of patients with acute cerebrovascular accidents. *Phys Ther*. 1992;72:781-793.

5   Denislic M, Meh D, Popovic M, Kos-Golja M. Small nerve fibre dysfunction in a patient with Sjögren's syndrome: neurophysiological and morphological confirmation. *Scand J Rheumatol*. 1995;24:257-259.

6   Beattie P. The use of an eclectic approach for the treatment of low back pain: a case study. *Phys Ther*. 1992;72:923-928.

7   Dunbar SB. A child's occupational performance: consideration of sensory processing and family context. *Am J Occup Ther*. 1999;53:231-235.

8   Santiesteban AJ. Isometric exercises and a simple appliance for temporomandibular joint dysfunction: a case report. *Phys Ther*. 1989;69:463-466.

9   McClure PW, Flowers KR. Treatment of limited shoulder motion: a case study based on biomechanical considerations. *Phys Ther*. 1992;72:929-936.

10 Gill-Body KM, Krebs DE, Parker SW, Riley PO. Physical therapy management of peripheral vestibular dysfunction: two clinical case reports. *Phys Ther*. 1994;74:129-142.

11 Cibulka MT. Management of a patient with forefoot pain: a case report. *Phys Ther*. 1990;70:41-44.

12 Carmick J. Clinical use of neuromuscular electrical stimulation for children with cerebral palsy, part 2: upper extremity. *Phys Ther*. 1993;73:514-527.

13 Flowers KR, McClure PW, McFadden C. Management of a patient with lacerations of the tendons of the extensor digitorum and extensor indicis muscles to the index finger. *Phys Ther*. 1996;76:61-66.

14 Fetters L, Kluzik J. The effects of neurodevelopmental treatment versus practice on the reaching of children with spastic cerebral palsy. *Phys Ther*. 1996;76:346-358.

Chapter 10:

Preparing for Peer Review

Some components of the case report are best tackled after the main body of the paper—the "who, what, where, when, how, and why"—is done. That's because those components serve the function of "tying up the loose ends." They may be the finishing touches, but they're important.

Title and Abstract

The title of a case report should be as short as possible, yet include all of the pertinent information. If your patients are soccer players, for example, don't refer to them as "athletes" in the title; refer to them as "soccer players." If the intervention was neurodevelopmental treatment, say so; don't call it "physical therapy."

Vague Title:

Use of Motor Learning With a Child with a Developmental Disability

Improved Title:

Use of Random Practice to Teach a Child With Myelodysplasia to Transfer From Wheelchair to Car

Vague Title:

Rehabilitation for Glenohumeral Joint Subluxation

Improved Title:

Use of Functional Electrical Stimulation to Reduce Glenohumeral Subluxation in a Patient Following Stroke

Although the abstract is the first element in an article, it's better if you write it last; that way, you can summarize what you wrote in the manuscript, highlighting the most important details. Avoid such statements as, "Outcomes will be discussed." Give the important details. Don't treat them as though they are secrets to be revealed only to those who read the entire article! This does not mean that abstracts have to be long. For most case reports, abstracts of no more than 150 words are sufficient.

For examples of abstracts, look at case reports in recent issues of the journal to which you plan to submit your report. *Physical Therapy* uses a structured abstract format, with topic headings clearly identified in boldface type. This not only helps readers quickly identify pertinent information, but helps you organize the abstract. Headings for a patient-related case report are: Background and Purpose, Case Description (which summarizes examination findings—including the pertinent history, systems review, and results of tests and measures—and intervention), Outcomes, and Discussion. Abstracts for case reports that do not involve patients should include Background and Purpose, Summary (of the key points), and Discussion.

Below is an example of a structured abstract from a patient-oriented case report published in *Physical Therapy*:

> **Background and Purpose.** Diabetic neuropathy can produce severe pain. The purpose of this case report is to describe the alteration of pain in a patient with severe, painful diabetic neuropathy following application of transcutaneous electrical nerve stimulation (TENS) to the low back. **Case Description.** The patient was a 73-year-old woman with pain in the left lower extremity over the lateral aspect of the hip and the entire leg below the knee. The pain prevented sound sleep. The intensity of pain was assessed with a visual analog scale. **Intervention.** The TENS (80 Hz) was delivered 1 to 2 hours a day and during the entire night through electrodes placed on the lumbar area of the back. **Outcomes.** Following 20 minutes of TENS on the first day of treatment, the patient reported a 38% reduction in intensity of pain. After 17 days, the patient reported no pain following 20 minutes of TENS and that she could sleep through the night. Application of TENS to the skin of the lumbar area may be an effective treatment for the pain of diabetic neuropathy.[1(p767)]

Formatting Your References

The rules of referencing are only slightly less complicated than celestial navigation.

The reference section immediately follows the discussion section. All sources of information cited in the text must be listed here. The rules of referencing are only slightly less complex than celestial navigation, but reference lists for case reports usually require knowing only how to reference journals and books. The accuracy of a reference list can reflect well or poorly on the rest of the manuscript in the eyes of editors and reviewers, so it is worth spending some time to be sure it reflects *well*.

How many authors should be listed? Should you put references in numerical or alphabetical order? Should all the words of book titles be capitalized? Which bit of punctuation goes where? How do you abbreviate state names? The best way to find out is to look at the reference lists of articles published recently in the journal to which you are submitting your case report. Style manuals also can be excellent sources of information. The manuals that may be especially useful are the *American Medical Association Manual of Style*,[2] which is used by *Physical Therapy* and many other health-related journals, and the *Publication Manual of the American Psychological Association*,[3] which is used by the *American Journal of Occupational Therapy* and other journals of interest to rehabilitation professionals. Instructions for authors sometimes specify the style that is used. Otherwise, just match your reference style to the samples provided by the journal articles—and remember to pay attention to all of those picky details!

Assembling Tables and Figures

When putting your manuscript together, place the tables, then the figures, after the reference list. As shown in Chapters 7, 8, and 9, tables and figures can be used to illustrate information that is difficult to describe or difficult for readers to grasp in text format. Tables and figures should not simply repeat information that is in the text; they should supplement the text. A usual way to incorporate tables or figures is to provide some background in the text, then refer the reader to the table or figure for the details.

Table titles and figure captions should give enough information so that readers can understand the tables or the figures without reading the text. This does not mean that titles and captions have to be a paragraph long! But they should include all of the pertinent details in a line or two. One example of a table title: "Measurements (in degrees) by Each Examiner of Foot Alignment and Range of Motion."[4] This title gives sufficient information to understand what the table is about without being too lengthy. As shown in **Table 20**,[5] the labeling of elements within the table also can help explain the data. Any words that are abbreviated for the sake of space should be footnoted and spelled out at the bottom of the table.

Table titles typically appear above the table, and figure captions should be listed separately on a single page that precedes the figures in the manuscript. Instructions for authors, style manuals, and examples in journal articles are all sources of inspiration and information for creating tables and figures.

Institute Your Own Review Process!

Once you've tied up all of the "loose ends," and before you submit your paper to a journal, ask colleagues to review your manuscript for you. They should be generally familiar with the concepts presented in the report, but they should *not* know the patient or be too familiar with your work. Be sure to tell them that you are not looking for praise, but that you want their help to identify every unclear word, weak transition, or omitted detail that the journal's reviewers are sure to

Table 20. Initial Evaluation Findings for Proximal Upper-Limb Strength[a,5]

Joint Movement	Left	Right
Shoulder		
Flexion	Normal	Fair minus
Extension	Good	Good
Abduction	Normal	Fair minus
Horizontal abduction	Normal	Normal
Medial rotation	Normal	Normal
Lateral rotation	Normal	Normal
Scapular		
Elevation	Normal	Normal
Adduction	Good	Good
Depression and adduction	Good	Good
Adduction and downward rotation	Normal	Normal
Abduction and upward rotation	Normal	Zero

[a]Manual muscle testing was performed using the system described by Daniels and Worthingham.[25]

notice. Remember: It's the praise of the reviewers that you want—not the praise of your friends.

While your colleagues are reading the manuscript, put your own copy away and let it get "cold" for at least 2 weeks. Resist the overwhelming temptation to send the manuscript off as soon as it is finished! Fresh eyes will make problems much clearer, and you'd rather find those problems and fix them than leave them to the reviewers in whose hands the fate of your manuscript will lie. The final step before submitting the manuscript is to read the instructions for authors again to make sure you have included everything that is requested.

Peer Review: A Survival Guide

Although the mechanics of peer review vary somewhat among journals, the process usually is similar to that used by *Physical Therapy*. The concept of peer review should be familiar to clinicians who have participated in both informal reviews (as part of everyday clinical practice) and formal reviews (as a component of quality improvement).

Just as peer review of clinical practice is intended to help clinicians as well as ensure high-quality care, peer review of manuscripts is intended to help authors as well as ensure high-quality articles. Manuscripts are not just "shot down" if they do not immediately meet publication standards. Editors work with authors to develop publishable manuscripts, using input from peer review. Understanding the review process used by *Physical Therapy* (**Figure 34**) may help alleviate any anxiety that you may have.

"What happens when my case report is received at the Editorial Office?" When a case report is submitted to *Physical Therapy*, it is logged into a database and sent to the Editor. As long as the manuscript meets minimal standards of readability and relevance and does not violate Journal policy (eg, prior publication), the Editor assigns the manuscript to two or three reviewers and an Editorial Board member (EBM) who have expertise in the content area. A copy also is sent to the Associate Editor for Case Reports.

Case reports receive a masked review, which means that the identities of the author and the reviewers are not intentionally revealed to each other. (The term "masked" is now used instead of "blind" because it is not always possible to completely conceal the identity of either the author or the reviewers, such as when authors cite their own previous work in the manuscript or reviewers make comments that only they are likely to make.)

"What do the reviewers do with my case report?" The EBM and the reviewers read the manuscript and comment on:

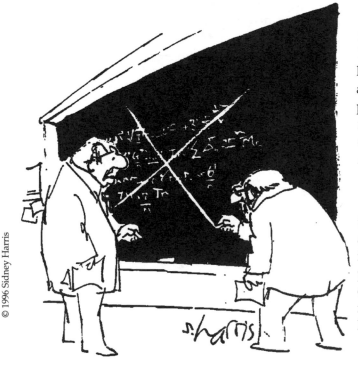

"That's it? That's peer review?"

```
┌─────────────────────────────────────────────┐
│        MANUSCRIPT REVIEW PROCESS:             │
│              CASE REPORTS                      │
└─────────────────────────────────────────────┘

┌──────────────────────────────────────────────────────┐
│  Editorial Office receives manuscript and sends copy to Editor  │
└──────────────────────────────────────────────────────┘
                         │
                         ▼
┌──────────────────────────────────────────────────────┐
│ • Editor confirms that manuscript is a case report and determines whether │
│   manuscript should be sent for review                 │
│ • Editor assigns Editorial Board member (EBM) and reviewers, based on expertise │
│ • Editorial Office sends copies of manuscript to EBM, reviewers, and │
│   Associate Editor                                     │
└──────────────────────────────────────────────────────┘
                         │
                         ▼
┌──────────────────────────────────────────────────────┐
│ • Reviewers complete review and send to Editorial Office │
│ • Editorial Office sends reviews to EBM                 │
└──────────────────────────────────────────────────────┘
                         │
                         ▼
┌──────────────────────────────────────────────────────┐
│ • Editorial Board member writes own review and a synopsis of reviewers' reviews, │
│   noting the reviewer suggestions that must be addressed, those that the author │
│   can decide to address or not address, and those that the EBM believes may │
│   make the paper worse                                 │
│ • Editorial Board member makes recommendation for disposition │
│ • Editorial Board member sends recommendation, reviews, and reviewer perfor- │
│   mance evaluations to Editorial Office                 │
└──────────────────────────────────────────────────────┘
                         │
                         ▼
┌──────────────────────────────────────────────────────┐
│ Editorial Office sends the EBM's synopsis and review, reviewers' reviews, and │
│    reviewer evaluations to Associate Editor (copy sent to Editor) │
└──────────────────────────────────────────────────────┘
                         │
                         ▼
┌──────────────────────────────────────────────────────┐
│ Associate Editor makes decision on manuscript:         │
│ • Accept (Editorial Office notifies author)            │
│ • Revise (Associate Editor writes letter to author, Editorial Office sends materials │
│   to author)                                           │
│ • No Decision ("Decision Pending") (Associate Editor writes letter to author, │
│   Editorial Office sends materials to author)          │
│ • Reject (Rewrite Encouraged) (Associate Editor writes letter to author, Editorial │
│   Office sends materials to author)                    │
│ • Reject (Rewrite Not Encouraged) (Associate Editor writes letter to author, │
│   Editorial Office sends materials to author)          │
└──────────────────────────────────────────────────────┘
```

Figure 34. *The peer-review process used by* Physical Therapy *for case reports.*

1. *Credibility*—A credible case report convincingly explains why it makes an important contribution to the professional literature and how it relates to other literature. As described in detail in this manual, a credible case report also describes appropriate collection and interpretation of information, clearly explains the intervention, discusses implications for clinical practice, and proposes research questions or hypotheses for future research.

2. *Organization and writing*—A good case report is coherently written in a tone that is appropriate for the audience, uses correct and contemporary terms, and organizes the content into the appropriate sections.

3. *Appropriateness for the journal*—Appropriate case reports have relevant content that makes a solid contribution to the field and has a clear relationship to existing knowledge.

The reviewers also are asked to make specific comments, paragraph by paragraph, as they go through the manuscript. They usually ask for clarification of anything that is unclear and offer suggestions for improvement. These comments are an excellent opportunity for the author to get input from peers with similar or greater expertise.

"When will I find out the results?" The reviewer comments are sent to the EBM, who writes a synopsis of the most important points of the reviews in addition to the EBM's own impressions of the manuscript. The reviews and the EBM synopsis, review, and recommendation about publication are sent to the Associate Editor for Case Reports. After reviewing the manuscript, the EBM's synopsis, and the two reviews, the Associate Editor makes a decision about the case report, communicates with the Editor, and writes a letter to the author. The entire process usually takes about 3 to 5 months.

One of four possible decisions can be made:

1. *Accept*—No changes are required; Journal staff will edit. This is a decision that even the most experienced and well-known writers have rarely seen and can only dream about! Revisions are almost always needed following the first submission of a manuscript. If the Associate Editor decides that the case report should be accepted with no further changes and the Editor agrees, the Editorial Office notifies the author.

2. *Revise*—The author needs to make minor to moderate changes before the case report can be accepted. **This is good news.** It means that no fatal flaws were detected during the review process and that, with some diligent attention to the comments of the EBM and the reviewers, the case report will probably be published.

3. *No Decision ("Decision Pending")*—The author must make revisions before a decision can be made. This category is used only when there are a small number of questions that have to be answered before the credibility of the case report can be judged.

4. *Reject*—The manuscript cannot be published in its current form. *Rejection usually does not mean that the case report will never be publishable.* Most often, rejection means that more-than-moderate revisions are needed before the manuscript can be published or before the credibility of the manuscript can be judged. In these instances, the author is encouraged to revise and resubmit the manuscript. A large number of the articles published in *Physical Therapy* (many by well-known authors) were rejected the first time around. Some manuscripts, though, have so many deficiencies that publication seems unlikely. In these cases, the author is not encouraged to rewrite and resubmit the manuscript. If the author thinks that the deficiencies can be overcome, the manuscript could still be revised and resubmitted.

The Editorial Office sends the Associate Editor's letter, the EBM's comments, and the reviews to the author. The identity of the author remains masked from the EBM, but the author is given the EBM's telephone number and e-mail address and is invited to communicate with the Editor, the Associate Editor for Case Reports, or the EBM about any questions. As hard as it may be to read some of the comments, the feedback can be a great learning opportunity, and, if the case report is eventually published, the process almost always results in a stronger article.

You may find it helpful to know that, just as there are stages of grieving, there are stages of dealing with feedback on manuscripts. As time passes, reactions to reading the reviews range from "What? Those idiots were either too stupid to understand or too lazy to read what I wrote!" to "Well, I probably could have described that procedure more clearly," to "Some of these suggestions really are pretty good." The process takes time, and it is important to anticipate and recognize it so that you don't give up in that initial blur of anger, hurt feelings, and frustration that can occur in response to reading suggestions for improving your hard work.

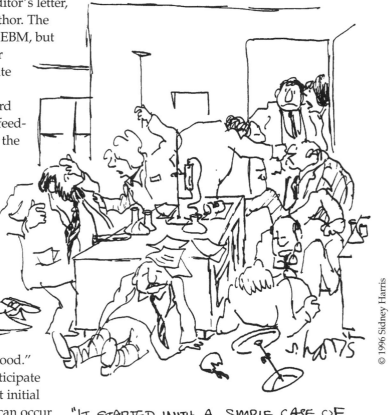

© 1996 Sidney Harris

"IT STARTED WITH A SIMPLE CASE OF PEER-REVIEW."

In an Editor's Note titled "The Ugly Side of Peer Review," *Physical Therapy* Editor Jules Rothstein[6] offered some insight into the process and made some suggestions about how authors can direct their emotions in a positive way. He also wrote, "Peer reviewers...become peer reviewers (for our Journal at least) only after they have been on the receiving end of the process, and most reviewers, including this Editor and the Editorial Board members, continue to publish and experience the process as recipients of reviews even as they review the works of others...." It may help you to know that even manuscripts written by EBMs—and the Editor—sometimes are rejected!

> It may help you to know that even manuscripts written by Editorial Board Members—and the Editor—sometimes are rejected!

"What happens when I resubmit my case report?" Resubmitted case reports that were "rejected" the first time around are treated as new manuscripts and repeat the process described above. Revised manuscripts that initially received a "no decision" or "revise" decision might go through the same process again or through a modified process. Following the initial review, the EBM specifies who should review a revised manuscript—all or one of the reviewers of the first version, or only the EBM. If reviews are requested, they are sent to the EBM, who again synthesizes the comments, adding the EBM's own impressions, and sends the synthesis and reviews to the Associate Editor for Case Reports. The Associate Editor again reads the case report, the EBM's recommendations, and the reviews. If the Associate Editor decides that the manuscript is ready to be accepted and the Editor agrees, the Editorial Office notifies the author and sends instructions for publication. If the Associate Editor decides that the manuscript is not ready to be accepted, the entire process may be repeated.

Careful attention to the questions and suggestions of the initial review, indicated either by appropriate revisions in the manuscript or explanations in a letter accompanying the revised manuscript, will help you avoid another round of reviews. To put things into perspective, the editors and EBMs of most journals are volunteers, with busy personal and professional lives of their own. Their requests and suggestions are intended to maintain the journal's standards in the most efficient manner possible; every review means that they as well as the author will have less time to spend on other important activities!

"After my manuscript is accepted, is that the end of the process for me"? Authors often are surprised to learn that accepted manuscripts almost always undergo more editing and revision. Following acceptance of a manuscript, the Associate Editor for Case Reports, the Editor, and Journal editorial staff review the manuscript to make copyedits and insert "author queries" that ask the author to clarify any unclear content and provide any missing information. Some queries arise because of the new material that may have been added to the manuscript as part of the revision process. Journal editorial staff then return the "marked up" manuscript to the author for approval of copyedits and responses to author queries.

Sometimes authors are frustrated by the need for further attention to the manuscript, but Journal Editors and staff are committed to making *Physical Therapy* as understandable as possible to its readership.[7]

The "Write" Stuff: Tips for Developing Writers

When going through school, most people who later become clinicians do not expect that they will also become authors. It's no wonder that many people who have wonderful cases to report are reluctant to try writing about them. Below are some suggestions to help get you started, help keep you going—and help the product meet writing standards that may not be obvious to developing writers.

- **If starting at the beginning is hard, start somewhere else.** It's easiest to start with what you know best, which usually is the description of the patient or patients, what you observed, what you did, or what happened.

- **Don't worry about how the first draft sounds; just get something on paper.** It's a whole lot easier to revise than it is to create.

- **Learn to use a computer if you don't already know how.** Writing for publication requires many revisions that are made immeasurably easier by using a computer as opposed to a pencil and paper or a typewriter.

- **Picture your reader as an advanced student or a colleague who is not in your area of practice.** Although the reviewers and EBMs will be familiar with the content area, they are responsible for ensuring that the report can be understood by a general rehabilitation audience. They will not read between the lines or make assumptions about missing information. Remember: It is much easier to take out unnecessary detail than it is to add details later.

- **Once you have revised the first draft—and second and third drafts!—let your manuscript sit in a quiet, dark place for a couple of weeks.** While the manuscript is "resting," ask your friends and colleagues to read it and give you honest feedback. Give it to colleagues who know the topic—and to those who do not. A colleague who knows the area well can check for accuracy, whereas colleagues who are less familiar with the area are more likely to note omitted or unclear details. Then, with your own fresh eyes and your colleagues' comments, go through the entire manuscript again and make needed revisions. Send it off to your chosen journal only after at least the fourth revision!

- **Beware of unintentional plagiarism.** Students and inexperienced writers often "half-copy" when they have trouble putting another author's flowing prose into their own words. Half-copying is what happens when you change a few words in a sentence or rearrange sentences within a paragraph, while retaining too much of the original source. Obviously some repetition of words and phrases from sources will occur (there are only so many ways of saying, for instance, that the quadriceps femoris muscle is a knee extensor), but if a paragraph follows the organization of a source paragraph closely and repeats a number of words and phrases, it should be rewritten. The easiest way to avoid unintentional plagiarism is to read and then set aside the articles, writing about what you gleaned from them.

- **Remember to use people-first terminology.** We work with people who have various conditions or problems, such as children with cerebral palsy (not "CP children") and people with brain injuries (not "the brain injured"). It is also important to refrain from using inaccurate, overly dramatic, or patronizing terminology, such as "stroke *victim*," "*confined* to a wheelchair," or "*suffering* from post-polio syndrome."

- **Use the terms "impairment," "functional limitation," and "disability" accurately.** As discussed in **Chapter 5**, these terms have specific meanings, depending on which disablement scheme is used, and should be used correctly to avoid any confusion on the part of the reader.

- **Use gender-neutral language, except when discussing a specific person or when sex is relevant.** Avoid awkward and distracting terms such as "his/her" or "s/he." The easiest way to do this is to reword a sentence to use a plural pronoun or a neutral noun equivalent or to change the voice. For example:

Avoid:

A therapist should observe how his/her patient moves.

Better:

Therapists should observe how their patients move.

Avoid:

> The patient worked as a mailman.

Better:

> The patient worked as a mail carrier.

Avoid attempting to solve the gender problem by using pronouns that do not agree with the subject, such as "When a person (singular) has poor posture, they (plural) are at risk." This could be corrected in several ways. The easiest way is to use a plural subject ("When people have poor posture ...").

■ **In general, make direct statements.** One common problem: The identity of the performer of an action is obscured because the writer uses passive voice. In the active voice, the subject of the sentence performs the action of the verb.

Passive voice:

> The patient's knee range of motion was measured. (*Who* measured the patient's knee range of motion?)

Rewritten in active voice:

> The first author measured the patient's knee range of motion.

■ **Resist the temptation to gratuitously scatter words that are meaningless, unnecessary, or imprecise.** "Functional," for example, should refer to a specific function; "within functional limits," "functional activities," and "functional status" are all meaningless without clearly specifying the function to which they refer. Other examples of problem terms: "accurately measure" (why would you report *in*accurate measurements?), "appropriately evaluate" (explain how you evaluated, and let the reader decide if its appropriate), "clinically important" (is it important only to a clinician, or is it also important in the patient's life?), and "pain symptoms" (pain *is* a symptom).

■ **Avoid ambiguous terms and jargon.** Try to avoid ambiguous terms and phrases such as "tone," "strength," "moderate assistance," and "a home exercise program was given." If you decide that you must use them, provide operational definitions. That is, how did you define them for the purposes of this case report? Some jargon is so much a part of our professional language that we do not recognize it as jargon, or we protest that "everyone knows what it means." As emphasized in Chapter 4, everyone probably does *not* know what it means, or different people may have different notions of what it means. Clearly communicate what you intend.

■ **Learn to be a better writer.** Well-written manuscripts have a "professional" look in the reviewer's eyes (and you know the importance of an anticipatory set!). Many books about writing can be found in public libraries and are worth scanning. Many are surprisingly entertaining. See the suggested readings.

Next: It's Up to You!

Writing a case report is hard work, but it will be worth it. You'll gain insights into the process of defining, measuring, and describing for communication with the larger world. And perhaps putting words on paper will become less mysterious or intimidating. Who knows what doors you'll open?

References

1 Somers DL, Somers MF. Treatment of neuropathic pain in a patient with diabetic neuropathy using transcutaneous electrical nerve stimulation applied to the skin of the lumbar region. *Phys Ther*. 1999;79:767-775.

2 Iverson C, Flanagin A, Fontanarosa PB, et al, eds. *American Medical Association Manual of Style*. 9th ed. Baltimore, Md: Williams & Wilkins; 1998.

3 *Publication Manual of the American Psychological Association*. 4th ed. Washington, DC: American Psychological Association; 1994.

4 Riddle DL, Freeman DB. Management of a patient with a diagnosis of bilateral plantar fasciitis and Achilles tendinitis: a case report. *Phys Ther*. 1988;68:1913-1916.

5 Watson CJ, Schenkman M. Physical therapy management of isolated serratus anterior muscle paralysis. *Phys Ther*. 1995;75:194-202.

6 Rothstein JM. The ugly side of peer review [editor's note]. *Phys Ther*. 1995;75:582-584.

7 Rothstein JM. Review the Journal! [editor's note]. *Phys Ther*. 1998;78:1260-1261.

Suggested Readings

Day RA. *How to Write and Publish a Scientific Paper*. 5th ed. Phoenix, Ariz: Oryx Press; 1998.

Day RA. *Scientific English: A Guide for Scientists and Other Professionals*. 2nd ed. Phoenix, Ariz: Oryx Press; 1995.

Lamott A. *Bird by Bird: Some Instructions on Writing and Life*. New York, NY: Anchor; 1995.

Publication Manual of the American Psychological Association. 4th ed. Washington, DC: American Psychological Association; 1994.

Appendix 1

Sample Author Guidelines:
Physical Therapy

Send submissions to:

The Editor

Physical Therapy

APTA

1111 N. Fairfax Street

Alexandria, VA 22314

Inquiries:

800/999-2782, ext 3187

ptjournal@apta.org

Manuscripts submitted to *Physical Therapy* should address issues of relevance to physical therapy and should do so in accordance with submission guidelines. The Editor reserves the right to return, without review, any manuscript that does not meet Journal criteria. All submissions accepted for peer review are privileged communications. Author identity is kept confidential from reviewers, unless otherwise indicated. All correspondence is sent to the first author named on the manuscript, unless otherwise requested.

Manuscript Categories

A manuscript is considered for review if it fits into one of the following categories of peer-reviewed articles.

Case Report: A report describing any element of practice not previously documented in the literature. Most case reports focus on a patient or a group of patients, but they also can focus on institutions, facilities, education programs, clinical sites, or other definable units. Issues addressed may include patient management, ethical dilemmas, use of equipment or devices, or administrative strategies. References are needed to support rationales and approaches. Author should supply a one-sentence description of the case in addition to an abstract. Extensive reviews of the literature are not appropriate. *Type of review:* Review by Associate Editor for Case Reports. Masked review by 2–3 reviewers and 1 Editorial Board member.

Research Report: Any original research, regardless of the methods used. Included in this category are studies using quantitative or qualitative methods and studies using single-subject designs. *Type of review:* Masked review by 2–3 reviewers and 1 Editorial Board member.

Technical Report: An original report that describes and documents the specifications or mechanical aspects of a device used by physical therapy practitioners in intervention or measurement. Evaluation of the device should be part of the report. References should be minimal, with major emphasis on the description of the methods used to evaluate the device. *Type of review:* Masked review by 2–3 reviewers and 1 Editorial Board member.

Literature Review: A critical analysis of literature on a specific topic of interest to physical therapists, written by acknowledged experts and by invitation only. Although the review may further a viewpoint or a theoretical approach, this should not be the major purpose of the paper. Authors may nominate themselves through communication with the Editor. *Type of review:* Nonmasked review by 2–3 reviewers and 1 Editorial Board member.

Perspective: A scholarly paper expounding on a specific clinical approach to patient care (on either a theoretical or practical basis) or addressing professional issues in physical therapy, health care, and related areas, written by acknowledged experts and by invitation only. Authors may nominate themselves through communication with the Editor. References should be sufficiently extensive to support the opinions put forth in the paper. *Type of review:* Nonmasked review by 2–3 reviewers and 1 Editorial Board member.

Update: A brief review of a topic of importance to physical therapy practice. Updates are highly focused and supported by the scientific literature. They do not present new data or perspectives or involve application to specific patients or groups of patients. Although references are required, extensive reviews of the literature are not appropriate. If literature is scarce on a given topic, the author may want to consider writing a case report. Length: Up to 12 double-spaced pages (not including references). No abstract required. *Type of review:* Review by Associate Editor for Updates. Nonmasked review by at least 1 content expert.

Exclusivity, Prior Disclosure

Physical Therapy accepts a manuscript for consideration with the understanding that the manuscript, including any original research findings or data reported in it, has not been published previously and is not under consideration for publication elsewhere, whether in print or electronic form. Reports of secondary analyses of data sets should specify the source of the data.

Prior disclosure of any part of the contents of any manuscript in a widespread and substantive form, print or electronic, may make the manuscript ineligible for publication in *Physical Therapy.* Note: Publication of abstracts and presentations at meetings do not constitute prior disclosure. Manuscripts that have been presented orally at a scientific meeting or at a professional forum should include a footnote alerting readers to that fact, and authors should notify the Editor in the cover letter of transmittal of any such oral presentations. Authors who need clarification of this policy should contact the Journal Editorial Office before releasing or distributing information from the manuscript.

Copyright

Authors agree to execute copyright transfer as requested (see form that follows). Manuscripts published in *Physical Therapy* become the property of APTA and may not be published elsewhere, in whole or in part, in print or electronic form, without the written permission of APTA, which has the right to use, reproduce, transmit, derivate, publish, and distribute the contribution, in the Journal or otherwise, in any form or medium.

Commercial/Financial Associations and Conflict-of-Interest

All funding sources supporting the work should be acknowledged in a footnote on the title page. All manuscripts must be accompanied by a disclosure statement (see form that follows), signed by all authors. This information will be held in confidence by the Editor during the review process and, if the paper is accepted for publication, will be shared with readers as appropriate.

Permissions

Protection of subjects. For Research Reports, on the title page, authors must name the institutional review board (or similar body) that approved the study. Authors also must include a statement in the "Method" section documenting informed consent of the subjects. The statement should indicate that the rights of human and animal subjects were protected.

Authors are encouraged to allow participants (subjects or patients) to see manuscripts of all types whenever the authors believe that the participants can assist in making the paper credible, in verifying the content of the paper, and in ensuring that participant confidentiality is maintained.

Photograph release. Authors must obtain and submit written permission to publish photographs in which subjects are recognizable. This statement must be signed by the subject, parent, or guardian.

Reprinted tables and figures. Authors must obtain and submit written permission from the original sources, in the name of APTA, to publish illustrations, photographs, figures, or tables taken from those sources.

Manuscript Preparation

Authors and reviewers should use their judgment in determining whether statements of hypotheses are necessary. The Journal welcomes papers that contribute to the literature, even if they report statistically nonsignificant findings. Authors of such papers should pay particular attention to the need to (1) justify the study, (2) make a case as to why the alternative hypothesis was viable before data were collected, and (3) address the possibility of a Type II statistical error. The reliability and validity of measurements used must be documented. Authors should specifically define all variables. Titles of articles should not be general or vague and should reflect measured variables.

For format and reference style, consult the American Medical Association [AMA] *Manual of Style*, 9th ed, published by Williams & Wilkins (Baltimore, Md). Do not use AMA style to format tables; instead, refer to recent issues of *Physical Therapy*.

All manuscripts must be submitted double-spaced, with pages numbered. Fifteen pages or fewer are preferred. Use 10- or 12-point font. State the purpose in the introduction. Refer to recent issues for examples of acceptable headings. Every manuscript must contain a title page, key words, and an abstract. Remember that most manuscripts received go through a masked review process; therefore, avoid mention of author names or affiliations except on the title page. If the manuscript is not submitted in the proper format, the

review process may be delayed until the format is corrected. Manuscript elements:

• *Title page*, including title, author name(s), and footnote of biographical data about the author(s). (See recent issues for examples.)

The Journal lists author credentials in the following sequence: professional credentials (eg, PT), terminal academic degree (eg, PhD), professional certification (eg, OCS), and honorary degree (eg, FAPTA). Include a notation in the footnote if the work was supported by a grant or other funding source or was adapted from a conference presentation. Because the review process is masked, authors should not include any author identification on inside text pages.

• *Key words* (up to five) that best represent the manuscript content. Editorial staff will use this list, along with other lists.

• *Abstract* of 150 words or fewer. Remember to double space. Research Report and Technical Report abstracts should include the following major headings: Background and Purpose, Subjects, Methods, Results, and Discussion and Conclusion. Abstracts for other types of papers should include purpose, summary of key points, and conclusions or recommendations. Abstracts for Case Reports should include Background and Purpose, Case Description, Outcomes, and Discussion. (Abstracts are not published with Updates.)

• *Manufacturer's information* in a footnote for all equipment and products mentioned in the text. Place at bottom of the page on which the item is mentioned, include full address with ZIP code, and use consecutive symbols (*, †, ‡, §, ||, #, **, ††, ‡‡, §§, ||||, ##).

• *Measurements*, expressed using the International System of Units. (English units may be given in parentheses.)

• *References*, indicated by numerical superscripts that appear consecutively in the text. Present references in consecutive order on a separate sheet at the end of the manuscript. Follow AMA style for references, with the following exception: In the reference list, include all authors' names for works with up to four authors; if there are five or more authors, list the first three names followed by "et al." Cite the reference number in the text each time an author is mentioned. Use *Index Medicus* for journal abbreviations. References should be listed in the order of appearance in the manuscript, not in alphabetical order.

• *Tables*, numbered consecutively and placed after the references. Refer to recent issues for acceptable tabular format.

• *Figures*, numbered consecutively and placed after the references and tables. Provide one original and three copies of each figure, with all legends typed on one sheet. Submit camera-ready material for line drawings, graphs, and charts. Lettering should be large, sharp, and clear, and abbreviations used with-

in figures should agree with Journal style. Send color photographs whenever possible, in sharp focus and with good contrast. Size: 12.7 by 17.8 cm (5 by 7 in) preferable. Write first author's last name and figure number on a gummed label, and place on back of the original set of figures. (Copies of figures should not be labeled.) Use arrow to indicate top of figure if not obvious. Do not write directly on the back of camera-ready material. Do not use paper clips or staples. Send figures protected between two pieces of cardboard. Note: Because the Journal does not return artwork to authors, you may want to retain copies.

• *Appendixes*, numbered consecutively and placed at the end of the paper. Use appendixes to provide essential material not suitable for figures, tables, or text.

People-First Language

Physical Therapy adheres to the use of "people-first" language. A subject should not be referred to by disability or condition (eg, "patients with stroke," not "stroke patients"), and terms that could be considered biasing or discriminatory in any way should be removed.

Submission Requirements

When submitting a new manuscript, include the following:

• One original and three copies of the paper
• A computer disk from an IBM or compatible PC
• One original and three copies of each figure
• Permission statements (protection of subjects, photograph release, permission to reprint tables and figures)
• Authorship, copyright, and financial disclosure statements, signed by all authors
• Cover letter indicating category of article and giving corresponding author's address, day and evening telephone numbers, fax number, and e-mail address

When submitting a revised manuscript, include the following:

• One original and two copies of the revised paper
• A computer disk from an IBM or compatible PC
• One original and two copies of each revised figure
• Cover letter stating that manuscript is a revision (provide manuscript number), explaining how review comments were addressed, and including any changes in corresponding author's address, telephone number(s), fax number, and e-mail address

Reprints

Authors are invited to order reprints of their articles. A reprint order form is sent to the corresponding author at the time of publication, along with a copy of the issue in which the article appears. Readers should contact the corresponding author of the article to obtain reprints.

AUTHORSHIP, COPYRIGHT TRANSFER, AND FINANCIAL DISCLOSURE

Title of manuscript: _____

Corresponding author: _____

Address: _____

_____

E-mail address: _____

All authors must sign below in order for their names to appear in the byline; all contributors must initial this form in order for their names to be listed in the rolling credits. Return all copies to Editor, *Physical Therapy*, 1111 North Fairfax Street, Alexandria, VA 22314-1488; 703/706-3169 (fax).

Authorship

The undersigned author or authors certify that they have made substantial contributions to (1) the conception and design or analysis and interpretation of data; (2) drafting or revising the manuscript critically for important intellectual content; and (3) final approval of the version to be published. All three of these conditions must be met. The author or authors further certify that they have participated sufficiently to take public responsibility for the work. They understand that acquisition of funding, collection of data, or general supervision of the research group by itself would not justify a claim of authorship. They affirm that the manuscript submitted is original and that neither this manuscript nor one with substantially similar content under their authorship has been published, nor is any such manuscript under consideration for publication elsewhere, except as described in an attachment. They understand that any report of secondary analyses of data sets should specify the source of the data.

The undersigned author or authors believe that the manuscript represents valid work. They have reviewed the final version of the submitted manuscript and approve it for publication. If requested, they will produce the data on which the manuscript is based for examination by the Editors or their designees.

Copyright Transfer

In compliance with the Copyright Revision Act of 1976, the undersigned author or authors warrant that they have sole ownership of the work submitted, that the work is original and has never been published, and that the author or authors have full powers to grant such rights.

In consideration of APTA's journal, *Physical Therapy*, taking action in reviewing and editing the submission, the undersigned author or authors hereby transfer, assign, or otherwise convey all copyright ownership to APTA. In addition, the author or authors hereby grant APTA's journal, *Physical Therapy*, the right to edit, revise, abridge, condense, and translate the foregoing work. They understand that they bear the responsibility for approving editorial changes. Copyright applies to publication in all print and electronic media.

Financial Disclosure

The undersigned author or authors certify (1) that they have no commercial/financial associations or conflicts of interest or (2) that they have disclosed, on a separate sheet, any affiliations (eg, employment, consultancies, stock ownership, honoraria, engagement as an expert witness, grants or patents received or pending, royalties), personal associations (including close family relationship), involvements (eg, as a director or officer), or other financial interests in any organization, entity, or person having a direct financial interest in the subject matter or the materials discussed in the manuscript.

Author(s) Signature:

_____   _____

_____   _____

_____   _____

_____   _____

WHICH OF THE FOLLOWING BEST DESCRIBE YOUR ROLE ON THE MANUSCRIPT?

Authors - please sign your name		Non-authors please print name and sign your initials
_____	Concept / idea / research design	_____
_____	Writing	_____
_____	Data collection	_____
_____	Data analysis	_____
_____	Project management	_____
_____	Fund procurement	_____
_____	Providing subjects	_____
_____	Providing facilities / equipment	_____
_____	Providing institutional liaisons	_____
_____	Clerical / secretarial support	_____
_____	Consultation (including review of manuscript before submitting)	_____

Appendix 2

Reliability and Validity of Measurements: Sample References

If you are told that, in a given study, two therapists measured range-of-motion impairments in patients with total knee replacement at hospital discharge and at 4, 8, and 12 weeks postdischarge and that certain intraclass correlation coefficients had been obtained, what do those numbers really tell you? Do you know, for instance, whether those patients are similar to yours? Do you know whether the therapists in the study had measurement skills that are similar to yours? *Unless you read the original study*, you cannot be confident that the reliability and validity findings apply to your case. Therefore, to be helpful to your readers, your case report needs to address reliability and validity based on your review of what the literature has to say about the measurements that you have chosen to use with a particular type of patient.

Measurement and outcomes are increasingly important aspects of practice, and new articles about reliability and validity are being published almost daily. This is particularly true when it comes to validity. In the following pages, we list references to some reliability and validity studies. To help you with your literature searches, we've organized the references according to topic area (cardiopulmonary, neurology, orthopedics, and pediatrics) and, when appropriate, anatomical region. We've also noted whether the studies relate to measurement of impairment, functional limitation, or disability. Studies are listed alphabetically by author name.

APTA's *Interactive Guide to Physical Therapist Practice*, Version 1.0,[1] includes a catalog of tests and measures with references and summaries of reliability and validity information. *Remember, however, that sources such as the Interactive Guide and this appendix are only places to start.* Studies vary in quality and approach, so you will always need to consult the original articles to determine whether they apply to your case report. For more on judging the appropriateness of validity and reliability studies, refer to APTA's *Standards for Tests and Measurements in Physical Therapy Practice.*[2]

References

1 *Interactive Guide to Physical Therapist Practice, With Catalog of Tests and Measures*. Version 1.0. Alexandria, Va: American Physical Therapy Association. In production.

2 *Standards for Tests and Measurements in Physical Therapy Practice*. Alexandria, Va: American Physical Therapy Association; 1991.

Cardiopulmonary[a]

IMPAIRMENT

Oxygen consumption ($\dot{V}O_2$)

- Becque MD, Katch V, Marks C, Dyer R. Reliability and within-subject variability of $\dot{V}e$, $\dot{V}CO_2$, heart rate and blood pressure during submaximal cycle ergometry. *Int J Sports Med*. 1993;14:220-223.
- Buono MJ, Borin TL, Sjoholm NT, Hodgdon JA. Validity and reliability of a timed 5 km cycle ergometer ride to predict maximum oxygen uptake. *Physiol Meas*. 1996;17:313-317.
- Cohen-Solal A, Zannad F, Kavanakis JG, et al. Multicentre study of the determination of peak oxygen uptake and ventilatory threshold during bicycle exercise in chronic heart failure: comparison of graphical methods, inter-observer variability and influence of the exercise protocol. The $\dot{V}O_2$ French Study Group. *Eur Heart J*. 1991;12:1055-1063.
- Covey MK, Larson JL, Wirtz S. Reliability of submaximal exercise tests in patients with chronic obstructive pulmonary disease. *Med Sci Sports Exerc*. 1999;31:1257-1264.
- Holland LJ, Bhambhani YN, Ferrara MS, Steadward RD. Reliability of the maximal aerobic power and ventilatory threshold in adults with cerebral palsy. *Arch Phys Med Rehabil*. 1994;75:687-691.
- Mador MJ, Rodis A, Magalang U. Reproducibility of Borg scale measurements of dyspnea during exercise in patients with COPD. *Chest*. 1995;107:1590-1597.
- Marciniuk DD, Watts RE, Gallagher CG. Reproducibility of incremental maximal cycle ergometer testing in patients with restrictive lung disease. *Thorax*. 1993;48:894-898.
- Melanson EL, Freedson PS, Hendelman D, Debold E. Reliability and validity of a portable metabolic measurement system. *Can J Appl Physiol*. 1996;21:109-119.
- Minor MA, Johnson JC. Reliability and validity of a submaximal treadmill test to estimate aerobic capacity in women with rheumatic disease. *J Rheumatol*. 1996;23:1517-1523.
- Noseda A, Carpiaux JP, Prigoginc T, Schmerber J. Lung function, maximum and submaximum exercise testing in COPD patients: reproducibility over a long interval. *Lung*. 1989;167:247-257.
- Pivarnik JM, Dwyer MC, Lauderdale MA. The reliability of aerobic capacity ($\dot{V}O_2max$) testing in adolescent girls. *Res Q Exerc Sport*. 1996;67:345-348.
- Wisloff U, Helgerud J. Evaluation of a new upper body ergometer for cross-country skiers. *Med Sci Sports Exerc*. 1998;30:1314-1320.

Ventilatory threshold
- Holland et al, 1994.

Heart rate
- Becque et al, 1993.
- Hwu YJ, Coates VE, Lin FY. A study of the effectiveness of different measuring times and counting methods of human radial pulse rates. *J Clin Nurs*. 2000;9:146-152.
- Noseda et al, 1989.

Blood pressure
- Becque et al, 1993.
- Fotherby MD, Potter JF. Reproducibility of ambulatory and clinical blood pressure measurements in elderly hypertensive subjects. *J Hypertens*. 1993;11:573-579.
- Mengden T, Hernandez Medina RM, Beltran B, et al. Reliability of reporting self-measured blood pressure values by hypertensive patients. *Am J Hypertens*. 1998;11:1413-1417.
- Mion D, Pierin AM. How accurate are sphygmomanometers? *J Hum Hypertens*. 1998;12:245-248.
- Reeves RA, Leenen FH, Joyner CD. Reproducibility of nurse-measured exercise and ambulatory blood pressure and echocardiographic left ventricular mass in borderline hypertension. *J Hypertens*. 1992;10:1249-1256.
- Zweiker R, Schumacher M, Fruhwald FM, et al. Comparison of wrist blood pressure measurement with conventional sphygmomanometry at a cardiology outpatient clinic. *J Hypertens*. 2000;18:1013-1018.

Perceived exertion (Borg Scale[b])
- Buckley JP, Eston RG, Sim J. Ratings of perceived exertion in braille: validity and reliability in production mode. *Br J Sports Med*. 2000;34:297-302.
- Eston RG, Williams JG. Reliability of ratings of perceived effort regulation of exercise intensity. *Br J Sports Med*. 1988;22:153-155.
- Groslambert A, Hintzy F, Hoffman MD, et al. Validation of a rating scale of perceived exertion in young children. *Int J Sports Med*. 2001;22:116-119.
- Lamb KL, Eston RG, Corns D. Reliability of ratings of perceived exertion during progressive treadmill exercise. *Br J Sports Med*. 1999;33:336-339.
- Mador et al, 1995.
- Whaley MH, Woodall T, Kaminsky LA, Emmett JD. Reliability of perceived exertion during graded exercise testing in apparently healthy adults. *J Cardiopulm Rehabil*. 1997;17:37-42.

Dyspnea
- Covey et al, 1999.
- Mador MJ, Kufel TJ. Reproducibility of visual analog scale measurements of dyspnea in patients with chronic obstructive pulmonary disease. *Am Rev Respir Dis*. 1992;146:82-87.
- Mahler DA, Faryniarz K, Lentine T, et al. Measurement of breathlessness during exercise in asthmatics: predictor variables, reliability, and responsiveness. *Am Rev Respir Dis*. 1991;144:39-44.
- Martinez JA, Straccia L, Sobrani E, et al. Dyspnea scales in the assessment of illiterate patients with chronic obstructive pulmonary disease. *Am J Med Sci*. 2000;320:240-243.
- Melanson et al, 1996.
- Powers J, Bennett SJ. Measurement of dyspnea in patients treated with mechanical ventilation. *Am J Crit Care*. 1999;8:254-261.

Arterial oxygen percent saturation (SpO_2)
- Escourrou PJ, Delaperche MF, Vissueaux A. Reliability of pulse oximetry during exercise in pulmonary patients. *Chest*. 1990;97:635-638.
- Gardner AW. Reliability of transcutaneous oximeter electrode heating power during exercise in patients with intermittent claudication. *Angiology*. 1997;48:229-235.
- Marciniuk et al, 1993.
- Orenstein DM, Curtis SE, Nixon PA, Hartigan ER. Accuracy of three pulse oximeters during exercise and hypoxemia in patients with cystic fibrosis. *Chest*. 1993;104:1187-1190.

Anaerobic threshold/Lactate threshold
- Belman MJ, Epstein LJ, Doornbos D, et al. Noninvasive determinations of the anaerobic threshold: reliability and validity in patients with COPD. *Chest*. 1992;102:1028-1034.
- Cohen-Solal et al, 1991.
- Marciniuk et al, 1993.
- Pfitzinger P, Freedson PS. The reliability of lactate measurements during exercise. *Int J Sports Med*. 1998;19:349-357.
- Zhou S, Weston SB. Reliability of using the D-max method to define physiological responses to incremental exercise testing. *Physiol Meas*. 1997;18:145-154.

Tidal volume
Ventilatory frequency
- Marciniuk et al, 1993.

Minute ventilation
- Becque et al, 1993.
- Covey et al, 1999.
- Mador et al, 1995.
- Marciniuk et al, 1993.
- Noseda et al, 1989.

---

[a]Reliability only, unless otherwise noted. Compiled with the assistance of Diane U Jette, PT, DSc.

[b]Skinner JS, Hustler R, Bergsteinova V, Buskirk R. The validity and reliability of a rating scale of perceived exertion. *Med Sci Sports*. 1973;5:94-96.

Lung sounds (includes validity)
- Brooks D, Thomas J. Interrater reliability of auscultation of breath sounds among physical therapists. *Phys Ther*. 1995;75:1082-1088.
- Brooks D, Wilson L, Kelsey C. Accuracy and reliability of specialized physical therapists in auscultating tape-recorded lung sounds. *Physiotherapy Canada*. 1993;45:21-24.

Ventilatory muscle endurance
- Larson JL, Covey MK, Berry J, et al. Discontinuous incremental threshold loading test: measure of respiratory muscle endurance in patients with COPD. *Chest*. 1999;115:60-67.

Maximal inspiratory pressure
- Aldrich TK, Spiro P. Maximal inspiratory pressure: does reproducibility indicate full effort? *Thorax*. 1995;50:40-43.
- Fiz JA, Montserrat JM, Picado C, et al. How many manoeuvers should be done to measure maximal inspiratory mouth pressure in patient with chronic airflow obstruction? *Thorax*. 1989;44:419-421.
- Larson JL, Covey MK, Vitalo CA, et al. Maximal inspiratory pressure: learning effect and test-retest reliability in patients with chronic obstructive pulmonary disease. *Chest*. 1993;104:448-453.

Spirometric measures
- Johns DP, Abramson M, Bowes G. Evaluation of a new ambulatory spirometer for measuring forced expiratory volume in one second and peak expiratory flow rate. *Am Rev Respir Dis*. 1993;147:1245-1250.
- Noseda et al, 1989.
- Studnicka M, Frischer T, Neumann M. Determinants of reproducibility of lung function tests in children aged 7 to 10 years. *Pediatr Pulmonol*. 1998;25:238-243.

FUNCTIONAL LIMITATION

Walk tests
- Gulmans VA, van Veldhoven NH, de Meer K, Helders PJ. The six-minute walking test in children with cystic fibrosis: reliability and validity. *Pediatr Pulmonol*. 1996;22:85-89.
- Guyatt GH, Sullivan MJ, Thompson PJ, et al. The 6-minute walk: a new measure of exercise capacity in patients with chronic heart failure. *Can Med Assoc J*. 1985;132: 919-923.
- Hamilton DM, Haennel RG. Validity and reliability of the 6-minute walk test in a cardiac rehabilitation population. *J Cardiopulm Rehabil*. 2000;20:156-164.
- King S, Wessel J, Bhambhani Y, et al. Validity and reliability of the 6 minute walk in persons with fibromyalgia. *J Rheumatol*. 1999;26:2233-2237.
- Larson JL, Covey MK, Vitalo CA, et al. Reliability and validity of the 12-minute distance walk in patients with chronic obstructive pulmonary disease. *Nurs Res*. 1996;45:203-210.
- Mercer TH, Naish PF, Gleeson NP, et al. Development of a walking test for the assessment of functional capacity in non-anaemic maintenance dialysis patients. *Nephrol Dial Transplant*. 1998;13:2023-2026.
- Montgomery PS, Gardner AW. The clinical utility of a six-minute walk test in peripheral arterial occlusive disease patients. *J Am Geriatr Soc*. 1998;46:706-711.
- Nakagaichi M, Tanaka K. Development of a 12-min treadmill walk test at a self-selected pace for the evaluation of cardiorespiratory fitness in adult men. *Appl Human Sci*. 1998;17:281-288.
- Noseda et al, 1989.
- Rejeski WJ, Foley KO, Woodard CM, et al. Evaluating and understanding performance testing in COPD patients. *J Cardiopulm Rehabil*. 2000;20:79-88.
- Solway S, Brooks D, Lacasse Y, Thomas S. A qualitative systematic overview of the measurement properties of functional walk tests used in the cardiorespiratory domain. *Chest*. 2001;119:256-270.
- Vitale AE, Jankowski LW, Sullivan SJ. Reliability for a walk/run test to estimate aerobic capacity in a brain-injured population. *Brain Inj*. 1997;11:67-76.

Physical function
- Cress ME, Buchner DM, Questad KA, et al. Continuous-scale physical functional performance in healthly older adults: a validation study. *Arch Phys Med Rehabil*. 1996;77: 1243-1250.

FUNCTIONAL LIMITATION AND/OR DISABILITY

St George's Respiratory Questionnaire
- Barr JT, Schumacher GE, Freeman S, et al. American translation, modification, and validation of the St George's Respiratory Questionnaire. *Clin Ther*. 2000;22:1121-1145.

Neurology

IMPAIRMENT

Balance
Validity
- Smithson F, Morris ME, Iansek R. Performance on clinical tests of balance in Parkinson's disease. *Phys Ther.* 1998;78: 577-592.

Berg Balance Scale
Reliability
- Berg KO, Williams JI, Wood-Dauphinee SL, Maki BE. Measuring balance in the elderly: validation of an instrument. *Can J Public Health.* 1992;83:7-11.

Validity
- Berg KO, Maki BE, Williams JI, et al. Clinical and laboratory measures of postural balance in an elderly population. *Arch Phys Med Rehabil.* 1992;73:1073-1080.

Chedoke-McMaster Stroke Assessment
Reliability
- Gowland C, Stratford P, Ward M, et al. Measuring physical impairment and disability with the Chedoke-McMaster Stroke Assessment. *Stroke.* 1993;24:58-63.

Validity
- Gowland et al, 1993.

Clinical gait assessment
Footprint analysis
Reliability
- Holden MK, Gill KM, Magliozzi MR, et al. Clinical gait assessment in the neurologically impaired: reliability and meaningfulness. *Phys Ther.* 1984;64:35-40.

Comorbidity scale
Validity
- Liu M, Tsuji T, Tsujiuchi K, Chino N. Comorbidities in stroke patients as assessed with a newly developed comorbidity scale. *Am J Phys Med Rehabil.* 1999;78:416-424.

Functional reach
Reliability
- Duncan PW, Weiner DK, Chandler J, Studenski S. Functional reach: a new clinical measure of balance. *J Gerontol.* 1990;45: 192-197.
- Giorgetti MM, Harris BA, Jette A. Reliability of clinical balance outcome measures in the elderly. *Physiother Res Int.* 1998;3:274-283.

- Rockwood K, Awalt E, Carver D, MacKnight C. Feasibility and measurement properties of the functional reach and the timed up and go tests in the Canadian study of health and aging. *J Gerontol A Biol Sci Med Sci.* 2000;55:M70-M73.

Validity
- Duncan et al, 1990.
- Rockwood et al, 2000.

Fugl-Meyer assessment[a]
Reliability
- Duncan PW, Propst M, Nelson SG. Reliability of the Fugl-Meyer assessment of sensorimotor recovery following cerebrovascular accident. *Phys Ther.* 1983;63: 1606-1610.
- Sanford J, Moreland J, Swanson LR, et al. Reliability of the Fugl-Meyer assessment for testing motor performance in patients following stroke. *Phys Ther.* 1993;73:447-454.

Validity
- Clarke B, Gowland C, Brandstater M, deBruin H. A re-evaluation of the Brunnström assessment of motor recovery in the lower limb. *Physiotherapy Canada.* 1983;35:207-211.

Muscle performance
Handheld dynamometry
Shoulder, elbow, wrist, hip, knee, ankle
Reliability
- Riddle DL, Finucane SD, Rothstein JM, Walker ML. Intrasession and intersession reliability of hand-held dynamometer measurements taken on brain-damaged patients. *Phys Ther.* 1989;69:182-194.

Validity
- Lamontagne A, Malouin F, Richards CL, Dumas F. Evaluation of reflex- and non–reflex-induced muscle resistance to stretch in adults with spinal cord injury using hand-held and isokinetic dynamometry. *Phys Ther.* 1998;78:964-975.

Isokinetic testing
Reliability
- Armstrong LE, Winant DM, Swasey PR, et al. Using isokinetic dynamometry to test ambulatory patients with multiple sclerosis. *Phys Ther.* 1983;63:1274-1279.
- Ayalon M, Ben-Sira D, Hutzler Y, Gilad T. Reliability of isokinetic strength measurements of the knee in children with cerebral palsy. *Dev Med Child Neurol.* 2000;42:398-402.

- Brosky JA Jr, Nitz AJ, Malone TR, et al. Intrarater reliability of selected clinical outcome measures following anterior cruciate ligament reconstruction. *J Orthop Sports Phys Ther.* 1999;29:39-48.
- Capranica L, Battenti M, Demarie S, Figura F. Reliability of isokinetic knee extension and flexion strength testing in elderly women. *J Sports Med Phys Fitness.* 1998;38:169-176.
- Porter MM, Vandervoort AA, Kramer JF. A method of measuring standing isokinetic plantar and dorsiflexion peak torques. *Med Sci Sports Exerc.* 1996;28:516-522.
- Tripp EJ, Harris SR. Test-retest reliability of isokinetic knee extension and flexion torque measurements in persons with spastic hemiparesis. *Phys Ther.* 1991;71:390-396.

Validity
- Lamontagne et al, 1998.

Multi-Directional Reach Test
Reliability
- Newton RA. Validity of the multi-directional reach test: a practical measure for limits of stability in older adults. *J Gerontol A Biol Sci Med Sci.* 2001;56:M248-M252.

Validity
- Newton, 2001.

Range of motion
Goniometry
Reliability
- Riddle DL, Rothstein JM, Lamb RL. Goniometric reliability in a clinical setting: shoulder measurements. *Phys Ther.* 1987;67:668-673.

Spasticity tests
- Priebe MM, Sherwood AM, Thornby JI, et al. Clinical assessment of spasticity in spinal cord injury: a multidimensional problem. *Arch Phys Med Rehabil.* 1996;77:713-716.

FUNCTIONAL LIMITATION

Barthel Index[b]
Reliability
- Roy CW, Togneri J, May E, Pentland B. An inter-rater reliability study of the Barthel Index. *Int J Rehab Res.* 1988;11:67-70.
- Shinar D, Gross CR, Mohr JP, et al. Inter-observer variability in the assessment of neurologic history and examination in the stroke data bank. *Arch Neurol.* 1985;42:557-565.

Validity
- Chester CS, McLaren CE. Somatosensory evoked response and recovery from stroke. *Arch Phys Med Rehabil.* 1989;70:520-525.

---

[a] Fugl-Meyer AR, Jaasko L, Leyman I, et al. The post-stroke hemiplegic patient: a method of evaluation of physical performance. *Scand J Rehabil Med.* 1975;7:13-31.

[b] Mahoney FI, Barthel DW. Functional evaluation: Barthel Index. *Md Med J.* 1965;14:61-65.

Barthel Index, Self-Rating
Reliability
- Hachisuka K, Ogata H, Ohkuma H, et al. Test-retest and inter-method reliability of the self-rating Barthel Index. *Clin Rehabil*. 1997;11:28-35.

Validity
- Hachisuka K, Okazaki T, Ogata H. Self-rating Barthel Index compatible with the original Barthel Index and the Functional Independence Measure motor score. *J UOEH*. 1997;19:107-121.

Berg Balance Scale
Validity
- Stevenson TJ, Garland SJ. Standing balance during internally produced perturbations in subjects with hemiplegia: validation of the balance scale. *Arch Phys Med Rehabil*. 1996;77:656-662.
- Thorbahn LD, Newton RA. Use of the Berg Balance Test to predict falls in elderly persons. *Phys Ther*. 1996;76:576-583.

Chedoke-McMaster Stroke Assessment
Reliability
- Gowland, et al, 1993.

Validity
- Gowland et al, 1993.

Clinical gait assessment
Footprint analysis
Reliability
- Holden MK, Gill KM, Magliozzi MR, et al. Clinical gait assessment in the neurologically impaired: reliability and meaningfulness. *Phys Ther*. 1984;64:35-40.

Functional Independence Measure (FIM)[c,d]
Reliability
- Ottenbacher KJ, Hsu Y, Granger CV, Fiedler RC. The reliability of the Functional Independence Measure: a quantitative review. *Arch Phys Med Rehabil*. 1996;77: 1226-1232.
- Roth E, Davidoff G, Haughton J, Ardner M. Functional assessment in spinal cord injury: a comparison of the modified Barthel Index and the Adapted Functional Independence Measure. *Clinical Rehabilitation*. 1990;4: 277-285.
- Stineman MG, Shea JA, Jette A, et al. The Functional Independence Measure: tests of scaling assumptions, structure, and reliability across 20 diverse impairment categories. *Arch Phys Med Rehabil*. 1996;77:1101-1108.

Validity
- Corrigan JD, Smith-Knapp K, Granger CV. Validity of the functional independence measure for persons with traumatic brain injury. *Arch Phys Med Rehabil*. 1997;78: 828-834.
- Granger CV, Deutsch A, Linn RT. Rasch analysis of the Functional Independence Measure (FIM) Mastery Test. *Arch Phys Med Rehabil*. 1998;79:52-57.
- Pollak N, Rheault W, Stoecker JL. Reliability and validity of the FIM for persons aged 80 years and above from a multilevel continuing care retirement community. *Arch Phys Med Rehabil*. 1996;77:1056-1061.
- Whiteneck GG. A Functional Independence Measure trial in SCI model systems. *ASIA Proceedings*. 1982:48.

Functional Independence Measure for Children (WeeFIM)
Reliability
- Ottenbacher KJ, Taylor ED, Msall ME, et al. The stability and equivalence reliability of the functional independence measure for children (WeeFIM). *Dev Med Child Neurol*. 1996;38:907-916.

Gait Abnormality Rating Scale
Reliaiblity
- VanSwearingen JM, Paschal KA, Bonino P, Yang JF. The modified Gait Abnormality Rating Scale for recognizing the risk of recurrent falls in community-dwelling elderly adults. *Phys Ther*. 1996;76:994-1002.

Validity
- VanSwearingen et al, 1996.

Gross motor function
Reliability
- Palisano R, Rosenbaum P, Walter S, et al. Development and reliability of a system to classify gross motor function in children with cerebral palsy. *Dev Med Child Neurol*. 1997;39:214-223.

Validity
- Palisano et al, 1997

Motor Assessment Scale (MAS)
Reliability
- Carr JH, Shepherd RB, Nordholm L, Lynne D. Investigation of a new motor assessment scale for stroke patients. *Phys Ther*. 1985;65: 175-180.
- Poole JL, Whitney SL. Motor assessment scale for stroke patients: concurrent validity and interrater reliability. *Arch Phys Med Rehabil*. 1988;69:195-197.

Validity
- Poole and Whitney, 1988.

PULSES Profile
Reliability
- Granger CV, Albrecht GL, Hamilton BB. Outcome of comprehensive medical rehabilitation: measurement by PULSES Profile and the Barthel Index. *Arch Phys Med Rehabil*. 1979;60:145-154.

Validity
- Granger et al, 1979.

Rivermead Mobility Index
Validity
- Hsieh CL, Hsueh IP, Mao HF. Validity and responsiveness of the Rivermead Mobility Index in stroke patients. *Scand J Rehabil Med*. 2000;32:140-142.

Timed "Up and Go"
Reliability
- Mathias S, Nayak USL, Issacs B. Balance in elderly patients: the "get up and go" test. *Arch Phys Med Rehabil*. 1986;67:387-389.
- Podsiadlo D, Richardson S. The timed "up and go": a test of basic functional mobility for frail elderly persons. *J Am Geriatr Soc*. 1991;39:142-148.

Validity
- Mathias et al, 1986.

FUNCTIONAL LIMITATION AND/OR DISABILITY

36-Item Short-Form Health Survey (SF-36)
Validity
- Anderson C, Laubscher S, Burns R. Validation of the Short Form 36 (SF-36) health survey questionnaire among stroke patients. *Stroke*. 1996;27:1812-1816.

Unified Parkinson's Disease Rating Scale
Validity
- Martinez-Martin P, Fontan C, Frades Payo B, Petidier R. Parkinson's disease: quantification of disability based on the Unified Parkinson's Disease Rating Scale. *Neurologia*. 2000;15:383-387.

---

[c] *Guide for the Uniform Data Set for Medical Rehabilitation (Adult FIM), Version 4.0.* Buffalo, NY: State University of New York at Buffalo/UB Foundation Activities Inc; 1993.

[d] *Guide for the Uniform Data Set for Medical Rehabilitation (Adult FIM), Version 5.1.* Buffalo, NY: State University of New York at Buffalo/UB Foundation Activities Inc; 1997.

Orthopedics[a]

IMPAIRMENT—Lumbar Spine

Range of motion (ROM)
Flexion
Modified Schöber method[b]
- Macrae IF, Wright V. Measurement of back movement. *Ann Rheum Dis.* 1969;28:584-589.

Single inclinometer method (with subject standing)
- Waddell G, Somerville D, Henderson L, Newton M. Objective clinical evaluation of physical impairment in chronic low back pain. *Spine.* 1992;17:617-628.

Double inclinometer method (with subject standing)
- Williams R, Binkley J, Bloch R, et al. Reliability of the modified-modified Schöber and double inclinometer methods for measuring lumbar flexion and extension. *Phys Ther.* 1993;73:26-37.

Fingertip-to-floor method
- Gauvin MG, Riddle DL, Rothstein JM. Reliability of clinical measurements of forward bending obtained using the modified fingertip-to-floor method. *Phys Ther.* 1990;70:443-447.

Extension
Attraction method
- Beattie P, Rothstein JM, Lamb RL. Reliability of the attraction method for measuring lumbar spine backward bending. *Phys Ther.* 1987;67:364-369.

Double inclinometer method
- Waddell et al, 1992.
- Williams et al, 1993.

Accessory motion testing
- Binkley J, Stratford PW, Gill C. Interrater reliability of lumbar accessory motion mobility testing. *Phys Ther.* 1995;75:786-795.
- Donahue MS, Riddle DL, Sullivan MS. Intertester reliability of a modified version of McKenzie's lateral shift assessments obtained on patients with low back pain. *Phys Ther.* 1996;76:706-716.
- Downey BJ, Taylor NF, Niere KR. Manipulative physiotherapists can reliably palpate nominated lumbar spinal levels. *Man Ther.* 1999;4:151-156.
- Hupli M, Sainio P, Hurri H, Alaranta H. Comparison of trunk strength measurements between two different isokinetic devices used at clinical settings. *J Spinal Disord.* 1997;10:391-397.

- Maher C, Adams R. Is the clinical concept of spinal stiffness multidimensional? *Phys Ther.* 1995;75:854-860.
- Maher C, Adams R. Reliability of pain and stiffness assessments in clinical manual lumbar spine examination. *Phys Ther.* 1994;74:801-811.
- Strender LE, Sjoblom A, Sundell K, et al. Interexaminer reliability in physical examination of patients with low back pain. *Spine.* 1997;22:814-820.
- Wilson L, Hall H, McIntosh G, Melles T. Intertester reliability of a low back pain classification system. *Spine.* 1999;24:248-254.

Gillet Test
- Meijne W, van Neerbos K, Aufdemkampe G, van der Wurff P. Intraexaminer and interexaminer reliability of the Gillet test. *J Manipulative Physiol Ther.* 1999;22:4-9.

Neurological testing
Straight leg raise (SLR)
Deep tendon reflex (DTR) test
- McCombe PF, Fairbank JCT, Cockersole BC, Pynsent PB. Reproducibility of physical signs in low back pain. *Spine.* 1989;14:908-918.

IMPAIRMENT—Cervical Spine

ROM
Goniometric method
CROM method
Visual estimate
- Fjellner A, Bexander C, Faleij R, Strender LE. Interexaminer reliability in physical examination of the cervical spine. *J Manipulative Physiol Ther.* 1999;22:511-516.
- Jordan K. Assessment of published reliability studies for cervical spine range-of-motion measurement tools. *J Manipulative Physiol Ther.* 2000;23:180-195.
- Smedmark V, Wallin M, Arvidsson I. Interexaminer reliability in assessing passive intervertebral motion of the cervical spine. *Man Ther.* 2000;5:97-101.
- Strender LE, Lundin M, Nell K. Interexaminer reliability in physical examination of the neck. *J Manipulative Physiol Ther.* 1997;20:516-520.
- Youdas JW, Carey JR, Garrett TR. Reliability of measurements of cervical spine range of motion—comparison of three methods. *Phys Ther.* 1991;71:98-106.

IMPAIRMENT—Other Joints

Muscle performance
Handheld dynamometry
Extremity
- Bohannon RW. Reference values for extremity muscle strength obtained by hand-held dynamometry from adults aged 20 to 79 years. *Arch Phys Med Rehabil.* 1997;78:26-32.

Shoulder and elbow
- Byl NN, Richards S, Asturias J. Intrarater and interrater reliability of strength measurements of the biceps and deltoid using a hand held dynamometer. *J Orthop Sports Phys Ther.* 1988;9:399-405.

Shoulder, elbow, wrist, hip, knee, and ankle
- Boiteau M, Malouin F, Richards CL. Use of a hand-held dynamometer and a Kin-Com dynamometer for evaluating spastic hypertonia in children: a reliability study. *Phys Ther.* 1995;75:796-802.
- Riddle DL, Finucane SD, Rothstein JM, Walker ML. Intrasession and intersession reliability of hand-held dynamometer measurements taken on brain-damaged patients. *Phys Ther.* 1989;69:182-194.
- Roebroeck ME, Harlaar J, Lankhorst GJ. The application of generalizability theory to reliability assessment: an illustration using isometric force measurements. *Phys Ther.* 1993;73:386-395.
- Roebroeck ME, Harlaar J, Lankhorst GJ. Reliability assessment of isometric knee extension measurements with a computer-assisted hand-held dynamometer. *Arch Phys Med Rehabil.* 1998;79:442-448.
- Walsworth M, Schneider R, Schultz J, et al. Prediction of 10 repetition maximum for short-arc quadriceps exercise from hand-held dynamometer and anthropometric measurements. *J Orthop Sports Phys Ther.* 1998;28:97-104.

Scapula
- Diveta J, Walker ML, Skiblinski B. Relationship between performance of selected scapular muscles and scapular abduction in standing subjects. *Phys Ther.* 1990;70:470-479.
- Personius KE, Pandya S, King WM, et al. Facioscapulohumeral dystrophy natural history study: standardization of testing procedures and reliability of measurements. The FSH DY Group. *Phys Ther.* 1994;74:253-263.
- Schenkman M, Laub KC, Kuchibhatla M, et al. Measures of shoulder protraction and thoracolumbar rotation. *J Orthop Sports Phys Ther.* 1997;25:329-335.

---

[a] Reliability only, unless otherwise noted.

[b] Schöber P. The lumbar vertebral column in backache. *Münchener Medizinisch Wochenschrift.* 1937;84:336-338.

Isokinetic testing

Shoulder rotation

- Frisiello S, Gazaille A, O'Halloran J, et al. Test-retest reliability of eccentric peak torque values for shoulder medial and lateral rotation using the Biodex isokinetic dynamometer. *J Orthop Sports Phys Ther.* 1994;19:341-344.

- Greenfield BH, Donatelli R, Wooden MJ, Wilkes J. Isokinetic evaluation of shoulder rotational strength between the plane of scapula and the frontal plane. *Am J Sports Med.* 1990;18:124-128.

Hip adduction

- Emery CA, Maitlans ME, Meeuwisse WH. Test-retest reliability of isokinetic hip adductor and flexor muscle strength. *Clin J Sport Med.* 1999;9:79-85.

Knee extension

- Kues JM, Rothstein JM, Lamb RL. Obtaining reliable measurements of knee extensor torque produced during maximal voluntary contractions: an experimental investigation. *Phys Ther.* 1992;72:492-504.

- Steiner LA, Harris BA, Krebs DE. Reliability of eccentric isokinetic knee flexion and extension measurements. *Arch Phys Med Rehabil.* 1993;74:1327-1335.

Arthrometer

- Ballantyne BT, French AK, Heimsoth SL, et al. Influence of examiner experience and gender on interrater reliability of KT-1000 arthrometer measurements. *Phys Ther.* 1995;75:898-906.

- Queale WS, Snyder-Mackler L, Handling KA, Richards JG. Instrumented examination of knee laxity in patients with anterior cruciate deficiency: a comparison of the KT-2000, Knee Signature System, and Genucom. *J Orthop Sports Phys Ther.* 1994;19:345-351.

BTE Work Simulator[c]

- McClure PW, Flowers KR. The reliability of BTE Work Simulator measurements for selected shoulder and wrist tasks. *J Hand Ther.* March 1992:25-28.

LIDO WorkSET[d]

- Hudak P, Hannah S, Knapp M, Shields S. Reliability of isometric wrist extension torque using the LIDO WorkSET for late follow-up of postoperative wrist patients. *J Hand Ther.* 1997;10:290-296.

Passive motion

- Hayes KW, Petersen C, Falconer J. An examination of Cyriax's passive motion tests with patients having osteoarthritis of the knee. *Phys Ther.* 1994;74:697-707.

Goniometry

- Eliasziw M, Young SL, Woodbury MG, Fryday-Field K. Statistical methodology for the concurrent assessment of interrater and intrarater reliability: using goniometric measurements as an example. *Phys Ther.* 1994;74:777-788.

- Elveru RA, Rothstein JM, Lamb RL, Riddle DL. Methods for taking subtalar joint measurements: a clinical report. *Phys Ther.* 1988;68:678-682.

- Gilliam J, Brunt D, MacMillan M, et al. Relationship of the pelvic angle to the sacral angle: measurement of clinical reliability and validity. *J Orthop Sports Phys Ther.* 1994;20:193-199.

- Holm I, Bolstad B, Lutken T, et al. Reliability of goniometric measurements and visual estimates of hip ROM in patients with osteoarthrosis. *Physiother Res Int.* 2000;5:241-248.

- LaStayo PC, Wheeler DL. Reliability of passive wrist flexion and extension goniometric measurements: a multicenter study. *Phys Ther.* 1994;74:162-176.

- Riddle DL, Rothstein JM, Lamb RL. Goniometric reliability in a clinical setting: shoulder measurements. *Phys Ther.* 1987;67:668-673.

- Rothstein JM, Miller PJ, Roettger RF. Goniometric reliability in a clinical setting: elbow and knee measurements. *Phys Ther.* 1983;63:1611-1615.

- Youdas JW, Bogard CL, Suman VJ. Reliability of goniometric measurements and visual estimates of ankle joint active range of motion obtained in a clinical setting. *Arch Phys Med Rehabil.* 1993;74:1113-1118.

Figure-8 method

- Mawdsley RH, Hoy DK, Erwin PM. Criterion-related validity of the figure-of-eight method of measuring ankle edema. *J Orthop Sports Phys Ther.* 2000;30:149-153.

Girth

- Soderberg GL, Ballantyne BT, Kestel LL. Reliability of lower extremity girth measurements after anterior cruciate ligament reconstruction. *Physiother Res Int.* 1996;1:7-16.

Knee Injury and Osteoarthritis Outcome Score (KOOS)

- Roos EM, Roos HP, Lohmander LS, et al. Knee Injury and Osteoarthritis Outcome Score (KOOS)—development of a self-administered outcome measure. *J Orthop Sports Phys Ther.* 1998;28:88-96.

Lachman test[e]

- Cooperman JM, Riddle DL, Rothstein JM. Reliability and validity of judgments of the integrity of the anterior cruciate ligament of the knee using the Lachman's test. *Phys Ther.* 1990;70:225-233.

Leg-length differences (includes validity)

- Beattie P, Isaacson K, Riddle DL, Rothstein JM. Validity of derived measurements of leg-length differences obtained by use of a tape measure. *Phys Ther.* 1990;70:150-157.

Lysholm Knee Stability Scale

- Lysholm J, Gillquist J. Evaluation of knee ligament surgery results with special emphasis on use of a scoring scale. *Am J Sports Med.* 1982;10:150-154.

McConnell classification

- Watson CJ, Propps M, Galt W, et al. Reliability of McConnell's classification of patellar orientation in symptomatic and asymptomatic subjects. *J Orthop Sports Phys Ther.* 1999;29:378-385.

McMurray test[f]

- Evans PJ, Bell GD, Frank C. Prospective evaluation of the McMurray test. *Am J Sports Med.* 1993;21:604-608.

Shoulder Pain and Disability Index (SPADI)

- Roach KE, Budiman-Mak E, Songsiridej N, Lertratanakul Y. Development of a shoulder pain and disability index. *Arthritis Care and Research.* 1991;4:143-149.

Valgus stress test

- McClure PW, Rothstein JM, Riddle DL. Intertester reliability of clinical judgments of medial knee ligament integrity. *Phys Ther.* 1989;69:268-275.

FUNCTIONAL LIMITATION

Activities of Daily Living Scale

- Irrgang JJ, Snyder-Mackler L, Wainner RS, et al. Development of a patient-reported measure of function of the knee. *J Bone Joint Surg Am.* 1998;80:1132-1145.

(Continued)

---

[c] BTE (Baltimore Therapeutic Equipment Co), 7455-L New Ridge Rd, Hanover, MD 21076.

[d] Loredan Biomedical Inc, 3650 Industrial Blvd, West Sacramento, CA 95691.

[e] Marshall JL, Wang JB, Furman W, et al. The anterior drawer sign: what is it? *Am J Sports Med.* 1975;3:152-158.

[f] McMurray TP. The semilunar cartilage. *Br J Surg.* 1942;29:407-414.

Orthopedics (Continued)

Anterior cruciate ligament injuries
- Neeb TB, Aufdemkampe G, Wagener JH, Mastenbroek L. Assessing anterior cruciate ligament injuries: the association and differential value of questionnaires, clinical tests, and functional tests. *J Orthop Sports Phys Ther*. 1997;26:324-331.

Back Pain Functional Scale
- Stratford PW, Binkley JM, Riddle DL. Development and initial validation of the back pain functional scale. *Spine*. 2000;25:2095-2102.

Cyriax "end feel" movement diagrams
- Chesworth BM, MacDermid JC, Roth JH, Patterson SD. Movement diagram and "end-feel" reliability when measuring passive lateral rotation of the shoulder in patients with shoulder pathology. *Phys Ther*. 1998;78:593-601.

Functional capacity evaluations
- King PM, Tuckwell N, Barrett TE. A critical review of functional capacity evaluations. *Phys Ther*. 1998;78:852-866.
- Lindstrom I, Ohlund C, Nachemson A. Validity of patient reporting and predictive value of industrial physical work demands. *Spine*. 1994;19:888-893.
- Smith RL. Therapists' ability to identify safe maximum lifting in low back pain patients during functional capacity evaluation. *J Orthop Sports Phys Ther*. 1994;19:277-281.

Functional Abilities Confidence Scale
- Williams RM, Myers AM. Functional Abilities Confidence Scale: a clinical measure for injured workers with acute low back pain. *Phys Ther*. 1998;78:624-634.

Iowa Level of Assistance Scale
- Shields RK, Enloe LJ, Evans RE, et al. Reliability, validity, and responsiveness of functional tests in patients with total joint replacement. *Phys Ther*. 1995;75:169-176.

Lysholm Knee Stability Scale
- Lysholm et al, 1982.

McKenzie low back pain classification
- Riddle DL, Rothstein JM. Intertester reliability of McKenzie's classifications of the syndrome types present in patients with low back pain. *Spine*. 1993;18:1333-1344.

Movement testing
- Fritz JM, Delitto A, Vignovic M, Busse RG. Interrater reliability of judgments of the centralization phenomenon and status change during movement testing in patients with low back pain. *Arch Phys Med Rehabil*. 2000;81:57-61.

Roland-Morris Disability Questionnaire
- Johansson E, Lindberg P. Subacute and chronic low back pain: reliability and validity of a Swedish version of the Roland and Morris Disability Questionnaire. *Scand J Rehabil Med*. 1998;30:139-143.
- Stratford PW, Binkley JM. A comparison study of the back pain functional scale and Roland Morris Questionnaire. North American Orthopaedic Rehabilitation Research Network. *J Rheumatol*. 2000;27:1928-1936.
- Stratford, et al. *Spine*. 2000.

Shoulder Pain and Disability Index (SPADI)
- Roach et al, 1991.

Standing flexion test
- Vincent-Smith B, Gibbons P. Inter-examiner and intra-examiner reliability of the standing flexion test. *Man Ther*. 1999;4:87-93.

FUNCTIONAL LIMITATION AND/OR DISABILITY

Activities of daily living
- Kwoh CK, Petrick MA, Munin MC. Interrater reliability for function and strength measurements in the acute care hospital after elective hip and knee arthroplasty. *Arthritis Care Res*. 1997;10:128-134.

Tests for return to function
- Alonso A, Khoury L, Adams R. Clinical tests for ankle syndesmosis injury: reliability and prediction of return to function. *J Orthop Sports Phys Ther*. 1998;27:276-284.

Disabilities of the Arm, Shoulder, and Hand (DASH) Outcome Questionnaire
- Atroshi I, Gummesson C, Andersson B, et al. The disabilities of the arm, shoulder and hand (DASH) outcome questionnaire: reliability and validity of the Swedish version evaluated in 176 patients. *Acta Orthop Scand*. 2000;71:613-618.

Gait analysis
- Fransen M, Crosbie J, Edmonds J. Reliability of gait measurements in people with osteoarthritis of the knee. *Phys Ther*. 1997;77:944-953.
- Krawetz P, Nance P. Gait analysis of spinal cord injured subjects: effects of injury level and spasticity. *Arch Phys Med Rehabil*. 1996;77:635-638.

Low back pain
- Fritz JM, George S. The use of a classification approach to identify subgroups of patients with acute low back pain: interrater reliability and short-term treatment outcomes. *Spine*. 2000;25:106-114.

- Van Dillen LR, Sahrmann SA, Norton BJ, et al. Reliability of physical examination items used for classification of patients with low back pain. *Phys Ther*. 1998;78:979-988.

Low back syndrome
- Delitto A. Are measures of function and disability important in low back care? *Phys Ther*. 1994;74:452-462.

McKenzie low back pain classification
- Razmjou H, Kramer JF, Yamada R. Intertester reliability of the McKenzie evaluation in assessing patients with mechanical low-back pain. *J Orthop Sports Phys Ther*. 2000;30:368-383.

Neck Disability Index
- Riddle DL, Stratford PW. Use of generic versus region-specific functional status measures on patients with cervical spine disorders. *Phys Ther*. 1998;78:951-963.

Resumption of Activities of Daily Living Scale
- Williams RM, Myers AM. A new approach to measuring recovery in injured workers with acute low back pain: Resumption of Activities of Daily Living Scale. *Phys Ther*. 1998;78:613-623.

Roland-Morris Disability Questionnaire
- Stratford PW, Binkley J, Solomon P, et al. Assessing change over time in patients with low back pain. *Phys Ther*. 1994;74:528-533.
- Stratford PW, Binkley J, Solomon P, et al. Defining the minimum level of detectable change for the Roland-Morris questionnaire. *Phys Ther*. 1996;76:359-365.

Tests of functional limitations associated with fibromyalgia syndrome
- Mannerkorpi K, Svantesson U, Carlsson J, Ekdahl C. Tests of functional limitations in fibromyalgia syndrome: a reliability study. *Arthritis Care Res*. 1999;12:193-199.

Shoulder Pain and Disability Index (SPADI)
- Heald SL, Riddle DL, Lamb RL. The shoulder pain and disability index: the construct validity and responsiveness of a region-specific disability measure. *Phys Ther*. 1997;77:1079-1089.
- Roddey TS, Olson SL, Cook KF, et al. Comparison of the University of California-Los Angeles Shoulder Scale and the Simple Shoulder Test with the shoulder pain and disability index: single-administration reliability and validity. *Phys Ther*. 2000;80:759-768.

Pediatrics

IMPAIRMENT

Isokinetic strength
Reliability
- Ayalon M, Ben-Sira D, Hutzler Y, Gilad T. Reliability of isokinetic strength measurements of the knee in children with cerebral palsy. *Dev Med Child Neurol.* 2000;42:398-402.

Movement Assessment of Infants (MAI)[a]
Reliability
- Haley SM, Harris SR, Tada W, Swanson MW. Item reliability of the Movement Assessment of Infants. *Physical and Occupational Therapy in Pediatrics.* 1986;6:21-38.
- Harris SR, Haley SM, Tada WL, Swanson MW. Reliability of observational measures of the Movement Assessment of Infants. *Phys Ther.* 1984;64:471-477.

Validity
- Dietz JC, Crowe TK, Harris SR. Relationship between infant neuromotor assessment and preschool motor measures. *Phys Ther.* 1987; 67:14-17.
- Harris SR. Early detection of cerebral palsy: sensitivity and specificity of two motor assessment tools. *J Perinatol.* 1987;7:11-15.
- Lydic JS, Short MA, Nelson DL. Comparison of two scales for assessing motor development in infants with Down's syndrome. *The Occupational Therapy Journal of Research.* 1983;3:213-221.

Muscle performance
Manual muscle testing
Shoulder abductors and external rotator; elbow and wrist flexors and extensors; hip flexors, extensors, and abductors; ankle dorsiflexors, plantar flexors, invertors, and evertors

Reliability
- Florence JM, Pandya S, King WM, et al. Clinical trials in Duchenne dystrophy: standardization and reliability of evaluation procedures. *Phys Ther.* 1984;64:41-45.

Physiological Cost Index
Validity
- Boyd R, Fatone S, Rodda J, et al. High- or low-technology measurements of energy expenditure in clinical gait analysis? *Dev Med Child Neurol.* 1999;41:676-682.

Range of motion
Goniometry—reliability only
Ankle dorsiflexion, popliteal angle, hip extension and abduction, scarf sign, elbow extension, and wrist extension
- Harris MB, Simons CJR, Ritchie SK, et al. Joint range of motion development in premature infants. *Pediatric Physical Therapy.* 1990;70:185-191.

Hip extension and abduction-extension, abduction-flexion, abduction, internal rotation, and external rotation; knee extension; ankle plantar flexion, inversion, and eversion
- Drews JE, Vraciu JK, Pellino G. Range of motion of the joints of the lower extremities of newborns. *Physical and Occupational Therapy in Pediatrics.* 1984;4:49-62.

"Contracture index" based on comparison of ROM with "normal" ROM
- Florence et al, 1984.

Shoulder abduction, elbow extension, wrist extension, hip extension, knee extension, ankle dorsiflexion, and iliotibial band
- Pandya S, Florence JM, King WM, et al. Reliability of goniometric measurements in patients with Duchenne muscular dystrophy. *Phys Ther.* 1985;65:1339-1342.

Shoulder flexion and abduction and elbow extension
- Harris SR, Smith LH, Krukowski L. Goniometric reliability for a child with spastic quadriplegia. *J Pediatr Orthop.* 1985;5:348-351.

Hip extension (Thomas test), straight leg raise (SLR), hip abduction, knee extension, and ankle dorsiflexion
- Stuberg WA, Fuchs RH, Miedaner JA. Reliability of goniometric measurements of children with cerebral palsy. *Dev Med Child Neurol.* 1988;30:657-666.

Hip abduction, hip extension, hip lateral rotation
- Ashton BB, Pickles B, Roll JW. Reliability of goniometric measurements of hip motion in spastic cerebral palsy. *Dev Med Child Neurol.* 1978;20:87-94.

FUNCTIONAL LIMITATION

Alberta Infant Motor Scales (AIMS)
Reliability
- Piper MC, Darrah J. *Motor Assessment of the Developing Infant.* Philadelphia, Pa: WB Saunders Co; 1993.

Validity
- Bartlett D. Primitive reflexes and early motor development. *J Dev Behav Pediatr.* 1997;18:151-157.
- Darrah J, Piper M, Watt MJ. Assessment of gross motor skills of at-risk infants: predictive validity of the Alberta Infant Motor Scale. *Dev Med Child Neurol.* 1998;40:485-491.
- Piper and Darrah, 1993.

Battelle Developmental Inventory
Reliability
- Newborg J, Stock JR, Wnek L, et al. *Battelle Developmental Inventory.* Chicago, Ill: Riverside Publishing; 1984.

Bayley Infant Neurodevelopmental Screener
Validity
- Aylward GP, Verhulst SJ. Predictive utility of the Bayley Infant Neurodevelopmental Screener (BINS) risk status classifications: clinical interpretation and application. *Dev Med Child Neurol.* 2000;42:25-31.

Bayley Scales of Infant Development (BSID)
Reliability
- Bayley N. *Bayley Scales of Infant Development.* New York, NY: Psychological Corporation; 1969.

Validity
- Harris, 1987.

Bayley Scales of Infant Development–Second Edition
Reliability
- Bayley N. *Bayley Scales of Infant Development.* 2nd ed. San Antonio, Tex: Psychological Corporation; 1993.

Gross motor function
Reliability
- Palisano R, Rosenbaum P, Walter S, et al. Development and reliability of a system to classify gross motor function in children with cerebral palsy. *Dev Med Child Neurol.* 1997;39:214-223.

Validity
- Palisano et al, 1997.

(Continued)

[a] Chandler LS, Andrews MS, Swanson MW. *Movement Assessment of Infants: A Manual.* Rolling Bay, Wash: Infant Movement Research; 1980.

Pediatrics (Continued)

Gross Motor Function Measure (GMFM)

Reliability

- Gowland C, Boyce WF, Wright V, et al. Reliability of the Gross Motor Performance Measure. *Phys Ther.* 1995;75:597-602.
- Russell D, Rosenbaum P, Gowland C, et al. *Gross Motor Function Measure Manual.* Hamilton, Ontario, Canada: McMaster University; 1990.

Validity

- Russell D, Palisano R, Walter S, et al. Evaluating motor function in children with Down syndrome: validity of the GMFM. *Dev Med Child Neurol.* 1998;40:693-701.
- Russell et al, 1990.

Functional Independence Measure for Children (WeeFIM)

Reliability

- Ottenbacher KJ, Taylor ED, Msall ME, et al. The stability and equivalence reliability of the functional independence measure for children (WeeFIM). *Dev Med Child Neurol.* 1996;38:907-916.

Kinematic, kinetic, and time distance parameters of gait

Reliability

- Steinwender G, Saraph V, Scheiber S, et al. Intrasubject repeatability of gait analysis data in normal and spastic children. *Clin Biomech.* 2000;15:134-139.

Peabody Developmental Motor Scales (PDMS)

Reliability

- Folio RM, Fewell R. *Peabody Developmental Motor Scales.* Chicago, Ill: Riverside Publishing; 1983.

Validity

- Palisano RJ. Concurrent and predictive validities of the Bayley Motor Scale and the Peabody Developmental Motor Scales. *Phys Ther.* 1986;11:1714-1719.

Peabody Developmental Motor Scales– Second Edition

Reliability

- Folio MR, Fewell RR. *Peabody Developmental Motor Scales.* 2nd ed. Austin, Tex; Pro-ed; 2000.

FUNCTIONAL LIMITATION AND/OR DISABILITY

Functional Independence Measure for Children (WeeFIM)

Reliability

- Ottenbacher KJ, Msall ME, Lyon N, et al. Functional assessment and care of children with neurodevelopmental disabilities. *Am J Phys Med Rehabil.* 2000;79:114-123.
- Ottenbacher KJ, Msall ME, Lyon NR, et al. Interrater agreement and stability of the Functional Independence Measure for Children (WeeFIM): use in children with developmental disabilities. *Arch Phys Med Rehabil.* 1997;78:1309-1315.
- Sperle PA, Ottenbacher KJ, Braun SL, et al. Equivalence reliability of the functional independence measure for children (WeeFIM) administration methods. *Am Journal Occup Ther.* 1997;51:35-41.

Goal Attainment Scaling (GAS)[b]

(Functional limitation or disability depends on the goal)

Validity

- Palisano RJ, Haley SM, Brown DA. Goal attainment scaling as a measure of change in infants with motor delays. *Phys Ther.* 1992;72:432-437.
- Stephens TE, Haley SM. Comparison of two methods for determining change in motorically handicapped children. *Physical and Occupational Therapy in Pediatrics.* 1991; 11:1-17.

Pediatric Evaluation of Disability Inventory (PEDI)

(Skills checklist, functional limitation; caregiver assistance scale, disability)

Reliability

- Haley SM, Coster WJ, Ludlow LH, et al. *Pediatric Evaluation of Disability Inventory (PEDI): Development, Standardization, and Administration Manual.* Boston, Mass: New England Medical Center Hospitals Inc; 1992.
- Ludlow, LH, Haley SM. Effect of context in rating of mobility activities in children with disabilities: an assessment using the Pediatric Evaluation of Disability Inventory. *Educ Psychol Meas.* 1996;56:122-129.

Validity

- Haley et al, 1992.

---

[b] Kiresuk T, Sherman R. Goal attainment scaling: a general method of evaluating comprehensive mental health programs. *Community Ment Health J.* 1968;4:443-453.

Appendix 3

Case Report Checklist

As you write, refer to this checklist to make certain that you are addressing all of the important components of a case report. You might want to check off the items on the list before you submit your case report for review.

Introduction

☐ Convincingly explains the importance of the topic, citing credible literature (primary sources, whenever possible).

☐ Cites credible literature to convincingly support the intervention that was selected (may be covered in the case description).

☐ Cites credible literature to convincingly support the importance of the outcome measurements that were used (may be covered in the case description).

☐ Leads clearly and logically to the purpose statement, which is made at the end of the introduction.

Case Description: Subject Description/History and Systems Review

☐ Explains why this patient was selected for the case report.

☐ Includes relevant medical diagnoses.

☐ Provides relevant history, including demographic characteristics and pertinent psychological, social, and environmental factors.

☐ Describes prior or current services related to the current episode of physical therapy.

☐ Explains comorbidities that may affect the prognosis, anticipated goals and expected outcomes, and plan of care.

☐ Describes the patient's (or family's) desired outcomes.

Case Description: Examination, Evaluation, Diagnosis, and Prognosis

☐ Clearly explains the rationale for using each test and measure.

☐ Explains the examination procedures so clearly and thoroughly that other clinicians could replicate them.

☐ Addresses the reliability and validity of the measurements (eg, cites published reliability studies, provides the results of your own mini-reliability study, or makes a presumptive argument).

☐ Clearly explains all examination data.

☐ Clearly explains the decision-making process that led from examination through the evaluation, diagnosis, and prognosis to the plan of care and the selection of the intervention.

Case Description: Intervention

☐ Explains the intervention so clearly and thoroughly that another clinician could replicate it.

☐ Clearly explains the rationale for changes that are made in the intervention over time.

☐ Clearly explains the chronology of interventions and the changes in treatment over time (ie, what happened over what period of time).

☐ Clearly explains the amount of intervention (eg, scheduled sessions, missed sessions, indicators of whether the patient actually participated in the home programs).

Outcomes Section

☐ Operationally defines the procedures used to obtain outcome measurements so that another clinician could replicate these procedures.

☐ Compares measured outcomes with the patient's initial status.

☐ Addresses the reliability and validity of outcome measurements (may be addressed under examination).

☐ Includes progress made toward the patient's desired outcomes.

Discussion

☐ Relates what happened to what others have reported in the literature.

☐ Avoids suggesting that the intervention caused the outcomes.

☐ Avoids generalizing to other patients.

☐ Gives good suggestions for future research.

Appendix 4

Case Reports in Physical Therapy, Occupational Therapy, and Other Rehabilitation Literature: Selected References

To help you as you think about your case report, we've created a reference list of case reports in the physical therapy, occupational therapy, and other rehabilitation literature published from 1997 to 2001. This is a selective list of recently published case reports and is not intended to be comprehensive. These example case reports may help you identify a topic or organize your own case report, but remember that they may lack the necessary detail to allow replication of the patient/client management.

The case reports from *Physical Therapy* were obtained by a hand search of recent issues. The list of case reports from the *Journal of Orthopaedic and Sports Physical Therapy* and *Archives of Physical Medicine and Rehabilitation* was generated from searches on PubMed (www.nlm.nih.gov), the Internet version of MEDLINE/ *Index Medicus,* using the journal title and the keywords "case report" and "physical therapy." The list from the occupational therapy literature was generated using the OT Search database (www.aota.org/otbibsys/index.asp) and the keyword "case report." If you decide to search the literature for case reports, keep in mind that some journals may use the term "case study" rather than "case report" to describe the same type of article (**See Chapter 1**).

Physical Therapy 1997-2001

- Almeida GL, Campbell SK, Girolami GL, et al. Multidimensional assessment of motor function in a child with cerebral palsy following intrathecal administration of baclofen. *Phys Ther.* 1997;77:751-764.

- Blanton S, Wolf SL. An application of upper-extremity constraint-induced movement therapy in a patient with subacute stroke. *Phys Ther.* 1999;79:847-853.

- Brach JS, VanSwearingen JM. Physical therapy for facial paralysis: a tailored treatment approach. *Phys Ther.* 1999;79:397-404.

- Carmick J. Use of neuromuscular electrical stimulation and a dorsal wrist splint to improve the hand function of a child with spastic hemiparesis. *Phys Ther.* 1997;77:661-671.

- Dal Bello-Haas V, Kloos AD, Mitsumoto H. Physical therapy for a patient through six stages of amyotrophic lateral sclerosis. *Phys Ther.* 1998;78:1312-1324.

- Ford-Smith CD. The individualized treatment of a patient with benign paroxysmal positional vertigo. *Phys Ther.* 1997;77:848-855.

- Fritz JM. Use of a classification approach to the treatment of 3 patients with low back syndrome. *Phys Ther.* 1998;78:766-777.

- Fritz JM, Erhard RE, Vignovic M. A nonsurgical treatment approach for patients with lumbar spinal stenosis. *Phys Ther.* 1997;77:962-973.

- Gill-Body KM, Popat RA, Parker SW, Krebs DE. Rehabilitation of balance in two patients with cerebellar dysfunction. *Phys Ther.* 1997;77:534-552.

- Gray JC. Diagnosis of intermittent vascular claudication in a patient with a diagnosis of sciatica. *Phys Ther.* 1999;79:582-590.

- Jones DL, Erhard RE. Diagnosis of trochanteric bursitis versus femoral neck stress fracture. *Phys Ther.* 1997;77:58-67.

- Kelo MJ, Riddle DL. Examination and management of a patient with tarsal coalition. *Phys Ther.* 1998;78:518-525.

- Kinney LaPier TL, Sirotnak N, Alexander K. Aerobic exercise for a patient with chronic multisystem impairments. *Phys Ther.* 1998;78:417-424.

- Laska T, Hannig K. Physical therapy for spinal accessory nerve injury complicated by adhesive capsulitis. *Phys Ther.* 2001;81:936-944.

- Lennon S. Gait re-education based on the Bobath concept in two patients with hemiplegia following stroke. *Phys Ther.* 2001;81:924-935.

- Maitland ME, Ajemian SV, Suter E. Quadriceps femoris and hamstring muscle function in a person with an unstable knee. *Phys Ther.* 1999;79:66-75.

- Maluf KS, Sahrmann SA, Van Dillen LR. Use of a classification system to guide nonsurgical management of a patient with chronic low back pain. *Phys Ther.* 2000;80:1097-1111.

- Mueller MJ, Smith KE, Commean PK, et al. Use of computed tomography and plantar pressure measurement for management of neuropathic ulcers in patients with diabetes. *Phys Ther.* 1999;79:296-307.

- Nussbaum EL. Low-intensity laser therapy for benign fibrotic lumps in the breast following reduction mammaplasty. *Phys Ther.* 1999;79:691-698.

- Olson VL. Whiplash-associated chronic headache treated with home cervical traction. *Phys Ther.* 1997;77:417-424.

- Peterson C. Exercise in 94°F water for a patient with multiple sclerosis. *Phys Ther.* 2001;81:1049-1058.

- Rine RM, Schubert MC, Balkany TJ. Visual-vestibular habituation and balance training for motion sickness. *Phys Ther.* 1999;79:949-957.

- Russek LN. Examination and treatment of a patient with hypermobility syndrome. *Phys Ther.* 2000;80:386-398.

- Somers DL, Somers MF. Treatment of neuropathic pain in a patient with diabetic neuropathy using transcutaneous electrical nerve stimulation applied to the skin of the lumbar region. *Phys Ther.* 1999;79:767-775.

- Vermeulen HM, Obermann WR, Burger BJ, et al. End-range mobilization techniques in adhesive capsulitis of the shoulder joint: a multiple-subject case report. *Phys Ther.* 2000;80:1204-1213.

- Weiss JM. Treatment of leg edema and wounds in a patient with severe musculoskeletal injuries. *Phys Ther.* 1998;78:1104-1113.

- Wong WP. Physical therapy for a patient in acute respiratory failure. *Phys Ther.* 2000;80:662-670.

- Zimny NJ. Clinical reasoning in the evaluation and management of undiagnosed chronic hip pain in a young adult. *Phys Ther.* 1998;78:62-73.

Selected Case Reports in Other Physical Therapy and Rehabilitation Literature

- Batavia M, Gianutsos JG, Kambouris M. An augmented auditory feedback device. *Arch Phys Med Rehabil.* 1997;78:1389-1392.

- Beissel MD. Role of manual therapy in the evaluation and treatment of a surgically stabilized pelvis. *J Orthop Sports Phys Ther.* 2000;30:453-465.

- Brach JS, VanSwearingen JM. Not all facial paralysis is Bell's palsy: a case report. *Arch Phys Med Rehabil.* 1999;80:857-859.

- Braverman DL, Kern HB, Nagler W. Recurrent spontaneous hemarthrosis associated with reflex sympathetic dystrophy. *Arch Phys Med Rehabil.* 1998;79:339-342.

- Braverman DL, Ku A, Nagler W. Herpes zoster polyradiculopathy. *Arch Phys Med Rehabil.* 1997;78:880-882.

- Brindle TJ, Coen M. Scapular avulsion fracture of a high school wrestler. *J Orthop Sports Phys Ther.* 1998;27:444-447.

- Brown A, Snyder-Mackler L. Diagnosis of mechanical low back pain in a laborer. *J Orthop Sports Phys Ther.* 1999;29:534-539.

- Brownstein B, Bronner S. Patella fractures associated with accelerated ACL rehabilitation in patients with autogenous patella tendon reconstructions. *J Orthop Sports Phys Ther.* 1997;26:168-172.

- Callahan MP, Pham T, Rashbaum I, Pineda H, Greenspan N. Cardiopulmonary rehabilitation in a patient with Noonan syndrome. *Arch Phys Med Rehabil.* 2000;81:230-232.

- Cibulka MT. Low back pain and its relation to the hip and foot. *J Orthop Sports Phys Ther.* 1999;29:595-601.

- Cottingham JT, Maitland J.A three-paradigm treatment model using soft tissue mobilization and guided movement-awareness techniques for a patient with chronic low back pain: a case study. *J Orthop Sports Phys Ther.* 1997;26:155-167.

- De Carlo M, Hamersly S. Decelerated rehabilitation after ACL reconstruction revisited. *J Orthop Sports Phys Ther.* 1998;27:238-239.

- De Carlo M, Shelbourne KD, Oneacre K. Rehabilitation program for both knees when the contralateral autogenous patellar tendon graft is used for primary anterior cruciate ligament reconstruction: a case study. *J Orthop Sports Phys Ther.* 1999;29:144-153.

- Divelbiss BJ, Kumar S. Isolated traumatic denervation of the extensor pollicis longus. *Arch Phys Med Rehabil.* 1997;78:783-785.

- Ferraro-Herrera AS, Kern HB, Nagler W. Autonomic dysfunction as the presenting feature of Guillain-Barre syndrome. *Arch Phys Med Rehabil.* 1997;78:777-779.

- Gann N, Nalty T. Vertical patellar dislocation: a case report. *J Orthop Sports Phys Ther.* 1998;27:368-370.

- George SZ. Differential diagnosis and treatment for a patient with lower extremity symptoms. *J Orthop Sports Phys Ther.* 2000;30:468-472.

- Gibson CJ, Poduri KR. Heterotopic ossification as a complication of toxic epidermal necrolysis. *Arch Phys Med Rehabil.* 1997;78:774-776.

・ Glasoe WM, Allen MK, Awtry BF, Yack HJ. Weight-bearing immobilization and early exercise treatment following a grade II lateral ankle sprain. *J Orthop Sports Phys Ther.* 1999;29:394-399.

・ Gocha VA. Modified axillary crutches for an adolescent with bilateral congenital transverse deficiencies of the radius and ulna and no hands. *Arch Phys Med Rehabil.* 1997;78:1165-1166.

・ Goriganti MR, Bodack MP, Nagler W. Pectoralis major rupture during gait training: case report. *Arch Phys Med Rehabil.* 1999;80:115-117.

・ Greenwood MJ, Erhard RE, Jones DL. Differential diagnosis of the hip vs. lumbar spine: five case reports. *J Orthop Sports Phys Ther.* 1998;27:308-315.

・ Guido J Jr, Voight ML, Blackburn TA, Kidder JD, Nord S. The effects of chronic effusion on knee joint proprioception: a case study. *J Orthop Sports Phys Ther.* 1997;25: 208-212.

・ Hardin JA, Voight ML, Blackburn TA, et al. The effects of "decelerated" rehabilitation following anterior cruciate ligament reconstruction on a hyperelastic female adolescent: a case study. *J Orthop Sports Phys Ther.* 1997;26:29-34.

・ Hartkopp A, Murphy RJ, Mohr T, et al. Bone fracture during electrical stimulation of the quadriceps in a spinal cord injured subject. *Arch Phys Med Rehabil.* 1998;79: 1133-1136.

・ Hastings MK, Mueller MJ, Sinacore DR, et al. Effects of a tendo-Achilles lengthening procedure on muscle function and gait characteristics in a patient with diabetes mellitus. *J Orthop Sports Phys Ther.* 2000;30:85-90.

・ Hausen HS, Lachmann EA, Nagler W. Cerebral diaschisis following cerebellar hemorrhage. *Arch Phys Med Rehabil.* 1997;78:546-549.

・ Henry A, Tunkel R, Arbit E, et al. Tethered thoracic cord resulting from spinal cord herniation. *Arch Phys Med Rehabil.* 1997;78: 530-533.

・ Holmes CF, Fletcher JP, Blaschak MJ, Schenck RC. Management of shoulder dysfunction with an alternative model of orthopaedic physical therapy intervention: a case report. *J Orthop Sports Phys Ther.* 1997;26:347-354.

・ Howard PD. Differential diagnosis of calf pain and weakness: flexor hallucis longus strain. *J Orthop Sports Phys Ther.* 2000;30: 78-84.

・ Hsieh LF, Liaw ES, Cheng HY, Hong CZ. Bilateral femoral neuropathy after vaginal hysterectomy. *Arch Phys Med Rehabil.* 1998;79:1018-1021.

・ Ingber RS. Shoulder impingement in tennis/racquetball players treated with subscapularis myofascial treatments. *Arch Phys Med Rehabil.* 2000;81:679-682.

・ Kern-Steiner R, Washecheck HS, Kelsey DD. Strategy of exercise prescription using an unloading technique for functional rehabilitation of an athlete with an inversion ankle sprain. *J Orthop Sports Phys Ther.* 1999;29: 282-287.

・ King L. Case study: physical therapy management of hip osteoarthritis prior to total hip arthroplasty. *J Orthop Sports Phys Ther.* 1997;26:35-38.

・ Kohzuki M, Abo T, Watanabe M, et al. Rehabilitating patients with hepatopulmonary syndrome using living-related orthotopic liver transplant: a case report. *Arch Phys Med Rehabil.* 2000;81:1527-1530.

・ Law LA, Haftel HM. Shoulder, knee, and hip pain as initial symptoms of juvenile ankylosing spondylitis: a case report. *J Orthop Sports Phys Ther.* 1998;27:167-172.

・ Liu S, Tunkel R, Lachmann E, Nagler W. Paraneoplastic cerebellar degeneration as the first evidence of cancer: a case report. *Arch Phys Med Rehabil.* 2000;81:834-836.

・ Mangione KK, McKee E, Hickey M, Hofmann M. Aerobic training in a patient with nonsevere aplastic anemia: a case report. *Arch Phys Med Rehabil.* 2000;81: 226-229.

・ Menck JY, Requejo SM, Kulig K. Thoracic spine dysfunction in upper extremity complex regional pain syndrome type I. *J Orthop Sports Phys Ther.* 2000;30:401-409.

・ Muller K, Snyder-Mackler L. Diagnosis of patellofemoral pain after arthroscopic meniscectomy. *J Orthop Sports Phys Ther.* 2000;30:138-142.

・ Nash MS, Nash LH, Garcia RG, Neimark P. Nonselective debridement and antimicrobial cleansing of a venting ductal breast carcinoma. *Arch Phys Med Rehabil.* 1999;80: 118-121.

・ Nawoczenski DA. Nonoperative and operative intervention for hallux rigidus. *J Orthop Sports Phys Ther.* 1999;29:727-735.

・ Pasquina PF, Dahl E. Total knee replacement in an amputee patient: a case report. *Arch Phys Med Rehabil.* 2000;81:824-826.

・ Patla CE, Abbott JH. Tibialis posterior myofascial tightness as a source of heel pain: diagnosis and treatment. *J Orthop Sports Phys Ther.* 2000;30:624-632.

・ Porter-Romatowski TL, Deckert J. Hemicorporectomy: a case study from a physical therapy perspective. *Arch Phys Med Rehabil.* 1998;79:464-468.

・ Quarrier NF, Wightman AB. A ballet dancer with chronic hip pain due to a lesser trochanter bony avulsion: the challenge of a differential diagnosis. *J Orthop Sports Phys Ther.* 1998;28:168-73.

・ Requejo SM, Kulig K, Thordarson DB. Management of foot pain associated with accessory bones of the foot: two clinical case reports. *J Orthop Sports Phys Ther.* 2000;30:580-591.

・ Russ DW. In-season management of shoulder pain in a collegiate swimmer: a team approach. *J Orthop Sports Phys Ther.* 1998;27:371-376.

・ Schmitt L, Snyder-Mackler L. Role of scapular stabilizers in etiology and treatment of impingement syndrome. *J Orthop Sports Phys Ther.* 1999;29:31-38.

・ Shamus JL, Shamus EC. A taping technique for the treatment of acromioclavicular joint sprains: a case study. *J Orthop Sports Phys Ther.* 1997;25:390-394.

・ Slipman CW, Lipetz JS, Jackson HB, Vresilovic EJ. Deep venous thrombosis and pulmonary embolism as a complication of bed rest for low back pain. *Arch Phys Med Rehabil.* 2000;81:127-129.

・ Stratford PW, Binkley JM. Applying the results of self-report measures to individual patients: an example using the Roland-Morris Questionnaire. *J Orthop Sports Phys Ther.* 1999;29:232-239.

・ Voorn R. Case report: can sacroiliac joint dysfunction cause chronic Achilles tendinitis? *J Orthop Sports Phys Ther.* 1998;27:436-443.

・ Wainner RS, Hasz M. Management of acute calcific tendinitis of the shoulder. *J Orthop Sports Phys Ther.* 1998;27:231-237.

・ Watanabe TK, O'Dell MW, Togliatti TJ. Diagnosis and rehabilitation strategies for patients with hysterical hemiparesis: a report of four cases. *Arch Phys Med Rehabil.* 1998;79:709-714.

・ Way MC. Effects of a thermoplastic foot orthosis on patellofemoral pain in a collegiate athlete: a single-subject design. *J Orthop Sports Phys Ther.* 1999;29:331-338.

・ Wilk BR, Fisher KL, Gutierrez W. Defective running shoes as a contributing factor in plantar fasciitis in a triathlete. *J Orthop Sports Phys Ther.* 2000;30:21-28.

Selected Case Reports from OT Search[a]: 1997-2001

- Canelon MF, Ervin EM. An on-site job evaluation performed via activity analysis. *Am J Occup Ther.* 1997;51:144-153.

- Cifu DX, Craig EJ, Pezzella N, Calabrese V. The rehabilitative management of acute severe combined demyelination: a case report. *NeuroRehabilitation.* 1997;9:237-243.

- Davis SE, Mulcahey MJ, Betz RR, et al. Outcomes of upper-extremity tendon transfers and functional electrical stimulation in an adolescent with C-5 tetraplegia. *Am J Occup Ther.* 1997;51:307-312.

- Dunbar SB. A child's occupational performance: considerations of sensory processing and family context. *Am J Occup Ther.* 1999;53:231-235.

- Gilin M. Above-elbow amputation: a case study in restoring function. *J Hand Ther.* 1998;11:278-283.

- Gillen G. Improving activities of daily living performance in an adult with ataxia. *Am J Occup Ther.* 2000;54:89-96.

- Gutman S. The transition through adult rites of passage after traumatic brain injury: preliminary assessment of an occupational therapy intervention. *Occupational Therapy International.* 1999;6:143-158.

- Gutman SA. Using a computer as an environmental facilitator to promote post-head injury social role resumption: a case report. *Occupational Therapy in Mental Health.* 2000;15:71-90.

- Head J, Patterson V. Performance context and its role in treatment planning. *Am J Occup Ther.* 1997;51:453-457.

- Kinnealey M. Princess or tyrant: a case report of a child with sensory defensiveness. *Occupational Therapy International.* 1998;5:293-303.

- Legault E, Rebeiro KL. Occupation as a means to mental health: a single-case study. *Am J Occup Ther.* 2001;55:90-96.

- Moyers PA, Stoffel VC. Alcohol dependence in a client with a work-related injury. *Am J Occup Ther.* 1999;53:640-645.

- Nakada M, Uchida H. Case study of a five-stage sensory reeducation program. *J Hand Ther.* 1997;10:232-239.

- O'Neill ME, Gwinn KA, Adler CH. Biofeedback for writer's cramp. *Am J Occup Ther.* 1997;51:605-607.

- Phillips ME, Katz JA, Harden RN. The use of nerve blocks in conjunction with occupational therapy for complex regional pain syndrome type I. *Am J Occup Ther.* 2000;54:544-549.

- Phillips ME, Bruehl S, Harden RN. Work-related post-traumatic stress disorder: use of exposure therapy in work-simulation activities. *Am J Occup Ther.* 1997;51:696-700.

- Reeves GD. Case report of a child with sensory integration dysfunction. *Occupational Therapy International.* 1998;5:304-316.

- Schultz-Krohn W, Cara E. Occupational therapy in early intervention: applying concepts from infant mental health. *Am J Occup Ther.* 2000;54:550-554.

- Yuen HK. Positive talk training in an adult with traumatic brain injury. *Am J Occup Ther.* 1997;51:780-783.

[a]A computerized database that contains bibliographic data and abstracts on occupational therapy and related subjects.

Appendix 5

Annotations to Three Published Case Reports

In this Appendix, we've annotated three case reports published in *Physical Therapy* to point out the components of a case report and to highlight how the authors addressed them. These examples are only three of the many that can be found in journals, so we encourage you to browse the literature to find other case reports that may be similar to the one you are preparing.

Because these case reports were published before the release of the second edition of the *Guide to Physical Therapist Practice*,[1] the terms used in them do not reflect the terminology that is now used in case reports written by physical therapists.

References

1 Guide to Physical Therapist Practice. 2nd ed. *Phys Ther.* 2001;81:9-744.

Case Report 1

This case report focuses on one patient, but it also describes a patient classification system.

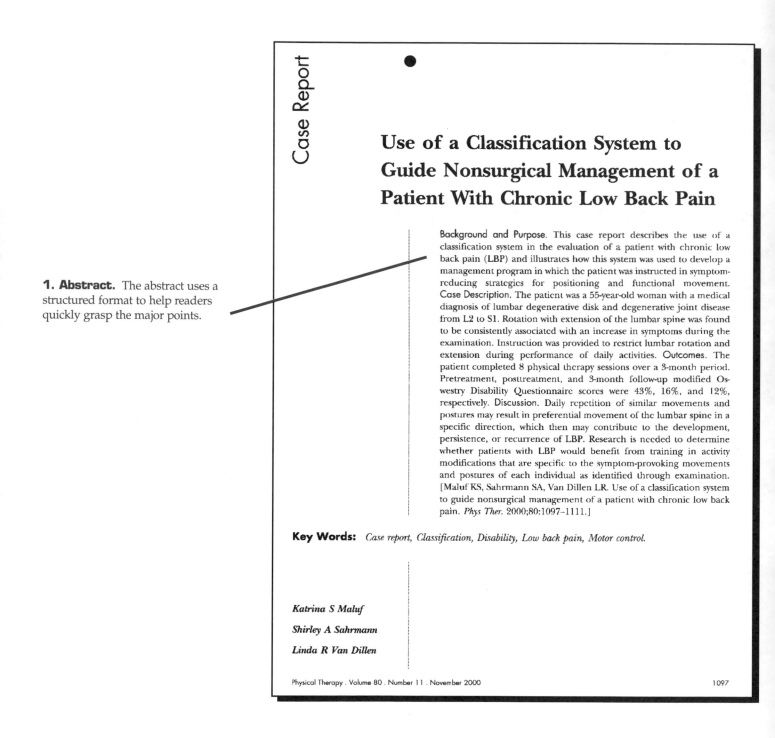

Case Report

1. Abstract. The abstract uses a structured format to help readers quickly grasp the major points.

Use of a Classification System to Guide Nonsurgical Management of a Patient With Chronic Low Back Pain

Background and Purpose. This case report describes the use of a classification system in the evaluation of a patient with chronic low back pain (LBP) and illustrates how this system was used to develop a management program in which the patient was instructed in symptom-reducing strategies for positioning and functional movement. **Case Description.** The patient was a 55-year-old woman with a medical diagnosis of lumbar degenerative disk and degenerative joint disease from L2 to S1. Rotation with extension of the lumbar spine was found to be consistently associated with an increase in symptoms during the examination. Instruction was provided to restrict lumbar rotation and extension during performance of daily activities. **Outcomes.** The patient completed 8 physical therapy sessions over a 3-month period. Pretreatment, posttreatment, and 3-month follow-up modified Oswestry Disability Questionnaire scores were 43%, 16%, and 12%, respectively. **Discussion.** Daily repetition of similar movements and postures may result in preferential movement of the lumbar spine in a specific direction, which then may contribute to the development, persistence, or recurrence of LBP. Research is needed to determine whether patients with LBP would benefit from training in activity modifications that are specific to the symptom-provoking movements and postures of each individual as identified through examination. [Maluf KS, Sahrmann SA, Van Dillen LR. Use of a classification system to guide nonsurgical management of a patient with chronic low back pain. *Phys Ther*. 2000;80:1097–1111.]

Key Words: *Case report, Classification, Disability, Low back pain, Motor control.*

Katrina S Maluf

Shirley A Sahrmann

Linda R Van Dillen

2. The introduction. The authors make it clear that *they* are the ones who believe that two issues contribute to the challenge of managing patients with low back pain. They avoid passive voice (eg, "Two issues, in particular, are believed to contribute to the challenge").

In the first few lines of the report, the authors state the two major topics of their case report: a classification system for low back pain, and the degree to which physical therapists address impairment and functional limitation in the management of patients with low back pain. In the second paragraph of the introduction, background information is given to support the authors' development of their own classification system, which they describe later in the article.

Despite being one of the most commonly treated disorders in outpatient physical therapy practice,[1] the management of low back pain (LBP) continues to be a challenge. We believe that 2 issues, in particular, contribute to this challenge. The first issue relates to the lack of an accepted classification system for LBP that is feasible to use and that is validated through research. The second issue relates to the conceptual distinction between physical impairment and functional limitation, and the degree to which each is addressed in the treatment of patients with low back–related disorders.

The need to classify patients into homogenous subgroups to better facilitate the management of LBP has received much attention in recent literature.[2–15] This need is reflected by the number of classification systems that have been proposed within the past 2 decades.[2–12] Riddle[13] provided a comprehensive review of the classification systems deemed most relevant to physical therapists, along with a discussion of issues related to LBP classification. There is no consensus regarding the most appropriate classification scheme to guide the rehabilitation of patients with LBP.[14] In the view of many authors, the ability to differentiate among various subgroups of patients with LBP would enhance both the clinical management and the scientific study of LBP.[14,15]

Measures of physical impairment such as range of motion, muscle force, and endurance are routinely assessed by physical therapists, with the goal of using the data obtained with these measures to help direct the management of patients with LBP.[1,16] However, as noted by Jette,[17] several major conceptual models indicate that physical impairments reflect only one aspect of the disablement process. Several authors[17–19] have suggested

There are potential benefits to using a classification approach to guide identification and treatment of symptom-provoking movements and postures.

that rehabilitation professionals must also consider functional limitations and disability. The terms "functional limitation" and "disability" will be considered together in this report and refer to an inability to perform the basic tasks of daily life and to fulfill one's social and occupational roles.[18] In a recent survey of patients with chronic LBP (*chronic LBP* in this study was defined as 8 or more episodes of recurrent LBP spaced at least 90 days apart within a 3-year period), difficulty performing everyday activities was the most frequently cited reason for seeking medical care.[20] However, in a national sample of over 2,300 outpatient physical therapy records, Jette et al[1] found that therapists cited independent function as a treatment goal for only 10.6% of all patients treated for LBP. Functional training was included in only 5.6% of the rehabilitation programs. A more recent study of physical therapy for LBP similarly revealed that the number of goals relating to range of motion (65%) and pain reduction (53%) outnumbered those relating to the facilitation of functional activity (20%).[21] Together, these studies suggest that physical therapists may tend to address physical impairments more readily than functional limitations in the treatment of patients with low back–related disorders.

Delitto[19] observed that clinicians may be more inclined to document measures of physical impairment com-

3. Disablement model. The definitions of "functional limitation" and "disability" and the reference cited (no. 18) indicate that the authors used the Nagi model of disablement as the conceptual framework for their patient/client management and as the framework for organizing their case report.

4. Operational definition. Here, the operational definition for *chronic low back pain*—as used in the study being cited—is made clear.

In this summary sentence, the authors help the readers understand the primary point of the paragraph. The first sentence of the next paragraph is a nice example of a smooth transition between paragraphs.

KS Maluf, MSPT, is Graduate Student, Movement Science Program, Program in Physical Therapy, Washington University School of Medicine, St Louis, Mo.

SA Sahrmann, PT, PhD, FAPTA, is Professor and Associate Director for Doctoral Studies, Program in Physical Therapy, Washington University School of Medicine, St Louis, Mo.

LR Van Dillen, PT, PhD, is Assistant Professor, Program in Physical Therapy, Washington University School of Medicine, Campus Box 8502, St Louis, MO 63110 (USA) (vandillenl@msnotes.wustl.edu). Address all correspondence to Dr Van Dillen.

All authors provided concept/project design, writing, and data analysis. Ms Maluf and Dr Van Dillen provided project management, and Dr Sahrmann, Dr Van Dillen, and Kate Crandell, PT, MSPT, provided consultation (including review of manuscript before submission). Ms Maluf provided data collection, and Dr Van Dillen provided subjects and facilities/equipment. The authors acknowledge Jennie Levin for help with photographs, Kate Crandell for valuable discussions regarding the management of the patient, and Michael Mueller, PT, PhD, for helpful comments on a previous draft of the manuscript.

This work was approved by the Human Studies Committee of Washington University School of Medicine.

This work was funded in part by National Institutes of Health-National Institute of Child Health and Human Development, National Center for Medical Rehabilitation Research, Grant No. 2 T32 HD07434-04A1 and Grant No. K01 HD01225-01A1.

This article was submitted July 20, 1999, and was accepted July 13, 2000.

This statement clearly is the *opinion*—not the peer-reviewed research findings— of the authors who are being cited. This is critical information for the reader.

5. Purpose of the case report.
The purpose statement usually is most appropriate at the end of the introduction. This purpose statement, however, came earlier in the article because one of the purposes of the case report was to describe the classification system, which belongs in the introduction.

As the introduction continues, the authors acknowledge that this is what they *believe*—they did not avoid using the first person ("I" or "we").

6. Reliability and validity. The authors acknowledge that the validity of the classification system has not yet been studied—and that is okay! They do need to address reliability, however, and they do so by giving the kappa values that were reported in a previous article that was published by two of the case report authors.

7. Using a table to summarize.
This is a good example of information that is easier to understand in tabular format than it would have been had the authors written about the signs and symptoms in the narrative.

8. Using examples from the literature to illustrate points.
The examples of a tennis player and a cyclist help readers understand the authors' protocol for examination of the lumbar spine.

---

pared with limitations of function based on the underlying assumption that correction of impairments will result in improved treatment outcomes. However, the link between physical impairment and decline in function in people with LBP remains unclear. Several research groups have failed to find an association between various impairment measures and subsequent development of LBP.[22–28] The absence of an established relationship between physical impairment and function in individuals with LBP suggests that limitations of function should be addressed directly in any therapeutic program that seeks to improve functional outcomes.

The purpose of this case report is 2-fold. First, we will describe the use of a classification system in the evaluation of a patient with chronic LBP. Second, we will demonstrate how this classification system was used to guide development of a treatment plan that included modification of symptom-producing motions and alignments of the lumbar spine during the performance of daily work, leisure, and self-care activities. In doing so, we hope to illustrate the potential benefits of using a classification approach to guide identification and treatment of the symptom-provoking movements and postures that are specific to each individual.

Conceptual Overview of LBP Classification Approach

The system of classification described in this report was designed in an effort to aid clinicians in identifying the primary movement problem toward which we believe physical therapy intervention should be directed. Therefore, each category of the classification system is named for the specific direction of spinal alignment or motion that is found to be consistently associated with an increase in LBP during testing. A summary of the signs and symptoms associated with each of the 5 categories proposed in this classification system is presented in Table 1.[12,29] The validity of data obtained with this classification system has not been demonstrated experimentally. The interrater reliability of data obtained for physical examination items used to classify patients according to this system has been reported previously (kappa≥.87 for 100% of items related to symptom production; kappa≥.42 for 72% of items related to alignment and movement signs).[12]

An underlying assumption of this approach is that the daily repetition of similar movements and postures can result in movement of the lumbar spine in a specific direction, which then may contribute to the development, persistence, or recurrence of mechanical LBP.[12] We believe that the direction of spinal motion associated with an increase in low back–related symptoms reflects movement strategies and postures that are repeated by a given individual throughout each day. For example, an

Table 1.
Mechanical Low Back Pain Classification Categories, With Associated Signs and Symptoms[29]

Category	Associated Signs and Symptom Behavior
Flexion	Tendency for the lumbar spine to move in the direction of flexion with movements of the spine and extremities. Lumbar spine alignment tends to be flexed relative to neutral[a] with the assumption of postures (ie, standing, sitting, supine, side lying, prone, quadruped). Symptoms occur or increase with the lumbar spine positioned or moved into flexion. Symptoms disappear or decrease with restriction[b] of lumbar flexion.
Extension	Signs and symptoms are similar to those described for flexion except that they occur with extension.
Rotation	Tendency for the lumbar spine to move in the direction of rotation with movements of the spine and extremities. Lumbar spine alignment tends to be rotated relative to neutral with the assumption of postures. Symptoms (often unilateral) occur or increase with the lumbar spine positioned or moved into rotation. Symptoms disappear or decrease with restriction of lumbar rotation.
Rotation with flexion	Tendency for the lumbar spine to move in the direction of rotation and flexion with movements of the spine and extremities. Lumbar spine alignment tends to be flexed and rotated relative to neutral with the assumption of postures. Symptoms (often unilateral) occur or increase with the lumbar spine positioned or moved into rotation and flexion. Symptoms disappear or decrease with restriction of lumbar rotation and flexion
Rotation with extension	Signs and symptoms are similar to those described for rotation with flexion except that they occur with rotation and extension.

[a] "Neutral" is defined as the position of the lumbar spine at which an inclinometer centered over each lumbar spinous process would result in a measure of 0 degrees, without rotation or side bending of any of the lumbar vertebrae.[12]
[b] Restriction of spinal motions and alignments is accomplished using verbal cues, active stabilization by the patient, and manual stabilization by the examiner.

avid tennis player may be inclined to develop a symptom causing predisposition for motion of the lumbar spine into a direction of extension and rotation, whereas a cyclist may be more likely to develop symptoms associated with lumbar flexion and rotation. Presumably, individuals may develop habitual movements and postures in response to functional activity demands that may contribute to LBP and that may be identified and corrected through the evaluation of alignments and motions of the lumbar spine.

To classify a patient as being in 1 of the 5 categories listed in Table 1, we believe that the clinician should attempt to identify a consistent pattern of signs

---

9. Using an appendix to provide a replicable description of examination procedures. The authors' examination protocol was too lengthy to publish in the Journal, but technology made it possible for readers to have access to that specific information via the Journal's Web site.

The authors continue to indicate that these are their beliefs, using the first person.

The studies referenced in this paragraph to support the reliability and validity of the verbal pain scale were conducted with patients who had low back pain—like the patient in this case report.

The authors describe the effect of the patient's low back–related symptoms on specific functional activities that are meaningful to the patient. They do not list only impairments or scores on tests of functional limitations.

The authors let the readers know that the patient is participating in a study that one of the authors is conducting and that part of the study results have been reported in the literature. In this way, readers find out that the case report is part of a larger body of knowledge. They also can read about the reliability study and watch for future reports.

(ie, direction-specific motions and alignments of the lumbar spine) and symptoms (ie, reproduction of low back–related complaints, including numbness, tingling, or pain in the back or lower extremities) in response to items performed in several different test positions (eg, standing, sitting). Due to the anatomical relationship between the spine and extremities, motions of the spine that occur during limb movement are evaluated in addition to overt spinal motions that occur during movement of the torso (eg, forward bending). Confirmation that the symptom-provoking spinal motion or alignment has been correctly identified occurs by restricting that motion or alignment and noting whether there is a reduction of symptoms (see Appendix in the full-text version of this article on the *Physical Therapy* Web site at http://www.apta.org/pt_journal).

In this system of classification, the primary direction of symptom-provoking spinal motion or alignment identified in the examination as causing symptoms is referred to as the *lumbar movement dysfunction.* We believe that once a patient has been classified according to the primary movement dysfunction, treatment strategies designed to limit direction-specific motions or alignments that increase the patient's low back–related symptoms can be implemented. We consider identification and correction of the lumbar movement dysfunction during work, leisure, and self-care activities to be a priority due to the presumed frequency with which these movements and postures are repeated throughout each day. We also believe that impairments in muscle force and joint flexibility should be addressed relative to their possible contribution to the lumbar movement dysfunction.

Case Description

Patient

The subject of this case report was a 55-year-old woman referred for physical therapy with a medical diagnosis of degenerative disk disease and degenerative joint disease of the lumbar spine. The radiography report described findings of decreased intervertebral disk space extending from L2 to S1, as well as decreased joint space and sclerotic changes in the facet joints at L2-3 and L4-5. The patient reported a 40-year history of recurrent LBP, with multiple episodes each year, and symptoms that typically persisted less than a week before resolving spontaneously. Previous management for the patient's current episode of LBP included approximately 12 physical therapy sessions at an unrelated facility. The patient reported these sessions to be marginally effective in reducing her low back–related symptoms at the time of treatment, with an exacerbation of symptoms occurring within 2 weeks of her final visit to that facility.

The patient's self-reported medical history included bladder neck suspension surgery performed in 1991 for the treatment of urinary incontinence, along with a history of cigarette smoking and high blood pressure. Medications included calcium supplements, Wellbutrin* (prescribed as an antidepressive agent), Premarin† (prescribed as a cholesterol-lowering agent), cyclobenzaprine (prescribed as a muscle relaxant), and ibuprofen. The patient reported taking the latter 2 medications infrequently for the relief of severe low back–related symptoms. The patient was self-employed as an insurance agent and worked approximately 40 hours per week from her home office. We were aware of no change in the patient's medications or employment during the course of treatment or during the 3-month follow-up period.

The symptoms for which the patient sought intervention began approximately 10 weeks prior to her first visit to our facility. Symptoms that persist for this duration are considered to be of a chronic nature by the Quebec Task Force for Spinal Disorders.[30] The patient reported that she had a constant ache across the central low back that fluctuated throughout the day. The average intensity of her symptoms was 6 on a verbal pain scale ranging from 0 to 10. The 11-point numeric rating scale of average pain intensity has been found to yield reliable measurements[31] and to be related to other measures of pain intensity when used by patients with LBP.[32] She was told that a rating of 0 should represent the absence of pain and a rating of 10 was the worst pain imaginable. The patient also noted an intermittent stabbing pain along her left posterior thigh and calf, which she said was exacerbated by twisting motions of the trunk. A tingling sensation was occasionally present in the left toes. The patient reported that the onset of her symptoms occurred after walking at a slow pace on a treadmill in her home for several minutes. The patient described herself as inactive, and she said that she had attempted to begin walking to help lose weight. She reported a gradual worsening of symptoms in the first few days after walking on her treadmill, with no notable improvement or decline of symptoms in subsequent weeks. She described having particular difficulty performing the following activities due to increased low back–related symptoms: brushing her teeth, rolling toward her left side, loading the dishwasher, getting into and out of her truck, and walking long distances, such as when grocery shopping.

The patient described in this case report was part of an ongoing clinical study of the effects of modifying

---

* Glaxo Wellcome Inc, 5 Moore Dr, Research Triangle Park, NC 27709.
† Wyeth-Ayerst Pharmaceuticals, Div of American Home Products Corp, PO Box 8299, Philadelphia, PA 19101.

---

10. Case description. As part of the case description, the next few paragraphs tell what the patient reported—without referring to her reports as "subjective," a modifier that suggests patient reports are somehow "unreliable."

Since this article was published, the Journal's policy is to use "patient," "participant," "student," "child," or other appropriate term instead of "subject."

Note that the authors said that they *presumed* that the patient held her breath to compensate for a lack of muscle control. They did not state this as "fact" without having evidence to support it.

11. Examination. This sentence describes the therapists' experience and training related to the classification system. Presumably, the study that is referenced gives more information about the training process.

12. Modifications to tests and measures. This section explains not only that the test items were modified, but how they were modified. This is important information for other clinicians who want to replicate the examination.

symptom-producing movements and postures during a physical examination being conducted by the third author. The patient was recruited from 1 of 6 outpatient physical therapy clinics participating in a previous study by our group.[12] With the exception of a notably higher Oswestry Disability Questionnaire[33] score (43% versus 24%), this patient exhibited characteristics similar to the patient population described in a previous report on the interrater reliability of data obtained by examiners administering physical examination items used in the classification of mechanical LBP.[12]

Examination
To classify the patient's lumbar movement dysfunction according to the system described above, the first author conducted posture and movement testing with the patient in the following positions: standing, sitting, supine, side lying, prone, and quadruped. The first author had limited experience (<6 months) with the proposed system of classification prior to receiving training, which was similar to that received by therapists participating in a previous study.[12] Briefly, training consisted of 5 individualized instruction sessions of 45 minutes to 1 hour duration with therapists having documented experience in the proposed classification system[12] and completion of a written examination on the content of a reference manual containing operational definitions of terms and standardized clinical examination procedures.

The patient's self-selected movement strategy or posture was assessed for signs of movement dysfunction during performance of each test item. Prior to each test, the patient assumed a reference position in which the intensity and location of the low back–related symptoms were assessed. For tests of alignment, the patient was asked to assume the test position for at least 10 seconds before noting any change in symptoms relative to symptoms in the reference position. For active movement tests, the patient was asked to indicate the point in the range of trunk or limb movement at which a change in symptoms occurred relative to symptoms in the reference position. The patient indicated whether the symptoms increased, decreased, or remained the same with each new position or movement, and descriptions of symptoms were noted. Any test that elicited an increase in the patient's symptoms was repeated, but was modified in an attempt to alleviate the symptoms. Modification of each test item involved restriction of the specific spinal motion or alignment that was observed during performance of the initial, symptom-provoking test. Restriction of symptom-producing spinal motions and alignments was accomplished using verbal cues, active stabilization by the patient, and manual stabilization by the examiner. Following each modified test item, the patient again was asked to indicate the status of her symptoms. Procedures

used in the examination of motions and alignments of the lumbar spine are described in further detail in the Appendix (shown in the full-text version of this article on the *Physical Therapy* Web site at http://www.apta.org/pt_journal). Findings from the examination of the patient are presented in Table 2.[12,30]

Active control of the alignment of the lumbar spine was facilitated by verbally and/or manually cueing the patient to contract her abdominal muscles just prior to and throughout the attainment of each modified test position or movement. She had difficulty using her abdominal muscles and often held her breath, which we presumed was to compensate for a lack of muscular control. Successful attempts at using the abdominal muscles, as identified through palpation, frequently resulted in complaints of cramping and pain localized to the pelvic region. The patient indicated that she had been experiencing such symptoms regularly in the 8 years since her bladder neck suspension surgery. The intensity of these symptoms could be reduced or eliminated by instructing the patient to reduce the effort of abdominal muscle contraction.

The first author also examined muscle force and joint flexibility to determine which physical impairments might contribute to the observed tendency for direction-specific motions and alignments of the lumbar spine. Pretreatment and posttreatment impairment measurements are summarized in Table 3.[29,34–38] The patient displayed no signs of neurological deficit, as assessed by light touch sensation and manual muscle testing of L1-S1 myotomes.[39] The straight-leg-raising test[30] was negative for signs of neural tension. Results of testing for nonorganic signs of magnified illness behavior as described by Waddell et al[40] also were negative. Neurologic and Waddell tests were used to identify the presence of nerve impairment and to rule out magnified illness behavior. Results were not used in classification of the patient's primary movement dysfunction.

The examiner believed that substitution using the hip flexors occurred during manual muscle testing of several lower-extremity muscle groups (Tab. 3). Hip flexor substitution was thought to be present when the extremity being examined moved from the desired manual muscle test position into a position of increased hip flexion. Excessive use of the hip flexors also was observed throughout the examination as the patient moved in her accustomed manner. For example, the patient's self-selected strategy for moving from a sitting position to a supine position was first to assume a long-sitting position and then to lower her upper body toward the support surface using no upper extremity assistance. This method, which presumably required eccentric contraction of the hip flexor muscles, was associated with an

13. Rationale for selecting tests and measures. The authors explain why they used the neurological and Waddell tests and how the findings contributed to their decision making.

14. Operational definition. In the next few paragraphs, the authors explain the observations that they believe indicate hip flexor substitution.

Table 2.
Findings From Examination of Alignments and Movements of the Lumbar Spine[a]

Test Item	Test Response With Self-Selected Alignments and Movements[b]	Test Response With Modified Alignments and Movements
Standing forward bending	No change in status of symptoms	
Return from forward bending	Large excursion into spinal extension prior to onset of hip extension (eg, return to upright position accomplished by leading with back rather than hips) ↑[c] in intensity of central LB[d] sxs	No signs of spinal extension Central LB sxs eliminated[c]
Standing lumbar extension	Lumbar extension ↑ in intensity of central LB sxs	No modified test
Side bending	Rotation of pelvis and lumbar spine in the horizontal plane when side bending toward left ↑ in intensity of central LB sxs	No signs of pelvic or lumbar rotation Central LB sxs eliminated
Sitting	Preferred position with lumbar spine aligned in extension and lateral side bend relative to neutral[e] ↓[c] in intensity of central LB sxs (relative to weight-bearing position in which lumbar spine was similarly aligned in extension)	
Sitting with lumbar spine flexed	No change in symptoms	
Sitting with lumbar spine extended	No change in symptoms	
Sitting active knee extension	No change in symptoms	
Supine hips and knees flexed	No change in symptoms	
Supine passive double knees to chest	No change in symptoms	
Supine hips and knees extended	No change in symptoms	
Supine active single knee to chest	Lumbar extension with initiation of right LE movement CW pelvic rotation with initiation of right LE movement ↑ in intensity of central LB sxs with initiation of right LE movement ↓ in intensity of central LB sxs during late phase of right LE movement as knee moved closer toward chest, reducing amount of lumbar extension	No signs of lumbar extension or pelvic rotation Central LB sxs eliminated
Supine active hip abduction and lateral rotation	No change in symptoms	
Side lying	Preferred position with hips and knees flexed >90° and lumbar spine aligned in flexion relative to neutral ↓ in intensity of central LB sxs	

increase in LBP. The patient also exhibited a habit that she referred to as "nervous legs," characterized by rapid bouncing movements of the lower extremities, apparently initiated at the hip. This habit was observed intermittently throughout the examination, most often when the patient was sitting or lying supine.

Classification and Intervention
Based on the signs and symptoms noted during the examination, we believed that the patient's primary movement dysfunction was lumbar rotation with extension (Tab. 4). We viewed decreased hip flexor length and excessive use of the hip flexor muscles during the performance of routine activities as impairments having the potential to contribute to rotation and extension of the lumbar spine with static postures and active movements of the spine and extremities. Our goal was to improve the patient's ability to perform functional activities, while minimizing the symptoms associated with rotation and extension of the lumbar spine.

During her initial visit, the patient was given instructions for activity modification based on the category to which she was assigned. The recommended strategies for activity modification are summarized in Table 5.[12] A feature common to each of these strategies was the specific

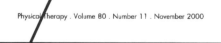

15. Explicit description of the decision-making process. This paragraph and Table 4 (page 183) explain the examination findings that led the authors to classify the patient as having lumbar rotation with extension.

16. Description of intervention. Beginning here and throughout the next two pages, the text, tables, and appendix all contribute to a description that would allow other clinicians to replicate the intervention.

Table 2.
Continued

Test Item	Test Response With Self-Selected Alignments and Movements[b]	Test Response With Modified Alignments and Movements
Prone	Lumbar extension ↑ in intensity of central LB sxs	No signs of lumbar extension ↓ in intensity of central LB sxs
Prone active knee flexion	No change in status of symptoms	
Prone active hip rotation	Lumbar extension and CCW pelvic rotation during movement of left hip into lateral rotation Change in location of sxs from central LB, to central LB and left posterior thigh	No signs of lumbar extension or pelvic rotation Left posterior thigh sxs eliminated No change in intensity of central LB sxs
Prone active hip extension	Lumbar extension and CCW pelvic rotation during left hip extension Lumbar extension and CW pelvic rotation during right hip extension Change in location of sxs from central LB in prone, to central LB and left posterior thigh during extension of each hip	No signs of lumbar extension or pelvic rotation with modified test for left and right hip extension Left posterior thigh and central LB sxs eliminated with modified test for left and right hip extension
Quadruped	Preferred position with lumbar spine aligned in extension and lateral side bend relative to neutral ↑ in intensity of central LB sxs	No signs of lumbar extension or lateral side bending Central LB sxs eliminated
Quadruped active arm lift	No change in symptoms	
Quadruped rocking backward	No change in symptoms	
Quadruped rocking backward in full flexion	No change in symptoms	
Quadruped rocking forward	No change in symptoms	

[a] Signs of direction-specific alignment or movement of the lumbar spine were recorded and modified only when associated with an *increase* in the patient's symptoms. Modification of each test item (third column) was accomplished with verbal cues, active stabilization by the patient, and manual stabilization by the examiner to specifically restrict the symptom-related alignments or motions (second column) listed for each item. A complete description of each test item is provided in the Appendix. Abbreviations: ↑=increase, ↓=decrease, LB=low back, sxs=symptoms, LE=lower extremity, CCW=counterclockwise (ie, forward rotation of the right hip with backward rotation of the left hip), CW=clockwise (backward rotation of the right hip with forward rotation of the left hip).

[b] "Self-selected alignments and movements" refers to alignments and movements of the lumbar spine that are observed when the patient initially assumes a test position (eg, sitting) or performs a test movement (eg, forward bending) using his or her preferred movement strategy with no further instruction from the examiner.

[c] An "increase" in symptoms is defined as pain or paresthesias that were either produced, increased in intensity, or moved distally from the lumbar spine with assumption of a test position or performance of a test movement. A "decrease" in symptoms is defined as pain or paresthesias that either diminished in intensity or moved proximally toward the lumbar spine with assumption of a test position or performance of a test movement. "Eliminated" is defined as the absence of symptoms that were present during assumption of a previous test position or performance of a previous test movement.

[d] "Central LB" refers to the region surrounding the spine extending from T12 to the gluteal fold.[29]

[e] "Neutral" is defined as that position of the lumbar spine at which an inclinometer centered over each lumbar spinous process would result in a measure of 0 degrees, without rotation or side bending of any of the lumbar vertebrae.[42]

discouragement of rotation and extension of the lumbar spine during daily activities. Along with addressing the activities that the patient identified as problematic, other tasks commonly associated with rotation and extension of the lumbar spine, such as reaching overhead or across the body, also were addressed (Tab. 5).

During subsequent visits, the patient was instructed in a home exercise program to address both functional limitations and specific physical impairments. The patient was encouraged to practice isolated limb movements while avoiding rotation or extension movements of the lumbar spine. This was accomplished through performance of the modified version of each movement test that resulted in symptoms during examination (Tab. 2), as described in the Appendix (shown in the full-text version of this article on the *Physical Therapy* Web site at http://www.apta.org/pt_journal). The importance of activity modification was emphasized by having the patient perform the majority of exercises both in isolation and during functional movement. For example, the patient was instructed to perform 10 to 15 daily repeti-

Table 3.
Pretreatment and Posttreatment Physical Impairment Measurements[a]

	Pretreatment	Posttreatment
Lumbar spine excursion range of motion (ROM) [°][b]		
Flexion	30°	80°
Extension	8°	45°
Side bend right	34°	31°
Side bend left	32°	24°
Muscle length [°] as indicated by ROM[c]		
Hamstrings (R/L)	70/78	76/67
Latissimus dorsi (R/L)	151/145	163/145
Hip flexors (R/L)[d]	−30/−20	0/−10
Muscle force[e]		
Hip medial rotators (R/L)[c]	4+/4	4+/4
Tensor fascia lata (R/L)[c]	3/3+	3/3+
Gluteus medius (R/L)[c]	3/4	3+/3+
Lower abdominals[f]	NT	2

[a] Flexibility and force tests performed for all major lower-extremity muscle groups. Measurements listed only for those tests that revealed limitations. Twelve-week time interval between pretreatment and posttreatment measurements.
[b] Spinal range-of-motion measurements reflect excursion of the lumbar spine from a position of upright standing and were obtained using the 2-inclinometer method with landmarks over the L1 and S2 spinous processes. Intrarater reliability for 3 examiners measuring 15 patients with low back pain has been reported to range from r=.13 to r=.85.[34]
[c] Tests performed as described by Kendall et al.[35] R=right, L=left. The average intrarater reliability for 4 examiners performing upper- and lower-extremity goniometric measurements on 12 male subjects without impairments has been reported to be r=.85.[36]
[d] The average intraclass correlation coefficient for indexing intrarater reliability for 2 examiners performing a modified version of the hip flexor length test as described by Kendall et al[35] on 10 subjects without impairments has been reported to be .82.[37]
[e] Muscle force grades were assigned using a modified Medical Research Council (MRC) grading scale,[38] with grades ranging from 0 to 5. Weighted kappa values to index the intrarater reliability for 4 examiners performing testing of proximal lower-extremity muscle groups according to the MRC scale in 102 patients with Duchenne muscular dystrophy ranged between .71 and .93.[38] Substitution of hip flexors noted on testing of hip medial rotator, tensor fascia lata, and gluteus medius muscles at pretreatment assessment only. (Note: all substitutions were corrected prior to assigning a manual muscle test grade.)
[f] Lower abdominal muscle force test performed as described by Sahrmann.[29] NT=not able to test because of pain.

Table 4.
Test Items for Which Patient's Symptoms Were Decreased or Eliminated With Restriction of Spinal Alignment or Movement[a]

Flexion	Extension	Rotation	Rotation With Flexion	Rotation With Extension
No lumbar flexion associated with an increase in symptoms	Return from forward bending Prone	Side bending (left)	No lumbar flexion with rotation associated with an increase in symptoms	Supine active single knee to chest (right) Active hip lateral rotation (left) Active hip extension (bilateral) Quadruped

[a] Test items listed according to the specific direction of spinal alignment or movement that was restricted during performance of the modified test for each item (see Tab. 2). Classification is determined based on the category having the majority of test items in which symptoms are increased. Priority in determining the low back pain classification category is given to those tests in which the examiner is able to decrease or eliminate symptoms by restricting the specific direction of spinal motion or alignment found to be associated with an increase in symptoms during the initial test.

tions of the forward bend exercise (Tab. 5), with additional instructions to use this same technique each time she bent forward throughout the day, such as when brushing her teeth. A brief description of each exercise and its functional correlate is provided in Table 5. The importance of maintaining a neutral or slightly flexed position of the lumbar spine through active use of abdominal muscles was emphasized. We believed that this position would prevent an increase in low back–related symptoms and facilitate strengthening of the abdominal muscles.

In addition to the exercise program, the patient was instructed in techniques that we believed would lengthen the hip flexors and improve gluteus medius muscle force production. While lying prone, the patient used a sheet positioned around her ankle to assist in passively flexing her knee to the point at which she perceived a gentle stretch in the anterior thigh. To avoid an increase in symptoms when positioned prone, the patient initially was instructed to position 2 pillows under her abdomen, but eventually was able to perform this stretch in the absence of pillows without an increase in LBP. In an effort to improve gluteus medius muscle

As they should, the authors state which statistics the researchers used in studies of the reliability of the Oswestry Disability Questionnaire. "Reproducibility" probably is the same as test-retest reliability, and inclusion of the reliability coefficients would have given readers more complete information.

Correlation coefficients of Oswestry Disability Questionnaire scores and scores on other tests— and the names of the "other accepted measures"—would be helpful in understanding the validity of these measurements.

17. Outcome description. In the following paragraphs, the descriptions of the patient's outcomes over time give a good picture of her status during and after the intervention.

Note use of the word "adherence" instead of "compliance." "Participation" is now preferred to "adherence."

The patient's improvements are easy to understand because the authors include her report of improvement in specific functional skills in addition to her scores on the Oswestry Disability Questionnaire.

The authors acknowledge a lack of documented reliability for many impairment measurements and appropriately suggest caution when interpreting small changes in measurements.

Follow-up—even a simple telephone call—can provide important information about how a patient is doing months after the intervention.

---

force, the patient was instructed in active hip lateral rotation and abduction performed while side lying. As with all other exercises, rotation and extension movements of the lumbar spine were specifically discouraged during the performance of these 2 exercises. Following instruction in gait modifications that we believed would reduce the magnitude of rotation of the pelvis and lumbar spine (Tab. 5), a walking program was prescribed to improve aerobic fitness. The patient reported that modifying her gait reduced her symptoms immediately following instruction. The patient declined referral to a urogynecologist regarding her symptoms of pelvic pain and cramping.

Outcomes

The patient completed 8 physical therapy sessions over a 3-month period. The first 3 sessions were spaced 1 week apart, with subsequent sessions once every 1 to 4 weeks. Her condition was assessed 3 months after discharge through a telephone interview and a mailed questionnaire. A modified Oswestry Disability Questionnaire[33] and a pain diagram were used to document patient-perceived progress once each month, with 1 exception due to an administrative oversight. Patient scores on the Oswestry Disability Questionnaire have been found to be reliable (Pearson r and intraclass correlation coefficients >.90)[33,41] as well as related to scores on other accepted measures of disability in patients with LBP,[12] an indication of construct validity of the questionnaire. Reproducibility of pain diagram responses in patients with chronic LBP has been documented.[43] Concordance between defined disorders associated with LBP and diagnoses based on pain diagram responses provides evidence of validity of the pain diagram as a clinical tool.[44] Physical impairment measurements were obtained by the first author during the patient's final therapy session for comparison with initial values.

During her initial visit, the patient received instruction in activity modification only. In the week following this visit, the patient noted a reduction in both the frequency and intensity of her symptoms. She reported a 75% decrease in the frequency of pain in the central low back region and a 40% reduction in the frequency of symptoms in the left lower extremity. She also reported that the average intensity of her symptoms was reduced from 6/10 to 3.5/10 on a verbal pain scale, with no symptoms present the day of her second session. When asked to describe her activities during the past week, the patient noted a substantial improvement in her ability to perform household chores and in her overall tolerance for physical activity. With the exception of sit-to-supine transfers, we observed adherence to all activity modifications taught in the initial therapy session throughout the second treatment session.

By her final therapy session, the patient no longer experienced lower-extremity symptoms. She noted symptoms localized to the central low back as typically being less than 3/10 when present, with approximately 75% to 80% of her week being symptom-free. She noted that the intensity of symptoms in the central low back region generally increased with increasing fatigue. The patient was able to independently demonstrate all prescribed exercises and activity modifications as instructed, without an increase in symptoms. She reported that she typically performed her home exercise program once daily, and was walking 3.5 to 4.5 minutes each day on her treadmill without an increase in low back–related symptoms.

The modified Oswestry Disability Questionnaire[33] contains items pertaining to both functional limitation and disability and was used in this case to document functional progress. The patient's pretreatment Oswestry score of 43% dropped to 16% by her final therapy session. As interpreted by Fairbank et al,[41] these scores reflect a transition in function from severe disability to minimal disability. In the 3 months following discharge from outpatient physical therapy, the patient did not experience an exacerbation of low back–related symptoms and continued to make functional improvements. Specific examples of functional improvement noted by the patient during the follow-up telephone interview at 3 months included the ability to brush her teeth, get into and out of her truck, and shop for over an hour without an increase in symptoms.

Less consistent changes were observed for measures of muscle force and joint flexibility (Tab. 3). Changes included what we believed to be indicators of increased length of the hip flexors, improved ability to use the abdominal muscles without an increase in pain, and an increase in spinal flexion and extension range of motion. Hamstring muscle flexibility and spinal side-bending range of motion declined over the course of treatment. Estimates of the intrarater reliability of data obtained for these physical impairment measures are provided in Table 3 to the extent that this information is available. However, due to the general lack of documented reliability for many of the physical impairment measures routinely used by clinicians, small changes in the measurements should be interpreted with caution.

Discussion

Numerous interventions are available for patients with low back–related disorders.[45] The challenge for physical therapists is to identify the most appropriate intervention for each patient, based on the findings from a standardized examination. This task is difficult because the etiology of LBP is unknown in the majority of cases[45]

Table 5.
Category-Specific Treatment Plan[a]

Activity	Functional Instruction[b]		Exercise Instruction[c]	
	Do:	Do Not:	Initial:	Progression:
Forward bending/return from forward bending (eg, brushing teeth, washing dishes)	Contract abdominals to support spine in neutral[d] or slightly flexed alignment[d] Flex at hip joints and maintain neutral alignment of lumbar spine while bending forward Extend at hip joints and maintain neutral alignment of lumbar spine while returning to the upright position	Arch LB when returning to the upright position	Same as modified forward bending/return from forward bending (see Appendix for patient position and instructions) [2]	Same as modified forward bending/return from forward bending without use of arms to support weight of upper both [3]
Supine ⇔ sit transfers and rolling	1. Bend knees by sliding 1 heel at a time toward body. Gently dig heel into support surface while sliding leg. Contract abdominals to support spine so that LB maintains contact with support surface throughout leg movement. Avoid arching LB with leg movement. 2. Roll onto side moving the entire body as a single unit. Avoid twisting. Use arms to push to upright sitting as legs drop over side of support surface at the same time. Reverse the technique to perform sit ⇒ supine transfers.	Move directly from supine to long-sitting by flexing at hip joints Lift both legs simultaneously from support surface Arch or twist LB when moving legs Use lumbar roll when sitting	Same as step 1 for supine ⇒ sit transfers Perform with 2 pillows placed under knee of stationary limb to help maintain pelvic and lumbar alignment [2]	Same as step 1 for supine ⇒ sit transfers Perform without pillows [3]
Vehicle transfers	Sit on edge of seat facing door and scoot as far back as possible, then pivot to face forward while using arms to help lift legs into vehicle	Twist trunk while getting into and out of vehicle		
Walking	Keep hips as level as possible Take smaller steps and reduce amplitude of arm swing to help avoid excessive twisting of pelvis Take frequent short breaks if walking long distances Move feet to turn body rather than twisting trunk		Single-limb stance: While standing on 1 leg, contract buttocks to maintain level pelvis and avoid bending trunk to either side Hold onto high counter or chair back to assist with balance Perform in front of mirror to monitor performance [3]	Single-limb stance: While standing on 1 leg, contract buttocks to maintain level pelvis and avoid bending trunk to either side Perform without support of arms [5]

Table 5.
Continued

Activity	Functional Instruction[b]		Exercise Instruction[c]	
	Do:	Do Not:	Initial:	Progression:
Overhead and cross-body reaching (eg, reaching for items located in overhead cabinets, reaching for items not directly in front of body, raising arms overhead to don/doff shirt, raising arms to wash or style hair)	Contract abdominals to support spine in neutral alignment when moving arms Whenever possible, stand directly in front of an item before reaching	Arch LB when reaching overhead Twist LB when reaching across body	1. While sitting in a straight-back chair, with LB supported, begin with shoulders and elbows bent to 90°, palms facing forward you and elbows facing forward. Raise both arms overhead while contracting abdominals so that LB maintains contact with support surface during arm motion. (3) 2. While sitting in a straight-back chair, with LB supported, begin with 1 arm overhead, holding a 0.94-kg (2-lb) weight. Lower arm down across body toward opposite hip. Contract abdominals so that LB and pelvis maintain contact with support surface. (6)	Perform exercise 1 while standing, with LB supported against a wall and pelvis tilted posteriorly (4) Perform exercise 2 while standing, with LB supported against a wall, and pelvis tilted posteriorly (7)
Sitting	Sit with LB either in neutral or slightly flexed alignment Use the chair back for support Support feet while sitting. Relax legs and let chair support the weight of thighs. Cross legs at ankles rather than at thighs to avoid pelvic rotation Take frequent breaks by standing up or performing a "push-up" from chair (ie, push down on arm rests to lift buttocks from chair seat)	Sit forward on edge of chair or place a lumbar roll behind LB Bounce legs repeatedly while sitting or let legs dangle unsupported	Posterior pelvic tilts while seated (2)	

[a] The patient was instructed to incorporate techniques for functional activity modification into performance of daily activities. In addition to exercises listed in table, the home exercise program (HEP) included performance of the modified version of each symptom-provoking movement test described in Table 2, as well as exercises to lengthen the hip flexors and improve gluteus medius muscle strength. The patient was initially instructed to perform 6 to 8 repetitions of each exercise, 2 to 3 times daily (with the exception of hip flexor stretch, which was performed twice daily for 3 to 5 repetitions, lasting 30 seconds each). Intermittent performance of a relatively low number of repetitions was chosen in order to avoid muscle fatigue and to optimize motor learning through random practice sessions. As the patient's endurance improved, the number of repetitions for each exercise was increased to 10 to 15 repetitions per session. A walking program was initiated in the third therapy session. LB low back.

[b] All functional instructions were provided during initial visit and were reviewed periodically across the 8 treatment sessions.

[c] Number in parentheses indicate at which visit the patient received instruction in each exercise (8 visits total). In general, exercises were progressed when the patient was able to perform at least 10 to 15 repetitions of initial exercise without verbal or manual cues from the therapist. In no case was an exercise progressed if the patient was unable to demonstrate the modified exercise as instructed and without an increase in symptoms. Upon discharge, the patient was encouraged to adhere to functional activity modifications indefinitely to prevent a recurrence of symptoms. We also suggested that she remain physically active by continuing her HEP and walking program at least once daily.

[d] "Neutral" is defined as that position of the lumbar spine at which an inclinometer centered over each lumbar spinous process would result in a measure of 0 degrees, without rotation or side bending of any of the lumbar vertebrae.[12]

18. The discussion. This paragraph briefly summarizes the major points of the introduction and the case description. The summary helps ensure that readers understand the major points, and it provides a context for the rest of the discussion section.

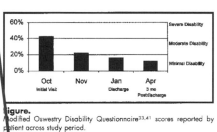

Figure.
Modified Oswestry Disability Questionnaire[33,41] scores reported by patient across study period.

and the relationship between physical impairment and disability in this population remains largely undefined.[19]

Our case report describes an intervention that was chosen based on the evaluation of spinal alignment with postures and spinal motions during active movement of both the spine and extremities. Given the documented lack of association between LBP and various traditional measures of physical impairment,[23] we sought to identify a particular pattern of spinal motions and alignments that appeared to be directly associated with a worsening of symptoms across several test positions. We then based intervention on modification of symptom-producing motions and alignments of the lumbar spine during the repetition of daily activities. Despite modest changes in measures of physical impairment (Tab. 3), the patient described in this case report exhibited what we consider a substantial and consistent reduction in low back–related functional limitations and disability (Figure) over the course of treatment. In addition, the most dramatic reduction in low back–related symptoms occurred following the first therapy session, in which the only treatment provided was category-specific instruction in activity modification.

Waddell et al[16] found a strong association between low back–related disability and fear-avoidance beliefs, or the extent to which patients avoid activity based on the anticipation of pain. Waddell et al suggested that restricting the activity of patients with LBP might serve only to reinforce fear-avoidance beliefs and increase the chances of subsequent disability. The benefits of maintaining customary activity levels in patients with LBP has been substantiated by the findings of Malmivaara et al.[47] These investigators found that subjects with LBP who were advised to continue their usual routine as tolerated recovered more quickly than those who were prescribed either 2 days of complete bed rest or back mobilizing exercises.

Teaching patients *specific* strategies to reduce the symptoms associated with movements can enable them to perform activities that they might otherwise avoid. We

believe that one of the primary advantages of the classification system described in this case report is that it allows physical therapists to make recommendations for activity modification that are specific to the symptom-provoking postures and movements of each patient. We propose that exercise prescription and generic postural instruction may be less effective in addressing restrictions of function in patients with LBP than is individualized instruction in symptom-reducing strategies for positioning and functional movement. The patient described in this report, for example, was instructed in ways to avoid rotation and extension of the lumbar spine during daily activities. The use of a lumbar roll is one example of a generic therapeutic modality that was discouraged in this case because it would have contributed to spinal extension, an alignment found to be associated with an increase in this patient's symptoms. Greater individualization of back care programs may be needed to facilitate patient adherence.[21] The patient described in this case report noted the greatest adherence to exercises and activity modifications that could be easily incorporated into her daily routine, such as those related to forward bending, walking, and sitting up in bed (Tab. 5).

The treatment approach described in this case report is founded on the notion that the repetition of direction-specific movements and postures of the lumbar spine can exacerbate low back–related symptoms and prolong recovery. The patient exhibited a consistent tendency toward lumbar rotation and extension, which was observed during examination of movements and postures across several positions as well as during the performance of functional tasks (eg, sit-to-supine transfers) and personal habits (eg, "nervous legs"). We have observed that the propensity for spinal motion to occur in a given direction varies among individuals, and we speculate that this variation may be partly related to individual variations in motor recruitment patterns. This idea is consistent with reports of high intersubject variability in trunk muscle activity patterns during a given movement.[48,49] Based on the results of an investigation into the effects of fatigue on trunk motion, Parnianpour et al[50] suggested that the loss of muscular coordination associated with fatigue may diminish spinal stability and allow loading of the spine in a more injury-prone pattern. The patient in this case report commented that she found it more difficult to control the position of her spine and pelvis when she was tired, and she associated an increase in her symptoms with fatigue.

We also have observed that variations in occupational and recreational activity demands appear to contribute to individual differences in direction-specific motions and alignments of the lumbar spine. We suggest that this may be related to changes in supportive structures of the

This paragraph and several that follow relate the authors' experiences with this case to other literature about patients with low back pain.

The authors are careful to say that their observations only suggest that their intervention may have influenced the patient's recovery. Case reports do not have the controls that research studies do, so authors cannot claim cause-and-effect relationships between interventions and outcomes.

This paragraph gives thoughtful and useful suggestions for future research. The authors did much more than simply suggest that researchers do studies with a larger number of subjects!

spine that occur with repeated stresses in a given direction over time. A relationship between repetitive spinal motion and LBP is suggested by epidemiologic studies that have identified repetition of non-neutral trunk postures as a risk factor for the development of LBP.[51] In addition, Gordon et al[52] have shown that repetitive loading of spinal segments positioned in a slight amount of flexion and rotation results in pathological changes in the intervertebral disk of the in vitro human spine.

Causal relationships cannot be established on the basis of a case report. Symptoms associated with disorders of the low back typically resolve within 6 weeks of onset, and only 5% of individuals have symptoms that persist longer than 3 months.[51] The LBP episode described in this case report began 10 weeks prior to the patient's initial therapy visit to our facility, which is beyond the time frame typically associated with natural resolution of LBP. Improvement in both functional ability and symptom reduction coincided with the initiation of treatment at our facility. The patient did not experience a recurrence of low back–related symptoms in the 3 months following discharge from our clinic, during which time she continued her home exercise program and activity modifications. Together, these observations suggest that our approach may have positively influenced the patient's recovery. This does not, however, rule out the possibility that the patient might have recovered spontaneously, or responded equally well to another therapeutic approach.

In any isolated case, there are several factors other than the intervention that might account for the observed outcomes. Aerobic training has been reported to be of benefit in the treatment of many disorders, including those related to the low back.[53] Based on reports of the efficacy of aerobic training, a walking program was prescribed during the third treatment session. It seems unlikely that the observed outcomes can be attributed to an improvement in aerobic conditioning, however, given that the patient remained unable to ambulate for more than 5 minutes at one time without becoming short of breath. It might be argued that improvements in hip flexor muscle length could be largely responsible for helping to reduce the patient's symptoms, as lower-extremity flexibility is a commonly addressed impairment in the treatment of LBP. To our knowledge, however, prospective studies have failed to demonstrate a consistent correlation between LBP and hip flexor tightness.[27,54] Because the psoas major muscle is known to impart substantial compressive forces on the lumbar spine,[55] it is conceivable that discouraging the active recruitment of this muscle may have influenced the observed outcome.

Further research is needed to determine the validity and clinical feasibility of the system of classification described in this case report. The theoretical assumptions on which the approach was founded should be investigated to determine construct validity. For instance, is it true that the lumbar spine can become predisposed to excessive movement in a given direction when subjected to repeated stresses in that direction? Examination of whether the proposed classification categories are mutually exclusive and appropriate for use in a rehabilitation context will be necessary to establish content validity. For example, can any patient referred to a physical therapist for the treatment of LBP be classified into 1 of the 5 proposed categories, or does this classification system describe a more limited patient population, such as those with chronic LBP? If the predictive validity of this system could be appropriately demonstrated, then we believe physical therapists could make a substantial contribution to preventative health care. Individuals could be screened for patterns of spinal motion and alignment that may increase the risk of developing mechanical LBP, and they could be provided with specific instruction regarding the modification of such patterns. Other areas of future research should include controlled clinical trials to establish the relative efficacy of individualized versus generic functional instruction, as well as to determine the optimal approach for improving rehabilitation outcomes for patients with LBP.

References

1 Jette AM, Smith K, Haley SM, Davis KD. Physical therapy episodes of care for patients with low back pain. *Phys Ther.* 1994;74:101–110.

2 Bernard TN Jr, Kirkaldy-Willis WH. Recognizing specific characteristics of nonspecific low back pain. *Clin Orthop.* April 1987:266–280.

3 Binkley J, Finch E, Hall J, et al. Diagnostic classification of patients with low back pain: report on a survey of physical therapy experts. *Phys Ther.* 1993;73:138–150.

4 Coste J, Paolaggi JB, Spira A. Classification of nonspecific low back pain, I: psychological involvement in low back pain: a clinical, descriptive approach. *Spine.* 1992;17:1028–1037.

5 Coste J, Paolaggi JB, Spira A. Classification of nonspecific low back pain, II: clinical diversity of organic forms. *Spine.* 1992;17:1038–1042.

6 Delitto A, Erhard RE, Bowling RW. A treatment-based classification approach to low back syndrome: identifying and staging patients for conservative treatment. *Phys Ther.* 1995;75:470–485.

7 Marras WS, Parnianpour M, Ferguson SA, et al. The classification of anatomic- and symptom-based low back disorders using motion measure models. *Spine.* 1995;20:2531–2546.

8 McKenzie RZ. *The Lumbar Spine: Mechanical Diagnosis and Therapy.* Waikanae, New Zealand: Spinal Publications Ltd; 1989.

9 Moffroid MT, Haugh LD, Henry SM, Short B. Distinguishable groups of musculoskeletal low back pain patients and asymptomatic control subjects based on physical measures of the NIOSH Low Back Atlas. *Spine.* 1994;19:1350–1358.

10 Roach KE, Brown MD, Albin RD, et al. The sensitivity and specificity of pain response to activity and position in categorizing patients with low back pain. *Phys Ther.* 1997;77:730–738.

11 Sikorski JM. A rationalized approach to physiotherapy for low-back pain. *Spine*. 1985;10:571–579.

12 Van Dillen LR, Sahrmann SA, Norton BJ, et al. Reliability of physical examination items used for classification of patients with low back pain. *Phys Ther*. 1998;78:979–988.

13 Riddle DL. Classification and low back pain: a review of the literature and critical analysis of selected systems. *Phys Ther*. 1998;78:708–737.

14 Borkan JM, Cherkin DC. An agenda for primary care research on low back pain. *Spine*. 1996;21:2880–2884.

15 Sahrmann SA. Diagnosis by the physical therapist—a prerequisite for treatment: a special communication. *Phys Ther*. 1988;68:1703–1706.

16 Battié MC, Cherkin DC, Dunn R, et al. Managing low back pain: attitudes and treatment preferences of physical therapists. *Phys Ther*. 1994;74:219–226.

17 Jette AM. Physical disablement concepts for physical therapy research and practice. *Phys Ther*. 1994;74:380–386.

18 Nagi S. Some conceptual issues in disability and rehabilitation. In: Sussman M, ed. *Sociology and Rehabilitation*. Washington, DC: American Sociological Association; 1965:100–113.

19 Delitto A. Are measures of function and disability important in low back care? *Phys Ther*. 1994;74:452–462.

20 McPhillips-Tangum CA, Cherkin DC, Rhodes LA, Markham C. Reasons for repeated medical visits among patients with chronic back pain. *J Gen Intern Med*. 1998;13:289–295.

21 Kerssens JJ, Sluijs EM, Verhaak PFM, et al. Back care instructions in physical therapy: a trend analysis of individualized back care programs. *Phys Ther*. 1999;79:287–295.

22 Bigos SJ, Battié MC, Spengler DM, et al. A longitudinal, prospective study of industrial back injury reporting. *Clin Orthop*. June 1992:21–34.

23 Bigos SJ, Battié MC, Fisher LD, et al. A prospective evaluation of preemployment screening methods for acute industrial back pain. *Spine*. 1992;17:922–926.

24 Battié MC, Bigos SJ, Fisher LD, et al. Anthropometric and clinical measures as predictors of back pain complaints in industry: a prospective study. *J Spinal Disord*. 1990;3:195–204.

25 Battié MC, Bigos SJ, Fisher LD, et al. The role of spinal flexibility in back pain complaints within industry: a prospective study. *Spine*. 1990;15:768–773.

26 Battié MC, Bigos SJ, Fisher LD, et al. Isometric lifting strength as a predictor of industrial back pain reports. *Spine*. 1989;14:851–856.

27 Hellsing AL. Tightness of hamstring and psoas major muscles: a prospective study of back pain in young men during their military service. *Ups J Med Sci*. 1988;93:267–276.

28 Waddell G, Main CJ, Morris EW, et al. Chronic low-back pain, psychologic distress, and illness behavior. *Spine*. 1984;9:209–213.

29 Sahrmann SA. *Diagnosis and Treatment of Movement Impairment Syndromes*. St Louis, Mo: Mosby; 2000.

30 Spitzer WO. Diagnosis of the problem (the problem of diagnosis). In: Scientific Approach to the Assessment and Measurement of Activity-Related Spinal Disorders: A Monograph for Clinicians' Report of the Quebec Task Force on Spinal Disorders. *Spine*. 1987;12(suppl):S16–S21.

31 Bolton JE. Accuracy of recall of usual pain intensity in back pain patients. *Pain*. 1999;83:533–539.

32 Strong J, Ashton R, Chant D. Pain intensity measurement in chronic low back pain. *Clin J Pain*. 1991;7:209–218.

33 Hudson-Cook W, Tomes-Nicholson K, Breen A. A revised Oswestry Disability Questionnaire. In: Roland MO, Jenner JR, eds. *Back Pain: New Approaches to Rehabilitation and Education*. New York, NY: Manchester University Press; 1989:187–204.

34 Williams R, Binkley J, Bloch R, et al. Reliability of the modified-modified Schober and double inclinometer methods for measuring lumbar flexion and extension. *Phys Ther*. 1993;73:33–44.

35 Kendall FP, McCreary EK, Provance PG. *Muscles: Testing and Function*. 4th ed. Baltimore, Md: Williams & Wilkins; 1993.

36 Boone DC, Azen SP, Lin CM, et al. Reliability of goniometric measurements. *Phys Ther*. 1978;58:1355–1390.

37 Van Dillen LR, McDonnell MK, Fleming DA, Sahrmann SA. Effect of knee and hip position on hip extension range of motion in individuals with and without low back pain. *J Orthop Sports Phys Ther*. 2000;30:307–316.

38 Florence JM, Pandya S, King WM, et al. Intrarater reliability of manual muscle test (Medical Research Council Scale) grades in Duchenne's muscular dystrophy. *Phys Ther*. 1992;72:115–126.

39 Hoppenfeld S. *Physical Examination of the Spine & Extremities*. East Norwalk, Conn: Appleton & Lange; 1976.

40 Waddell G, McCulloch JA, Kummel E, Venner RM. Nonorganic physical signs in low-back pain. *Spine*. 1980;5:117–125.

41 Fairbank JC, Couper J, Davies JB, O'Brien JP. The Oswestry low back pain disability questionnaire. *Physiotherapy*. 1980;66:271–273.

42 Stratford PW, Binkley J, Solomon P, et al. Assessing change over time in patients with low back pain. *Phys Ther*. 1994;74:528–533.

43 Ohnmeiss DD. Repeatability of pain drawings in a low back pain population. *Spine*. 2000;25:980–988.

44 Mann NH, Brown MD, Enger I. Expert performance in low-back disorder recognition using patient pain drawings. *J Spine Disord*. 1992;5:254–259.

45 van Tulder MW, Koes BW, Bouter LM. Conservative treatment of acute and chronic nonspecific low back pain: a systematic review of randomized controlled trials of the most common interventions. *Spine*. 1997;22:2128–2156.

46 Waddell G, Newton M, Henderson I, et al. A Fear-Avoidance Beliefs Questionnaire (FABQ) and the role of fear-avoidance beliefs in chronic low back pain and disability. *Pain*. 1993;52:157–168.

47 Malmivaara A, Hakkinen U, Aro T, et al. The treatment of acute low back pain: bed rest, exercises, or ordinary activity? *N Engl J Med*. 1995;332:351–355.

48 McGill SM. Electromyographic activity of the abdominal and low back musculature during the generation of isometric and dynamic axial trunk torque: implications for lumbar mechanics. *J Orthop Res*. 1991;9:91–103.

49 Hodges PW, Richardson CA. Inefficient muscular stabilization of the lumbar spine associated with low back pain: a motor control evaluation of transversus abdominis. *Spine*. 1996;21:2640–2650.

50 Parnianpour M, Nordin M, Kahanovitz N, Frankel V. The triaxial coupling of torque generation of trunk muscles during isometric exertions and the effect of fatiguing isoinertial movements on the motor output and movement patterns. *Spine*. 1988;13:982–992.

51 Frymoyer JW. Back pain and sciatica. *N Engl J Med*. 1988;318:291–300.

Case Report 2

This case report focuses on one patient.

1. Title. The title clearly conveys what the case report is about. *Physical Therapy* is now using the term "case report," instead of "case study," to differentiate case descriptions from qualitative research using a case study approach.

2. Abstract. This report was published before 1996, when the journal started using a structured format for abstracts. Headings of Background and Purpose, Case Description, Outcomes, and Discussion would be appropriate.

3. Rationale for the case. The first paragraph suggests that the case will involve intervention for patients with limited passive range of motion of the shoulder, for which no studies have clearly established the best intervention.

4. Support for the approach to the case. The next several paragraphs give rationale for needing to know whether patients have structural or nonstructural changes in periarticular structures as a basis for intervention.

This section gives rationale for differentiating intervention based on whether limitation is a result of structural or nonstructural changes.

Treatment of Limited Shoulder Motion: A Case Study Based on Biomechanical Considerations

This article describes the management of a 57-year-old female patient following a fracture and dislocation of the right humeral head. The treatment of the patient involved the use of thermal agents, manual therapy, continuous passive motion, and splinting of the arm in an elevated position. We describe an approach to treatment of limited shoulder motion that is focused on identifying and applying tension to restricting structures rather than restoration of translatory gliding movements of the humeral head. Our treatment approach is based on recent data from biomechanical studies that challenge the concave-convex theory of arthrokinematic motion first described by MacConaill. We believe that tension in capsular tissues, rather than joint surface geometry, may control the translatory movements of the humeral head. The rationale for treatment involving low-load prolonged stress to tissues in the form of continuous passive motion and splinting is discussed as well as potential limitations of more brief forms of stress such as joint mobilization and manual stretching. [McClure PW, Flowers KR. Treatment of limited shoulder motion: a care study based on biomechanical considerations. Phys Ther. 1992;72:929–936.]

Key Words: *Joint instability; Kinesiology/biomechanics, upper extremity; Manual therapy; Shoulder joint; Upper extremity, shoulder.*

Philip W McClure
Kenneth R Flowers

Various treatment approaches have been described for limited shoulder passive range of motion (PROM).[1–4] These approaches include various forms of manual therapy, electrotherapy, active exercises, and various forms of passive stretching.[1–4] There have been no well-controlled studies that have clearly established the most effective type of treatment.

We believe that proper treatment should be based on an understanding of the cause of limited range of motion (ROM). We classify causes of limited shoulder ROM into two categories. The first category of limited ROM results from structural changes in the periarticular structures. These changes include shortening of capsules, ligaments, or muscles as well as adhesion formation. These structural changes generally result from a combination of inflammation and immobilization.[5] The second category of limited ROM is caused by problems not associated with structural changes in the periarticular tissues. An example of nonstructural problems leading to decreased ROM would be pain (and associated protective muscle contractions to prevent painful movements) or the presence of a loose body within the joint space.[4] Muscle weakness could result in decreased active range of motion (AROM); how-ever, weakness alone should not cause a limitation of PROM. Our classification system does not address the situation in which only AROM is limited. We believe the distinction between the two types of problems with PROM is important because they involve different treatment strategies.

We believe that treatment of limited PROM attributable to structural changes should be geared toward applying tension in an effort to cause elongation of the restricting tissues.[6–8] This contrast to treatment of limited ROM attributable to nonstructural changes, we believe, should focus on relieving the problem producing the limitation. For example, an acutely inflamed joint with associated pain and protective muscle action should be treated with modalities oriented toward decreasing inflammation and relieving pain.[9]

PW McClure, PT, OCS, is Assistant Professor, Department of Orthopedic Surgery and Rehabilitation, Hahnemann University, MS 502, Broad and Vine Streets, Philadelphia, PA 19102 (USA). Address correspondence to Mr McClure.

KR Flowers, PT, CHT, is Director, Valley Forge Hand Rehabilitation, Phoenixville, PA 19453.

Physical Therapy/Volume 72, Number 12/December 1992

929/97

The authors then tell us how they decide whether a patient has structural or nonstructural changes. They provide operational definitions of the potentially ambiguous terms "loss of passive motion in the capsular pattern" and "capsular end feel."

Findings from the history and physical examination that lead us to hypothesize that PROM is limited because of structural changes are

1. A history of trauma followed by immobilization.[5]

2. A history of restricted motion greater than 3 weeks.[5]

3. Loss of passive motion in a capsular pattern.[10] (For the shoulder, greatest percentage of limitation of lateral (external) rotation followed by abduction.)

4. A capsular end-feel.[10] (A *capsular end-feel* is defined as a firm halt to passive movement with only a slight degree of give to further force.)

5. No pain with resisted isometric contractions with the joint in a neutral position.[10]

We believe that if either of the first two findings is present, then structural changes are very likely. We believe that the last three possible findings are helpful in confirming the presence of structural changes but are not sufficient evidence by themselves.

The purposes of this article are to discuss some biomechanical considerations that can be used to guide evaluation and treatment of limited shoulder ROM and to describe the management of a patient with limited shoulder ROM following a fracture and dislocation of the humerus. This article discusses limited shoulder ROM presumed to be due to structural changes in the periarticular structures.

The Concave-Convex Rule and Arthrokinematic Studies

MacConaill[11] appears to have been one of the first authors to discuss the arthrokinematic movements (movements of joint surfaces relative to one another) occurring at the glenohumeral joint. His descriptions of the movements occurring at joint surfaces were based on mechanical models rather than direct measurements. He stated that "in abduction of the humerus, the humeral head not only rolls upwards but also slides downwards upon the curved glenoid surface of the scapula."[11(p30)] More generally he stated that when a convex surface moves on a concave surface, "the direction of the slide that accompanies a roll is *opposite* to that of the roll."[11(p29)]

Kaltenborn[1] used MacConaill's descriptions[11] to propose an "indirect method" for determining the appropriate direction to apply a gliding mobilization technique that he called the *concave-convex rule*. According to the concave-convex rule, sliding of the humeral head occurs in the direction opposite movement of the humerus. For example, the head of the humerus should slide inferiorly during abduction and anteriorly during lateral rotation or horizontal adduction. Other authors[12,13] describing manual therapy techniques have since used the concave-convex rule for determining the appropriate direction of gliding mobilization.

Data are now available from studies that have measured the translatory movement of the humeral head during various physiologic movements of the arm.[14-16] These data challenge the concave-convex rule of arthrokinematic motion.

Poppen and Walker[14] studied movements of the humeral head during abduction of the arm in the scapular plane (30° anterior to the frontal plane) using radiographs. Radiographs were taken at 0, 30, 60, 90, 120, and 150 degrees of arm elevation on 12 healthy volunteers and 15 patients. The authors found the following:

> From 0 to 30 degrees, and often from 30 to 60 degrees, the humeral ball moved upwards on the glenoid face by about 3 millimeters. Thereafter it remained constant, moving only one millimeter or at the most two millimeters upward or downward between each successive position.[14(p199)]

In healthy subjects, the mean translation (±SD) for each 30-degree change in position was 1.09±0.47 mm. Seven subjects demonstrated "excessive" translation, and all of these subjects had a history of either instability or rotator-cuff tear. *Excessive translation* was defined as greater than one standard deviation from the mean translation for each 30-degree change in position. All subjects with abnormal translation demonstrated over 2 mm of translation of the humeral head.

Howell et al[15] studied humeral head movement during various amounts of horizontal abduction of the arm with and without lateral rotation. The four positions used were (1) maximum horizontal abduction and lateral rotation, (2) maximum horizontal abduction with no rotation, (3) 90 degrees of abduction (frontal plane) with full lateral rotation, and (4) 80 degrees of flexion with full medial (internal) rotation. They used a radiographic technique on 20 healthy volunteers and 12 patients with clinical evidence of anterior glenohumeral instability. All 12 patients had a history of recurrent dislocation or subluxation and demonstrated a positive anterior apprehension test result. The apprehension sensation was such that it prevented patients from maximally extending and laterally rotating the arm. All healthy subjects demonstrated a posterior translation of the humeral head of 3.9±0.8 mm when the arm was fully horizontally abducted and laterally rotated (position 1). For the healthy subjects, there was less average translation for the other positions, but the translation was still in a posterior direction. The values were 0.3±0.5 mm for position 2, 0.1±0.5 mm for position 3, and 0.4±0.4 mm for position 4. Patients with anterior instability were positioned similarly except that full lateral rotation was not combined with full horizontal abduction because of the patients' inability to stay in that position. Seven of the 12 patients demonstrated anterior translation when positioned in maximum horizontal abduction (3.3±0.6 mm) and also in position 3 (3.6±0.7 mm). The other 5 patients demonstrated a mean translation of less than 0.3 mm in all posi-

---

5. Purpose of the case report.

This paragraph clearly states two purposes of the case report. The first purpose is to provide the reader with a conceptual basis for the authors' management of patients with limited range of motion of the shoulder. The second purpose is to illustrate the application of that conceptual basis to the management of a patient presumed to have limited range of motion of the shoulder due to structural changes. It also would have been acceptable for the authors to include the conceptual (or theoretical) basis for this management in the previous paragraphs and to conclude the entire introduction section with only the second purpose statement.

6. Rationale for the intervention.
The next section gives theoretical rationale for the intervention. The authors provide a more extensive review of literature than is usually necessary because they are casting doubt on a traditional, widely accepted construct. Case reports that support theory usually have a shorter and less detailed review of related literature.

Note the operational definition of "excessive translation" in the following paragraph. Without it, would you have known what the authors meant?

9. The final paragraph of the introduction brings the reader back to the case by summarizing the rationale for the approach to patient/client management that the authors used with the patient described in the next section of the report.

tions. The healthy subjects, therefore, demonstrated translatory motion in the opposite direction to that predicted by the concave-convex rule. Only patients with instability demonstrated translation in the direction predicted by the concave-convex rule.

Harryman et al[16] studied the humeral head translation in cadaver specimens with a device that measured motion with 6 degrees of freedom. The glenohumeral motions studied were the following: flexion, extension, lateral rotation, medial rotation, and "cross-body movement." All joints were tested under the following conditions: capsule intact, capsule vented to the air with a needle, and tightening of the posterior capsule with a suturing technique. Both flexion and medial rotation resulted in anterior translation of the humeral head, whereas extension and lateral rotation both resulted in posterior translation of the humeral head. The translation associated with the cross-body movement was variable and did not show a consistent direction. Mean values and ranges for translation were as follows (a negative value indicates posterior translation): flexion (3.79±3.8 mm, −0.44 to 10.94), medial rotation (1.01±2.4 mm, −1.47 to 5.64), extension (−4.92±2.6 mm, −1.9 to −9.7), lateral rotation (−1.68±1.8 mm, −4.81 to 1.17), and cross-body movement (−0.14±2.8 mm, −3.92 to 2.91).

Venting the capsules increased mean translation for all movements, but these increases were all less than 2 mm. Tightening of the posterior capsule caused a significant shift toward greater anterior translation with all movements, especially flexion and the cross-body movement. The authors explained this finding by suggesting that a tight posterior capsule forces the humeral head anteriorly.

The results of these studies seem to challenge the concave-convex theory of arthrokinematic motion. The motion of the humeral head seems to be primarily of a spin-type motion with translation occurring mostly at end-ranges. The amount of translation also seems to be increased with

both capsular laxity[14,15] and capsular tightening.[16]

The explanation put forth by Harryman et al[16] seems to offer a plausible basis for understanding translatory movement of the humeral head. In essence, they suggest that as a portion of the glenohumeral capsule becomes taut, the humeral head is forced in an opposite direction by the taut capsule. This theory could explain the data of Howell et al,[15] who found posterior translation during maximal lateral rotation and horizontal abduction in healthy subjects. As the anterior capsule became taut because of lateral rotation and horizontal abduction, the humeral head could have been pushed posteriorly. In patients with anterior laxity, anterior rather than posterior translation was observed. The lack of posterior translation could be explained by the laxity in the anterior capsule. Therefore, the direction and amount of humeral head translation may be primarily a function of tissue tension rather than joint surface geometry.

We believe that when limited ROM is thought to be due to a structural change in the periarticular tissues, the therapist should consider what structures could potentially limit that ROM. Selection of a stretching technique should then be based on what type of maneuver will best put tension on the restricting tissue.

For example, consider a patient who has limited lateral rotation of the glenohumeral joint. Authors advocating joint mobilization suggest performing anterior glides (anterior translation of the humeral head on the glenoid cavity) based on the concave-convex theory.[1,12,13] The data of Howell et al,[15] however, suggest that posterior glide is the normal translatory movement occurring during lateral rotation. Ironically, we would also use anterior gliding (rather than posterior gliding), but for a different reason. Anterior glides probably place more tension on the anterior capsule than does posterior gliding, and the anterior capsule is known to restrain

lateral rotation.[17,18] To summarize, we believe treatment decisions should be based on consideration of the structures limiting motion and how to best put tensile stress on these structures rather than restoring a translatory motion that does not really occur during physiologic movement.

This may seem like a purely academic issue; however, it can have implications for treatment. There are many ways of placing tensile stress on tissues besides a gliding-type joint mobilization. If the emphasis is taken away from restoring a particular gliding motion, other forms of stretching such as AROM and PROM, continuous passive motion (CPM), and splinting become logical choices for the treatment of limited ROM. These techniques are not only appropriate, they also have the advantage of not requiring direct care from a therapist. Some stretching techniques can be done independently by patients; therefore, they can be performed more frequently and for longer periods than can therapist-conducted treatments. Home programs thus allow greater amounts of time to be spent on stretching restricting tissues. We have previously suggested that prolonged tensile stress can improve limited ROM more than can short-duration joint mobilization procedures.[2] Threlkeld (see article in this issue) points out that length changes in connective tissues produced by joint mobilization procedures are probably transient, although this question has not been studied directly. Other authors[19,20] also support the notion that the mechanical effects of brief forms of stretching on connective tissue are short-lived. The following case study illustrates how this thinking influences our treatment approach to limited shoulder motion.

Case Study

History

A 57-year-old female medical secretary fell on an icy pavement, sustaining a Neer two-part fracture with avulsion of the greater tuberosity of

Physical Therapy/Volume 72, Number 12/December 1992

931 / 99

7. The introduction continues. After the relatively lengthy review of literature, the following paragraphs help the reader to understand how it applies to the case.

8. In the next paragraphs, the authors describe the application of the principles that they have drawn from the literature to a patient who has limited range of motion associated with structural change in periarticular tissues.

10. Subject description. The subject and the history are described succinctly.

Table. *Chronological Description of Treatment and Passive Range of Motion (PROM)*

Weeks Postinjury	Treatment	PROM (°) Flexion	PROM (°) Abduction[a]	PROM (°) Lateral Rotation[b]
0	Fracture/dislocation			
6	Moist heat, ultrasound, pendulum, low-grade manual therapy, ice post-exercise (visits three times per week)	80	60	5
6+day	Increase to high-grade manual therapy, continuous passive motion, home program (three times per day): pendulum, wand, ice	80	60	5
8	Allow gentle activities of daily living	100	75	15
10	Reduce visits to twice per week, discontinue ultrasound, add elevation splint 1 hour four times per day	105	85	20
12	Discontinue all treatment in clinic, continue to monitor outcome of home program, add strengthening, increase splint time to 2 hours four times per day	130	105	40
13	No change	140	120	50
14	No change	155	145	65
15	No change	165	160	65
16	No change	165	165	70
25	Patient discharged	175	170	80

[a]Abduction measured with the arm 40° to the coronal plane.

[b]Lateral rotation measured with the arm by the side.

her right (dominant) proximal humerus.[21] The history obtained in the emergency department suggested a concomitant anterior dislocation. Her husband, who is a physician, reported that he manually reduced the dislocation at the scene of the fall. There was no prior history of dislocation. She was evaluated by an orthopedic surgeon in the emergency department, and her arm was immobilized in a sling combined with a swathe to hold the arm in medial rotation. After 6 weeks of immobilization, she was referred to physical therapy with the goal of increasing shoulder ROM.

Evaluation

The patient's primary complaint was restricted motion with difficulty in activities that required reaching above the level of her head. Her primary goal was to regain sufficient motion to allow for independence with dressing, hair care, and household activities (eg, cooking, cleaning, gardening). She was not participating in athletics

or other strenuous recreational activities at the time of her injury.

The initial physical therapy evaluation occurred 6 weeks postinjury. The patient was unable to actively flex or abduct her arm horizontally. Passive flexion and abduction were limited to 80 and 60 degrees, respectively (see Table and Figure for all ROM data). There was no pain when she was resting the arm. Pain was elicited as the end-ranges of all passive motions were approached. The pain was confined to the anterolateral shoulder area, with no radiation proximally or distal to the insertion of the deltoid muscle. Motions in all directions were limited by capsular end-feel.[10] No atrophy was noted upon inspection by the therapist. Manual muscle testing of the shoulder muscles was not performed. Forces produced by shoulder flexion, abduction, and medial and lateral rotation were tested isometrically with the patient's arm by her side in a position of neutral rotation. The patient was able to produce moderate resistance to all motions without pain. The elbow, wrist, and digits all had full AROM, based on visual inspection, and had no gross weakness, based on the isometric testing. There was no noticeable deficit of sensibility. Cervical spine AROM did not appear limited and was pain-free.

Treatment and Results

Initial physical therapy began 6 weeks postinjury and consisted of application of hydrocollator packs for 20 minutes to the anterior aspect of the patient's shoulder while she lay supine with her arm resting at her side and with her elbow flexed 90 degrees. The moist heat was followed by 5 minutes of continuous ultrasound* at 1.5 W/cm². The ultrasound was directed to the anterior shoulder area while the patient's humerus was held by the therapist (KRF) at its comfortable end-range of lateral rotation in an effort to increase the compliance of the tissues passing across the anterior aspect of the glenohumeral joint. Immediately following the ultrasound, pendulum exercise was performed with a 0.91-kg (2-lb) wrist cuff

*Intellect 200, Chattanooga Corp, PO Box 4287, Chattanooga, TN 37405.

12. The results of the physical therapist examination are clearly described, including screening to rule out involvement of muscle and other joints.

13. Intervention and outcomes.
The authors chose to report their intervention and outcomes in the same section, probably because they believed that it was the clearest way to describe the intervention, which was modified over time in response to changes in the patient. Other case report writers find it easier to write separate intervention and outcomes sections.

The table summarizes the intervention and the passive range-of-motion measurements (impairment) over time.

This paragraph describes the initial intervention with such clarity and detail that another therapist could replicate it. Note the operational definition of "low-grade gliding movements."

11. Examination. In their first paragraph, the authors state the patient's primary complaint and and the patient's goals and desired outcomes, toward which the examination was directed.

The home program is described so that it also could be replicated. Self-report or other means to indicate whether the patient carried out the home exercise program would have been useful information.

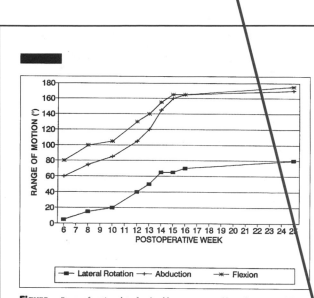

Figure. *Range-of-motion data for shoulder movements of lateral rotation, abduction, and flexion in 57-year-old female patient following fracture and dislocation of right humeral head.*

14. The description of the intervention continues. This paragraph describes when range-of-motion measurements were taken and provides rationale and an operational definition for "preconditioning."

In the following paragraphs, the authors reveal their rationale for modifying the intervention, describe the modified intervention in such a way that it could be replicated, and give another operational definition (for "high-grade gliding movements").

for 3 minutes. Pendulum exercise consisted of the patient leaning forward supported by her uninvolved left arm and allowing her right arm to dangle. The patient produced a pendulum-type movement by shifting her trunk forward and back, thus attempting to keep the shoulder muscles as relaxed as possible. The pendulum exercise was followed immediately by manual therapy, consisting of low-grade anterior and inferior gliding movements. We define *low-grade gliding movements* as those that do not approach the end of the available range of gliding. Our gliding movements were delivered for approximately 3 minutes each with the patient positioned supine and her glenohumeral joint in the neutral position. The purpose of the pendulum exercise and gliding techniques was to decrease pain and promote gentle stretching of periarticular tissues.

All ROM measurements were taken at this point in the session to ensure that the connective tissue had been preconditioned.[22] Preconditioning occurs with cyclic loading and unloading of connective tissues. *Preconditioning* is the phenomenon in which increases in tissue deformation occur when a given load is applied cyclically. A tissue is said to be preconditioned when tissue deformation reaches a steady state and continued cyclic loading produces no additional deformation.[22] We believe ROM measurements are more reliable and meaningful when taken with the periarticular tissues "preconditioned" (as after exercise) rather than "cold," particularly when ROM measurements taken several days apart are compared to determine changes in ROM.

The patient was evaluated the next day to assess the reaction to the prior day's intervention. As there was no increase in pain or evidence of inflammation, or any loss or gain of

ROM, the vigor of the program was increased. The manual therapy was more aggressive, consisting of more forceful (ie, high-grade) anterior and inferior gliding movements. We define *high-grade gliding movements* as those that take the joint to the available end-range. A 30-minute session of CPM was added following the manual therapy. With the patient seated, a CPM device[†] oscillated the patient's arm between 60 and 80 degrees in the plane of the scapula. The purpose of the high-grade anterior and inferior gliding movements and the CPM was to apply end-range tensile stress to the restricting periarticular tissues. A relatively limited excursion was used with the CPM device to maximize the time the joint was at or near the end-range of motion.

A home exercise program was taught to the patient. The home exercise program consisted of 3 minutes of pendulum exercise followed by 3 minutes of overhead wand exercises, which moved the arm into forward flexion from the supine position. The exercise was followed by 15 minutes of ice to the anterior aspect of the shoulder. The patient was instructed to do the home exercise program three times daily. The patient was told to wear the sling at all times when she was not exercising. The swathe that held the arm medially rotated, however, was removed. The patient was told to avoid activities that involved lifting or resisted motions of the right arm. Active range of motion of the elbow, wrist, and hand was performed for 10 minutes daily to maintain full motion of these joints.

The patient was treated in this manner for six visits over a 2-week period. At 8 weeks postinjury, the patient's ROM increased modestly (20° of flexion, 15° of abduction, and 10° of lateral rotation). The patient was encouraged to wean herself from use of the sling immobilizer over the next 2 weeks. She did this without significant pain. Also at 8 weeks postinjury, she was permitted to perform any activities of daily living that did not result in sharp or lasting pain. For example, she was able to handle

[†]Invacare Corp, 899 Cleveland St, Elyria, OH 44036.

Physical Therapy/Volume 72, Number 12/December 1992

933/101

The authors continue to clearly reveal their clinical decision-making process in the following paragraphs. They provide rationale for further modification of the intervention, based on reexamination of the patient and reevaluation of the findings, based on the literature, and based on their own experiences.

The authors continue to describe changes in the intervention over time and the rationale for the changes.

This paragraph is a good discussion of how range of motion was measured and of the reliability of the measurements. Rationale for not taking certain measurements also is given. This information could easily have been placed in the section on the initial examination, where it would have clarified both the measurements and their quality.

Today, the *Physical Therapy* Editorial Board would probably ask the authors to modify their statement that passive range of motion was the most important outcome measure. Limitation of active range of motion (impairment) prevented the patient from accomplishing her goals, which involved activities of daily living (functional limitation) and actions, tasks, or activities for her required role as a homemaker (disability). The authors mentioned the patient's goals and outcomes at the beginning of the section in which they discussed the examination. They are mentioned again at the end of this section, but they should have been highlighted, with range-of-motion measurements secondary.

The following sentences are an example of citing literature to support the reliability of a measurement.

The ultimate outcome is nicely described in disability terms. The 1-year and 5-year outcomes are particularly informative.

---

table utensils, help with bathing, and type for short periods. She was told not to drive or lift heavy objects.

Ten weeks after her injury, the patient's motion was improving more slowly than we desired, based on our experience. Because of this, the amount of time spent with the joint at end-range was increased. This decision was also based on considerations of the changes that occur with wound healing and scar formation. As a scar matures, the rate of collagen degradation and synthesis slows.[23] Because the scar is less dynamic, we consider the joint restrictions less amenable to change and we are therefore more aggressive in our treatment (ie, increasing time at end-range).

The patient's home program was increased by the addition of a static, end-range, abduction splint of the type previously described by the authors.[7] The splint was fabricated by one of us (KRF) out of thermoplastic material and an adjustable aluminum rod that was created by cutting an adjustable cane. The splint allows the arm to be held at its comfortable end-range of abduction in the plane of the scapula without attempting to control the scapula itself. Initially, the splint was worn 1 hour four times per day. Before dispensing the splint, the patient was tested for signs of suprahumeral impingement by simultaneously flexing and medially rotating her arm, which did not provoke pain.[24] Clinic visits were reduced to twice per week, and the ultrasound was discontinued. The ultrasound was discontinued because it did not appear to be making a difference in the patient's ROM or her perception of stiffness.

Twelve weeks after the injury, the patient's ROM gains had reached desired levels. Clinic visits were reduced to one per week, and all modalities, including manual therapy, were discontinued. Based on previous experience, we felt that the amount of

time spent at the end-range of motion accomplished by use of the splint would be sufficient. Decisions as to what constitutes adequate gains in ROM are clinical judgments based on experience rather than attainment of specific gains in ROM. Decisions to decrease clinical visits were based on our belief that increases in ROM are directly related to time at the end-range of motion that the patient could accomplish independently using the splint and her exercise program.

The therapeutic program 12 weeks after injury, therefore, consisted only of using the splint and a strengthening program for the rotator cuff that was added. Strengthening was performed using a double strand of yellow Thera-Band®‡ for 10 repetitions each of medial rotation, lateral rotation, and abduction. Each set of repetitions was done once daily from the standing position, starting with the patient's arm at her side. Ice was applied after exercise when the patient felt it necessary to reduce pain.

The time the splint was worn was progressively increased over the next 2 weeks, based on the patient's tolerance, to a maximum daily schedule of 2 hours, four times per day. Monitoring of pain and ROM were the only subsequent physical therapy activities. Sixteen weeks after injury, visits were reduced to once per month. The patient was discharged 25 weeks after her injury.

Passive range of motion was the most important outcome measure because of the patient's primary complaint of lost motion rather than of pain or weakness. Range of motion was measured during each visit by the same therapist, and AROM was never visibly different than PROM. The ROM measurements were taken with the patient positioned supine. A large plastic goniometer was used, with the measurements recorded to the nearest 5-degree increment. The supine position was chosen to facilitate relax-

ation. Lateral rotation was measured with the patient's arm at her side, and abduction was measured with her humerus positioned in the plane of the scapula. This position is believed to most closely approximate the normal plane of arm elevation during function.[25] Riddle et al[26] have demonstrated good reliability of shoulder ROM measurements even when the technique used was not standardized. Medial rotation was not measured with a goniometer. We have since learned to describe medial rotation, as suggested by the American Academy of Shoulder and Elbow Surgeons,[27] by measuring how far superior the patient can place the thumb on the spine. Unfortunately, we only monitored medial rotation visually and did not quantify this motion. Although medial rotation was limited initially, functional medial rotation (ability to tuck in shirt and fasten bra) appeared to increase by 12 weeks postinjury. No attempt was made to stabilize the scapula during ROM measurements. Measurements, therefore, reflect shoulder girdle ROM, not pure glenohumeral motion. Based on observation, the limitation of motion and subsequent gains occurred primarily at the glenohumeral joint. There was no limitation of passive scapulothoracic motion, based on our manual tests. The acromioclavicular joint and the sternoclavicular joint could have potentially contributed to motion restrictions. We do not feel that passive restrictions at these joints during either physiological motion or accessory motion testing can be reliably measured in a clinical examination.

Twenty-five weeks after her injury, the patient had achieved almost full pain-free PROM (Table and Figure). She was independent in activities of daily living including dressing, bathing, cooking, typing, and lifting the types of objects she was able to lift prior to her injury. At 1-year and 5-year follow-ups, she had no complaints of pain and she had full function and ROM.

‡The Hygenic Corp, 1245 Home Ave, Akron, OH 44310.

The following paragraph is a nice example of decision making based on the authors' own clinical experiences and beliefs. Literature support is not always available for intervention decisions, so clinicians' beliefs and experiences appropriately serve as rationale. When writing a case report, this rationale must be clearly presented.

15. Discussion. In this section, the authors do a good job of linking theory back to their case description. The discussion anticipates questions that other clinicians would ask and provides rationale for doing what they did in response to those questions.

In this paragraph, the phrases "in our opinion" and "in our view" allow the authors to speculate about stretching—without suggesting that their case report proved what they believe.

16. Conclusion. The conclusion highlights the authors' major theoretical points.

The final sentence strays a little beyond the boundaries of a case report, but could easily be modified: *"For this reason, we recommend* that intervention should focus on...."

Discussion

Initially, manual therapy was used to decrease pain and thereby facilitate relaxation in this patient.[28] For this purpose, low-grade gliding movements were selected and performed with the patient's arm at her side in a neutral position. We do not believe we can accurately discern between four grades of amplitude for gliding mobilization as described by Maitland.[29] We believe that only one distinction needs to be made, that is, the distinction between movements that take the periarticular tissues to end-range, which we call high-grade movements, and movements that do not take periarticular tissues to end-range, which we call low-grade movements. We use low-grade mobilization when trying to decrease pain, based on the theory of neurophysiologic modulation of pain produced by mild mechanical stimuli.[30] For the stiff joint, we use high-grade mobilization in order to apply end-range tensile stress to restricting periarticular structures.

In our opinion, any form of stretching dependent on therapist technique, such as high-grade mobilization, has limited application because, as Brand has noted, "any elongation of tissue accomplished by stretch will shorten again once the force is relaxed."[31(p849)] Therefore, in our view, the increase in tissue length produced by a brief session of high-grade mobilization serves only to temporarily deform the tissue rather than to produce a permanent length change. This temporary elongation achieves the "preconditioned" states of the joint structures.[22] Although this temporary elongation may be very useful for facilitating further exercise and function, permanent elongation of a tissue is probably accomplished through another mechanism—remodeling.

Remodeling, unlike the transient viscoelastic phenomenon of stress relaxation, is probably a subtle rearrangement of the collagen and cross-links within the connective tissue over time. This is the desired biological response to gentle, prolonged tensile stress.[8,19,20,31] We often prefer splints to stimulate remodeling because of the long end-range times afforded by splinting.

At 10 weeks postinjury, when the initial improvement of ROM had slowed, our emphasis shifted to increasing the end-range stress. This was accomplished with the end-range splint. Likewise, at 12 weeks, we tried to maximize the total time spent at the end-range of ROM by increasing the time the patient wore the splint.

In the splint, no attempt is made to control the scapula, allowing the humerus to come to a comfortable position at its available end-range. When the joint is taken to the point of limitation, tensile stress is being applied to the restricting structures. Because we believe that there are sufficient research data to suggest that inferior gliding is not a component of elevation, there is no provision for the motion in the splint. Our experience indicates that patients who show no signs of suprahumeral impingement prior to the application of the splint do not develop subsequent impingement problems.

Conclusion

We have discussed the management of a patient with limited shoulder ROM. Many of our treatment decisions were based primarily on clinical experience rather than direct scientific data. We believe that limited motion attributable to adaptive shortening of periarticular tissues is most effectively treated by methods that hold the joint at or near the end-range of motion for prolonged periods of time. Treatment of limited shoulder motion should be focused on identifying and applying tension to restricting structures rather than restoration of translatory gliding movements of the humeral head.

Acknowledgment

We thank Kelley Fitzgerald, PT, for his help with editing this manuscript.

References

1 Kaltenborn FM. *Mobilization of the Extremity Joints.* Oslo, Norway: Olaf Noris Bokhandel Universitetsgaten; 1980.

2 McClure PW, Flowers KR. Treatment of limited shoulder motion using an elevation splint. *Phys Ther.* 1992;72:57–62.

3 Rizk TE, Christopher RP, Pinals RS, et al. Adhesive capsulitis: a new approach to its management. *Arch Phys Med Rehabil.* 1983;64: 29–33.

4 Neviaser RJ, Neviaser TJ. The frozen shoulder: diagnosis and management. *Clin Orthop.* 1987;223:59–64.

5 Akeson WH, Amiel D, Abel M, et al. Effects of immobilization on joints. *Clin Orthop.* 1987; 219:28–37.

6 Flowers KR, Michlovitz SL. Assessment and management of loss of motion in orthopedic dysfunction. *Postgraduate Advances in Physical Therapy.* 1988;2-8:1–11.

7 Light KE, Nuzik S, Personius W, Barstrom A. Low-load prolonged stretch vs high load brief stretch in treating knee contractures. *Phys Ther.* 1984;64:330–333.

8 Arem AJ, Madden JW. Effects of stress on healing wounds: intermittent noncyclical tension. *J Surg Res.* 1976;20:93–102.

9 Michlovitz SL. Cryotherapy: the use of cold as a therapeutic agent. In: Michlovitz SL, ed. *Thermal Agents in Rehabilitation.* Philadelphia, Pa: FA Davis Co; 1986:87–90.

10 Cyriax JH. *Textbook of Orthopaedic Medicine, Volume I: Diagnosis of Soft Tissue Lesions.* 6th ed. Baltimore, Md: Williams & Wilkins; 1975.

11 MacConaill MA, Basmajian JV. *Muscles and Movements: A Basis for Human Kinesiology.* Baltimore, Md: Williams & Wilkins; 1969.

12 Kisner C, Colby LA. *Therapeutic Exercise: Foundations and Techniques.* Philadelphia, Pa: FA Davis Co; 1985.

13 Wadsworth CT. *Manual Examination and Treatment of the Spine and Extremities.* Baltimore, Md: Williams & Wilkins; 1988.

14 Poppen NK, Walker PS. Normal and abnormal motion of the shoulder. *J Bone Joint Surg [Am].* 1976;58:195–201.

15 Howell SM, Galinat BJ, Renzi AJ, Marone PJ. Normal and abnormal mechanics of the glenohumeral joint in the horizontal plane. *J Bone Joint Surg [Am].* 1988;70:227–232.

16 Harryman DT, Sidles JA, Clark JM, et al. Translation of the humeral head on the glenoid with passive glenohumeral motion. *J Bone Joint Surg [Am].* 1990;72:1334–1343.

17 Turkel SJ, Panio MW, Marshall JL, Girgis FG. Stabilizing mechanisms preventing anterior dislocation of the glenohumeral joint. *J Bone Joint Surg [Am].* 1981;63:1208–1217.

18 Terry GC, Hammon D, France P, Norwood LA. The stabilizing function of passive shoulder restraints. *Am J Sports Med.* 1991;19:26–34.

19 Brand PN. *Clinical Mechanics of the Hand.* St Louis, Mo: CV Mosby Co; 1984:68.

20 Peacock EE. *Wound Repair.* 3rd ed. Philadelphia, Pa: WB Saunders Co; 1984:273–274.

21 Neer CS. Displaced proximal humeral fractures, part I: classification and evaluation. *J Bone Joint Surg [Am].* 1970;52:1077.

Case Report 3

This case report is longer than many because it separately describes two patients with different types of vestibular problems. Most multiple-patient case reports have patients with similar problems and combine them into a single description. The case descriptions within this report are consistent across the two patients, so comments are made on the report of the first patient only.

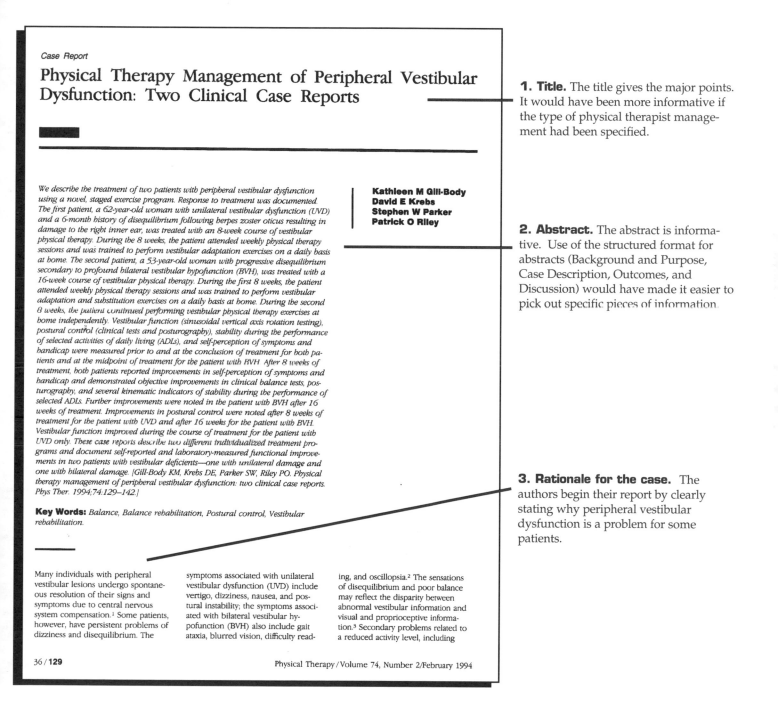

Case Report

Physical Therapy Management of Peripheral Vestibular Dysfunction: Two Clinical Case Reports

We describe the treatment of two patients with peripheral vestibular dysfunction using a novel, staged exercise program. Response to treatment was documented. The first patient, a 62-year-old woman with unilateral vestibular dysfunction (UVD) and a 6-month history of disequilibrium following herpes zoster oticus resulting in damage to the right inner ear, was treated with an 8-week course of vestibular physical therapy. During the 8 weeks, the patient attended weekly physical therapy sessions and was trained to perform vestibular adaptation exercises on a daily basis at home. The second patient, a 53-year-old woman with progressive disequilibrium secondary to profound bilateral vestibular hypofunction (BVH), was treated with a 16-week course of vestibular physical therapy. During the first 8 weeks, the patient attended weekly physical therapy sessions and was trained to perform vestibular adaptation and substitution exercises on a daily basis at home. During the second 8 weeks, the patient continued performing vestibular physical therapy exercises at home independently. Vestibular function (sinusoidal vertical axis rotation testing), postural control (clinical tests and posturography), stability during the performance of selected activities of daily living (ADLs), and self-perception of symptoms and handicap were measured prior to and at the conclusion of treatment for both patients and at the midpoint of treatment for the patient with BVH. After 8 weeks of treatment, both patients reported improvements in self-perception of symptoms and handicap and demonstrated objective improvements in clinical balance tests, posturography, and several kinematic indicators of stability during the performance of selected ADLs. Further improvements were noted in the patient with BVH after 16 weeks of treatment. Improvements in postural control were noted after 8 weeks of treatment for the patient with UVD and after 16 weeks for the patient with BVH. Vestibular function improved during the course of treatment for the patient with UVD only. These case reports describe two different individualized treatment programs and document self-reported and laboratory-measured functional improvements in two patients with vestibular deficients—one with unilateral damage and one with bilateral damage. [Gill-Body KM, Krebs DE, Parker SW, Riley PO. Physical therapy management of peripheral vestibular dysfunction: two clinical case reports. Phys Ther. 1994;74:129–142.]

Kathleen M Gill-Body
David E Krebs
Stephen W Parker
Patrick O Riley

Key Words: Balance, Balance rehabilitation, Postural control, Vestibular rehabilitation.

Many individuals with peripheral vestibular lesions undergo spontaneous resolution of their signs and symptoms due to central nervous system compensation.[1] Some patients, however, have persistent problems of dizziness and disequilibrium. The symptoms associated with unilateral vestibular dysfunction (UVD) include vertigo, dizziness, nausea, and postural instability; the symptoms associated with bilateral vestibular hypofunction (BVH) also include gait ataxia, blurred vision, difficulty reading, and oscillopsia.[2] The sensations of disequilibrium and poor balance may reflect the disparity between abnormal vestibular information and visual and proprioceptive information.[3] Secondary problems related to a reduced activity level, including

---

1. Title. The title gives the major points. It would have been more informative if the type of physical therapist management had been specified.

2. Abstract. The abstract is informative. Use of the structured format for abstracts (Background and Purpose, Case Description, Outcomes, and Discussion) would have made it easier to pick out specific pieces of information.

3. Rationale for the case. The authors begin their report by clearly stating why peripheral vestibular dysfunction is a problem for some patients.

5. Purpose of the case report. The authors' statement that there have been no detailed descriptions of intervention programs and outcomes for patients with vestibular dysfunction implies the purpose of their case report.

4. Support for the approach. The next several paragraphs define "vestibular physical therapy" and give rationale for the intervention approach, including the anatomical and physiological basis.

6. This paragraph describes some of the medical examination of each patient prior to referral for physical therapy. The authors probably placed the information here because it is common to both patients—who are described separately in the subsequent sections—thus avoiding repetition. In other case reports, this information could be included in a history/examination section.

---

muscle weakness, limited endurance, and loss of flexibility, can further impair postural responses.[4] For patients with persistent symptoms, pharmacologic management appears to benefit only a small number[5] and surgical management is appropriate for even fewer patients.[6] Because the individual's ability to move in the environment without experiencing dizziness or loss of balance is severely impaired, overall functional abilities and quality of life are compromised.

Vestibular physical therapy is an exercise approach that has developed over the past several years to help manage the persistent functional problems associated with peripheral vestibular dysfunction.[7-10] Exercise programs, aimed at remediating the problems of dizziness, gaze instability, and balance dysfunction, are designed for each patient based on the patient's signs, symptoms, and functional limitations. A different type of treatment is utilized based on whether the patient exhibits absent versus reduced vestibular function.[7]

For patients with residual vestibular function, the treatment program, denoted the adaptation approach, is similar to that described by Cawthorne in the 1940s for patients with persistent symptoms from vestibular dys-

function.[11] The brain's ability to adapt to changes in demand or changes in sensory information received is key to this treatment approach.[12] By providing stimuli that induce adaptation of the vestibular system, such as combining movement of an image across the retina with head movement, compensation within the central nervous system is thought to be promoted.[7] For patients with unilaterally reduced or abnormal vestibular function, such as the first patient reported here, the adaptation approach is utilized.

For patients with no remaining vestibular function, a substitution approach is used. In this approach, the patient is encouraged to rely on visual and proprioceptive information to stabilize gaze and maintain postural stability in place of vestibular information.[3] For patients with bilaterally reduced (but not absent) vestibular function, such as the second patient reported here, a combined approach (incorporating exercises to foster both adaptation and substitution) is utilized, as it cannot be determined whether central nervous system adaptation to the maximum possible extent has already occurred. Vestibular physical therapy, as described in this case report, is currently offered in various centers across the United States, and some general information is available re-

garding patient response to the treatment approach in terms of subjective symptoms and self-rated disability.[13]

Horak et al[14] recently reported preliminary results regarding the relative effectiveness of vestibular rehabilitation, general conditioning exercises, and vestibular suppressant medication on reducing dizziness and imbalance. Their results suggest that although all three treatment approaches reduce dizziness, only vestibular rehabilitation improves balance (as measured by duration of unilateral stance and posturography).[14] To date, however, no one has both described a specific treatment program in detail and reported data regarding patient response to treatment in terms of whole-body movement analysis, clinical balance testing, posturography, symptoms of dizziness and disequilibrium, and perceived level of disability for an individual patient or series of patients with vestibular dysfunction.

The medical workup for each patient just prior to referral to physical therapy consisted of a neurological examination by a neurologist, vestibular testing including an electronystagmogram with caloric stimulation, sinusoidal vertical axis rotation, visual vestibular interaction rotation, and posturography testing utilizing the Equitest™ system.*[15,16] Each patient also underwent a three-dimensional movement analysis in our biomotion laboratory. A full-body kinematic and kinetic analysis of key activities of daily living (ADLs) (standing, free and paced gait, walking in place, ascending steps, and rising from a chair) was completed.[17,18] The motion analysis system is described in detail elsewhere.[17-19] This system consists of an 11-segment, 66-degree-of-freedom, full-body (head, arms, trunk, pelvis, thighs, shanks, and feet) kinematic model; two force plates; and software to integrate the kinematic and kinetic data.[18] SELSPOT II hardware[+] and a TRACK kinematic data-analysis software package[‡] are used to acquire and analyze the three-dimensional full-body kinematic data. Floor reaction forces are acquired from two Kistler platforms[§] and processed on

KM Gill-Body, PT, is Neurological Clinical Specialist, Physical Therapy Services, Massachusetts General Hospital, Fruit St, Boston, MA 02114 (USA), and Assistant Professor, MGH Institute of Health Professions, 101 Merrimac St, Boston, MA 02114. Address all correspondence to Ms Gill-Body.

DE Krebs, PhD, PT, is Associate Professor, MGH Institute of Health Professions, Director, Massachusetts General Hospital Biomotion Laboratory, Boston, MA 02114, Instructor, Harvard Medical School, Boston, MA 02138, and Lecturer, Massachusetts Institute of Technology, Cambridge, MA 02139.

SW Parker, MD, is Chief of Otoneurology, Massachusetts General Hospital, and Assistant Professor of Neurology, Harvard Medical School.

PÖ Riley, PhD, is Assistant Technical Director, Massachusetts General Hospital Biomotion Laboratory, and Lecturer, Massachusetts Institute of Technology.

This work was supported by the National Institute for Disability and Rehabilitation Research, DOE, grant H133G00025.

This article was submitted December 31, 1992, and was accepted September 21, 1993.

*NeuroCom International Inc, 9570 SE Lawnfield Rd, Clackamas, OR 97015.

[†]Selective Electronics Co, Partille, Sweden.

[‡]Developed at the Massachusetts Institute of Technology, Cambridge, MA 02139.

[§]Type 9281A, Kistler Instruments AG, Winterthur, Switzerland.

the same computer as the kinematic data. Kinematic and kinetic data are sampled at 153 Hz and digitally filtered. Dynamic stability is quantified using the kinematics of the center of gravity (COG) and center of pressure (COP) as well as standard time-distance parameters (ie, double support time, average velocity, and so forth). The COG-COP moment arm, the horizontal separation between the COG and COP, is used to quantify the dynamics of each activity.[18,20]

Unilateral Vestibular Dysfunction

History

A 62-year-old right-handed woman was referred to physical therapy with a diagnosis of right-sided vestibular damage due to a herpes zoster oticus. The patient history included an initial onset of a right posterior headache followed by right facial paralysis the next day. On the day after onset of paralysis, the patient was extremely unsteady, had difficulty walking, and was hospitalized. After 5 days, lesions of herpes zoster were noted in the right ear and the patient was treated with acyclovir and prednisone. Two weeks later, at the time of discharge from the hospital, she was still unable to walk without assistance. Over the next 5 months, the patient noted some improvements in her facial palsy and balance ability. At the time the patient was seen at our hospital (6 months after the initial onset of symptoms), she reported persistent unsteadiness; difficulty walking out-of-doors; some ringing and buzzing in the right ear; and the inability to return to work as a city tour guide due to her inability to stand on a moving bus, walk in a straight line, or maintain balance in busy environments. These problems had been unchanged for the preceding 3 months.

Prerehabilitation Findings

Examination by the neurologist revealed full extraocular movements with no spontaneous or gaze nystagmus. The patient reported that an audiogram performed 4 months ear-

lier had shown high-frequency hearing loss in the right ear. Hearing was intact to watch tick bilaterally, and a repeat audiogram was not performed. Facial sensation was intact, and there was a mild right facial droop. Patellar and Achilles tendon reflexes were brisk and symmetrical. Coordination and strength (tested by performing resisted isometric contractions of the shoulder flexors, elbow flexors and extensors, finger flexors, hip flexors, knee extensors, and ankle dorsiflexors) were intact in all extremities. A Romberg test was negative with sway. The patient was able to stand on foam with eyes closed, but appeared very unsteady and repeatedly fell backward. Gait appeared stable, with normal-sized steps and good arm swing. Tandem gait appeared moderately unsteady, with a tendency to fall to either side after a few steps. Positional testing (Hallpike maneuver both with and without head turning) revealed no nystagmus or dizziness. There was no spontaneous, gaze, post–head-shaking, or positional nystagmus behind Frenzel lenses.

An electronystagmogram revealed an 87% reduced right caloric response (total peak slow-phase velocity after warm and cool stimulation of the right and left ears was 2° and 29°/s, respectively) and left-beating positional nystagmus (eye movements with a fast component to the left and a slow component to the right). Sinusoidal vertical-axis rotation (SVAR) with a peak velocity of 50°/s at frequencies from 0.01 to 1.0 Hz revealed mildly decreased gains (slow-phase eye velocity/chair velocity[21]) of the vestibular ocular reflex in the lower frequencies of rotation to the following extent: between 2.0 and 2.5 standard deviations below the mean at 0.01 Hz and between 1.0 and 2.0 standard deviations below the mean at 0.02 to 0.05 and 0.1 Hz (as compared with healthy subjects) (Fig. 1). The SVAR also revealed increased phase leads (the relationship between the onset of the rotation-induced nystagmus and the angular velocity of the chair movement; an increased phase lead is seen with damage to the vestibular system) of greater than 2.5

standard deviations from the mean at 0.01, 0.02, and 0.05 Hz. Finally, there was a left preponderance (ie, more left than right) of rotation-induced nystagmus of greater than 2.5 standard deviations at 0.01, 0.02, 0.05, 0.10, 0.20, 0.50, and 1.0 Hz (ie, at all frequencies of rotation). There was good fixation suppression on visual vestibular interaction testing, and optokinetic nystagmus was normal. Details regarding SVAR testing and interpretation of the raw data obtained to compute gain, phase, and symmetry are described elsewhere.[22] These test results, combined with the examination and symptoms, are consistent with a poorly compensated unilateral vestibular lesion on the right side.

Posturography testing revealed excessive sway and falls on a sway-referenced platform with eyes closed and moderate sway with one fall on a sway referenced platform with eyes fixed on a sway-referenced visual surround (Fig. 2). To achieve sway-referencing, the patient's anterior-posterior body sway is used to produce a rotation of the platform or the visual surround in a plane collinear with the patient's ankles at a gain of 1.0 (ie, at a speed that matches the patient's body sway); these maneuvers are intended to alter joint sensory information (proprioception) by keeping the angle between the foot and the leg constant when the platform is sway-referenced, or to provide conflicting visual information when the visual surround is sway-referenced.

During the initial physical therapy examination, the patient's sensation for light touch (of the lower leg and foot) and proprioception (of the knees, ankles, and toes) were intact. Proprioception was tested by having the patient identify the position of each joint as it was moved in different directions while her eyes were closed. Deep tendon reflexes were brisk and symmetrical. Manual muscle testing (of the shoulder girdle; hip extensors and abductors; knee flexors and extensors; and ankle dorsiflexors, plantar flexors, invertors, and ever-

7. Subject description. The history and the chronology of the first patient's problem are clearly described.

8. Patient's outcome statement. The patient's desired outcome is suggested in the following sentence. The authors have organized her complaints within a disablement framework. Impairments include unsteadiness and ringing and buzzing in her ears; functional limitations are difficulty in walking out-of-doors and inability to stand on a moving bus, walk in a straight line, and maintain balance in busy environments; and disability is inability to work as a tour guide.

9. Examination. The authors use the subheading "Prerehabilitation Findings" to cover information obtained from patient report, physicians' reports, and physical therapist examination.

Note how the authors describe how proprioception was tested.

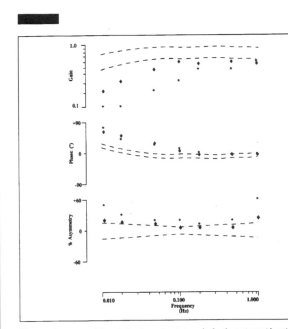

Figure 1. *Sinusoidal vertical-axis rotation test results for the patient with unilateral vestibular dysfunction before (∗) and after (♦) treatment. Gain (the ratio of peak slow-phase eye velocity to peak chair velocity), phase (the interval between the stimulus and the response), and asymmetry (the percentage of difference between the peak slow-component eye velocities to the right and left) are displayed. Testing was performed at seven frequencies of rotation (0.01, 0.02, 0.05, 0.10, 0.20, 0.50, and 1.00 Hz). The dashed lines represent the mean values (±1 standard deviation) across all frequencies of rotation for healthy subjects. This patient's test results demonstrated decreased low-frequency gains and increased low-frequency phase leads both before and after treatment. Asymmetry was reduced following treatment, consistent with central nervous system adaptation to vestibular damage.*

tors) showed Normal (5/5) strength in all muscle groups except for the right-sided facial musculature, in which weakness was evidenced by minimal muscle contractions during attempts to smile, grimace, and purse lips. Heel-to-shin movements, finger-to-nose movements, and rapid alternating movements of the forearm were performed quickly, accurately, and smoothly, bilaterally. Active range of motion of the spine, shoulders, hips, knees, and ankles was full except for rotation and lateral flexion at the cervical spine, which was reduced by half. The patient reported a pulling sensation in the posterior cervical and upper trapezius muscle regions bilaterally during active cervical lateral flexion and rotation movements. Pursuit and saccadic eye movements could be performed fully and without symptoms. The patient reported that she had slightly blurred vision in the right eye. She reported not having vertigo or dizziness. She also reported the sensation of disequilibrium frequently (more than once per month but not continuously) at an intensity of 4/10 (10 being the highest level of intensity imaginable).

The patient scored 14 out of a possible 100 on the Dizziness Handicap Inventory (DHI)[23] (100 = the highest level of handicap), reporting problems in three of the nine items related to functional activities and in four of the seven items related to physical activities. The DHI, originally devised to measure perception of handicap in individuals with benign paroxysmal positional vertigo, is used in our clinic for all patients with vestibular dysfunction to objectively document perception of handicap related to dizziness or balance problems.

Clinical balance assessment revealed that the patient could stand with her eyes closed and her feet together for 60 seconds (measured with a digital stopwatch), but it demonstrated a significantly increased ankle sway (sway was observed and not measured). Unilateral stance with eyes open could be performed for 7 seconds, and the patient was unable to perform unilateral stance with her eyes closed. The patient could perform tandem stance for 60 seconds with her eyes open and for 5 seconds with her eyes closed. Stance on foam with eyes open could be performed for 60 seconds without difficulty; with eyes closed, stance on foam could be performed for 20 seconds with a marked ankle sway. Tandem gait with eyes open could be performed for a maximum of five steps. The patient adopted a forward-bent posture during standing and walking activities. Gait was wide based and characterized by an immobile trunk, no arm swing, and gaze fixation on the floor. The patient was unable to ambulate in a straight line at any speed; rather, she moved in a side-to-side path (to both sides) as she moved forward. Turns (90°) were performed slowly and with multiple small steps. During attempts to ambulate while rotating her head from side to side, the patient's speed of gait decreased and she crossed one foot over the other repeatedly.

Rehabilitation

The vestibular adaptation treatment program that the patient received consisted of exercises and activities outlined under phase 1 through

10. Intervention. The following paragraphs and Table 1 (on page 202) describe the intervention and its progression in such detail that it could be replicated by another clinician. Note how much easier it is to grasp the rationale and activities of the intervention program from the table than it would have been from the text of the article. The table was also probably easier to write than a narrative.

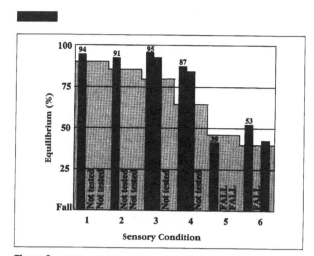

Figure 2. *Baseline (week 0) posturography (sensory organization) test results for patient with unilateral vestibular dysfunction. (Note: Equitest™ system was used.) Equilibrium score represents the angular difference between the patient's calculated maximum anterior-posterior center of gravity and the theoretical maximum displacement of 12.5 degrees; the result is expressed as a percentage between 0% and 100%, with 0% indicating sway exceeding the limits of stability and 100% indicating perfect stability. Numerical equilibrium scores for the best performance for each trial are indicated above the vertical bars. Shaded areas represent norms for performance; scores above the shaded areas represent normal test scores. Sensory conditions: 1=fixed platform, eyes open/fixed visual surround; 2=fixed platform, eyes closed; 3=fixed platform, eyes open/sway-referenced visual surround; 4=sway-referenced platform, eyes open/fixed visual surround; 5=sway-referenced platform, eyes closed; 6=sway-referenced platform, eyes open/sway-referenced visual surround. Not tested=repeat trials not performed; standard testing procedures are to perform only one trial for sensory conditions 1 through 3, unless the patient is observed to have a large amount of sway or falls, and to perform three trials for sensory conditions 4 through 6, unless patient appears to have successfully completed the test in fewer trials. Fall=patient fell during trial.*

phase 3 in Table 1. The patient performed phase 1 of the program during the first 2 weeks of treatment, phase 2 during weeks 3 through 6, and phase 3 during weeks 7 and 8. The patient progressed to each new phase during weekly visits to the physical therapy clinic as her performance on the previous phase improved to the point at which the individual exercises could be performed easily and without an increase in the perception of disequilibrium. Correct posture and alignment were emphasized during all of standing and walking activities. A brief explanation of the rationale for each activity in the treatment program is included in Table 1 and is based primarily on the

work of Herdman[7] and Shumway-Cook and Horak.[8,10] The patient was instructed to perform the exercises at least one time per day at home and to note daily the exercises she performed, number of repetitions, and any difficulties she experienced using a standard patient compliance tool in use at our clinic. The patient completed daily exercise logs indicating that she was compliant with the daily home program (ie, she performed the exercises 6–7 days per week over the course of the entire treatment period). The patient reported completing the daily exercise program once per day during weeks 1 through 3 and twice per day during weeks 4 through 8. After 8 weeks of treatment, the

patient was reevaluated in the clinic and in the biomotion laboratory utilizing the same measures as those used during the initial assessment. Repeat SVAR testing and posturography were also performed.

The vestibular adaptation treatment program (Tab. 1) designed for this patient was based on the following interpretation of the patient's condition:

1. The patient's decreased cervical range of motion could be related to her voluntarily holding her head still during gait and other functional activities; decreased cervical range of motion and alignment could impair postural responses[10] and were therefore worth addressing in treatment.

2. The patient's primary problem of impaired postural stability was related to her vestibular hypofunction on the right side, as supported by the posturography test results of difficulty with sensory conditions 5 and 6 (Fig. 2).

3. The patient clearly demonstrated some ability to utilize vestibular information for postural control in situations in which accurate visual and proprioceptive information were not available (ie, sensory conditions 5 and 6 could be partially performed on some trials).

Postrehabilitation Findings

At the conclusion of the 8-week period of treatment, the patient reported a slight decrease in the intensity of her sensation of disequilibrium (3/10) and improvements in four physical and two functional activities previously reported to be problematic on the DHI (Tab. 2). No items on the DHI were reported to be worse. Clinical balance assessment revealed no change in ability to perform unilateral stance with eyes open or eyes closed. Tandem stance with eyes closed could be performed for 20 seconds (improved from 5 seconds). Stance with eyes closed and with feet together on the floor and on foam could be per-

In the next section, the authors describe the clinical reasoning process that led to the intervention. If this section had appeared before the description of the intervention, the flow of the article might have been improved.

11. Outcome. The authors report impairment, functional limitation, and disability measurements following 8 weeks of intervention. Table 2, on the next page, is a good example of using a table to clarify outcomes. The list of specific Dizziness Handicap Inventory items that changed is much more informative than an overall score or other numerical data. Notice that throughout this section the authors describe the outcomes using the same measurements that they reported for the initial examination.

The authors illustrate the use of a patient log to provide information about the extent to which patients carry out a home exercise program.

Table 1. *Vestibular Rehabilitation Treatment Program and Its Rationale for Patient With Unilateral Vestibular Dysfunction*

Rationale	Treatment Activity[a]
Phase 1	
1. Encourage active extraocular movements	Extraocular movements, self-selected speed
2. Enhance vestibular adaptation	Visual fixation, EO, stationary target, slow head movements, near targets
3. Encourage resetting of VOR gain	Imaginary visual fixation, EC, small head movements, self-selected speed
4. Promote utilization of somatosensory and vestibular inputs for postural control	Static stance, EO and EC, feet together, arms outstretched, book on head
5. Improve dynamic postural control utilizing all sensory inputs	Gait with narrowed base of support, EO
6. Improve dynamic postural control utilizing all sensory inputs	March in place slowly, EO
7. Decrease cervical musculature tightness	Active neck range of motion, all directions, slow movements
Phase 2	
1. Promote use of VOR at various speed head movements	Visual fixation, EO, stationary target, fast and slow movements, near targets
2. Enhance vestibular adaptation by inducing retinal slip	Visual fixation, EO, moving target in opposite direction, slow head movements
3. Promote utilization of somatosensory and vestibular inputs for postural control	Static stance, semitandem, EO and EC, arms close to body, book on head
4. Promote use of somatosensory inputs for postural control	Static stance on foam surface, EO, book on head
5. Improve dynamic postural control utilizing somatosensory inputs	Gait with narrowed base of support, EO, book on head
6. Improve dynamic postural control utilizing somatosensory inputs	Gait with normal base of support, EO, book on head
7. Decrease cervical muscle tightness	Active neck range of motion, all directions, slow movements
Phase 3	
1. Enhance vestibular adaptation	Visual fixation, EO, stationary target, fast and slow head movements, near and far targets
2. Enhance vestibular adaptation	Visual fixation, EO, moving target, slow and fast head movements
3. Promote use of somatosensory and vestibular inputs for postural control	Static stance on foam surface, EC, with and without book on head
4. Improve dynamic postural trol utilizing vestibular and somatosensory inputs	Gait with narrowed base of support, EC, with and without book on head
5. Improve dynamic postural control when head is moving utilizing all sensory inputs	Gait with normal base of support, fast head movements
6. Improve dynamic postural control utilizing somatosensory and vestibular inputs	March in place slowly, EO and EC, with and without book on head
7. Decrease cervical muscle tightness	Active neck range of motion, all directions, slow movements

[a]EO=eyes open; EC=eyes closed; VOR=vestibular ocular reflex.

Table 2. *Self-Reported Changes on the Dizziness Handicap Inventory[23] for Patient With Unilateral Vestibular Dysfunction[a]*

Physical/Functional Factors (0- to 8-Week Changes)

+   Fewer restrictions on travel for business or pleasure

+   Ability to move head quickly

+   Ability to do job and household responsibilities

++   Ability to walk down the aisle of a supermarket

++   Ability to walk down a sidewalk

+   Ability to bend over

[a]+=item rated as "a little improved"; ++=item rated as "much improved."

formed without any observable increase in sway for 60 seconds. Tandem gait with eyes open could be performed for seven steps (improved from five steps). The patient's active cervical range of motion was full, and she no longer reported any feelings of muscular pulling during active cervical movements. Posture was improved, as noted by a more erect stance and only a minimally displaced forward head. During observation of gait, her base of support appeared normal and she demonstrated some arm swing and trunk rotation. She was able to walk in a straight line without difficulty but continued to stagger to the side if she attempted to turn quickly. She was able to ambulate in a straight path without slowing her speed of gait while rotating her head from side to side with only occasional cross steps.

Repeat sinusoidal vertical-axis rotation testing revealed less asymmetry of rotation-induced nystagmus (values were 2.5 standard deviations below the norm only at two frequencies of rotation—0.01 and 0.02 Hz), consistent with some central adaptation to the damage to the right inner ear (Fig. 1). Repeat posturography testing revealed an improvement in the patient's ability to stand on a sway-referenced platform with eyes closed

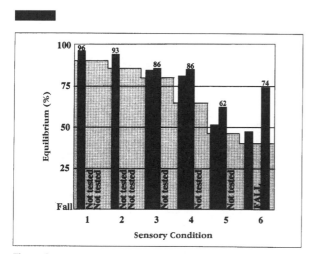

Figure 3. *Posttreatment (week 8) posturography (sensory organization) test results for patient with unilateral vestibular dysfunction.*

and with eyes fixed on a sway-referenced visual surround (Fig. 3). With eyes closed (sensory condition 5), the improvement consisted of no falls and less sway. With eyes open and fixed on a sway-referenced visual surround (sensory condition 6), the improvement consisted of less sway. Comparing the best performance on each trial, there was a 59% improvement (ie, less sway) on sensory condition 5 and a 28% improvement on sensory condition 6, as compared with the pretreatment posturography test.

The three-dimensional movement analysis revealed several changes indicative of improved postural stability (Tab. 3). The patient demonstrated reduced COG displacements during quiet standing with feet together and with eyes open and closed, which is a marker of improved balance control.[18] During preferred pace (or free) gait, velocity increased and double support time decreased, indicating that the patient spent more time in single-limb stance and moved more quickly during gait. The maximum COG-COP moment arm increased

during free gait and preferred pace chair rise, indicating that the patient was able to increase the distance between the body's COP and COG—another marker of a higher level of stability.[18] Reduced medial-lateral COG excursion occurred along with reduced head displacements (relative to the room) in all directions and reduced head accelerations in the flexion-extension and lateral flexion directions, indicating that the patient walked in a more stable manner even when the speed of gait was controlled.

Bilateral Vestibular Hypofunction

History

A 53-year-old woman was referred to physical therapy with a diagnosis of BVH for a trial of physical therapy to help improve her balance, function, and activity level. The patient history, obtained through self-report, included 20 years of intermittent vertigo and the recent onset of worsening disequilibrium. The patient reported brief episodes of dizziness intermit-

tently over the preceding 6 years, which usually followed a cold or flying in an airplane and would last a few days at a time. Four months prior to evaluation, the patient noted the onset of a persistent "floating" sensation made worse by head movements and following two upper respiratory infections. The patient complained of feeling unsteady while walking and of being nauseated and fatigued. All of these symptoms had been unchanged for 4 months prior to referral to physical therapy. The etiology of vestibular damage was unclear but believed to be due to either sequential unilateral damage (such as might be seen with viral labrynthitis) or a degenerative process involving only the vestibular portion of the inner ear or eighth cranial nerve.

Prerehabilitation Findings

Examination by a neurologist revealed full extraocular movements with no spontaneous or gaze nystagmus. The patient's hearing was normal bilaterally. There was normal strength (tested via isometric resisted contractions in the same muscle groups that were tested in the patient with UVD) in all extremities and no limb ataxia. Vibration and position sensation were present at the toes. A Romberg test was negative. Tandem gait was done well while the patient was walking forward and backward with eyes open. Positional testing revealed no nystagmus and only momentary dizziness in left and right ear down positions. There was no spontaneous, gaze, post–head-shaking, or positional nystagmus behind Frenzel lenses.

An audiogram was normal. The only abnormality on the electronystagmogram was very small (nearly absent) caloric responses bilaterally. Sinusoidal vertical-axis rotation with a peak velocity of 50°/s revealed extremely low gains (more than 3 standard deviations below normal) of the vestibular-ocular reflex at frequencies of 0.01, 0.02, 0.05, and 0.1 Hz, with values below 0.1 (Fig. 4). At higher frequencies of rotation, there was some remaining function, with gains only slightly below normal. Visual

The authors now go on to describe the second patient, following the same format as they used to describe the first patient. If the patients had been similar, both patients could have been described at the same time. We'll skip a few pages now to the discussion section.

12. Discussion. The discussion starts with a summary of the interventions and outcomes for the two patients. Notice that the patient reports of improvement are given as much credence as the measurements of postural stability.

Table 5. *Self-Reported Changes on Dizziness Handicap Inventory[2,3] for Patient With Bilateral Vestibular Hypofunction[a]*

Physical/Functional Factors

0- to 8-Week Changes	9- to 16-Week Changes	Emotional Factors
+ Ability to look up	+ Ability to look up	+ Less feeling of embarrassment in front of others
+ Ability to move head quickly	+ Ability to move head quickly	+ Less fear that others think individual is intoxicated
++ Ability to walk down aisle of supermarket	+ Ability to walk down aisle of supermarket	− Ability to participate in social activities
++ Ability to do job	+ Ability to walk down a sidewalk	− Feelings of depression

[a] +=item rated as "a little improved"; ++=item rated as "much improved"; −=item rated as "a little worse."

stance duration time combined with an increased velocity of gait, indicating that she took longer strides. Reduced medial-lateral COG excursion occurred along with a variety of changes in head displacement (relative to the room) and reduced head accelerations in all directions. The patient's head displacements increased in some directions (flexion-extension and rotation), whereas a marked decrease was seen in the lateral direction. Finally, COG-COP maximum moment arm increased during paced chair rise.

Findings at Follow-up

At the conclusion of the 16-week treatment period, the patient reported no symptoms of dizziness and only occasional perceptions of disequilibrium at an intensity of 5/10. On the DHI, she reported further improvements (since the 8-week period) in four physical activities and in two items related to emotional health (Tab. 5). No items were reported as worsened since the 8-week test period. The only change in static balance noted was an improvement in her ability to stand on a foam support (60 seconds) with eyes open. Dynamic balance had improved in that tandem gait could be performed consistently for 10 consecutive steps

without difficulty. Walking in a straight line for 6.1 m with head rotation from side to side could be performed without any cross steps.

There was no change in SVAR testing from the initial test or the 8-week test, indicating that no change occurred in this patient's baseline vestibular function. On posturography testing, the patient demonstrated less sway when standing on a sway-referenced platform with eyes open and closed and with eyes fixed on a sway-referenced visual surround (Fig. 6). Comparing the best performance among all trials for each sensory condition from pretreatment to posttreatment at 16 weeks, an 8% improvement (ie, less sway) was noted in sensory condition 4, a 39% improvement was noted in sensory condition 5, and a 65% improvement was noted in sensory condition 6. In addition, the patient demonstrated consistent performance and normal sway when standing on a fixed platform with eyes open looking at a sway-referenced visual surround (sensory condition 3).

On three-dimensional movement analysis of ADL tasks, the patient demonstrated continued or further changes in performance (with a few exceptions), indicative of further improvements in postural stability (Tab.

6). Improvements in performance were only partially sustained during the 9- to 16-week period of treatment for anterior-posterior COG excursion with feet together and eyes closed, medial-lateral COG excursion during free gait, double support and stance duration during paced gait, and COG-COP maximum moment arm during paced chair rise. Performance was still, however, improved over baseline for these factors. Head displacements during paced gait in the flexion-extension and lateral flexion directions were reduced, whereas head displacements in the rotation direction were slightly higher. Head accelerations during paced gait were reduced in all directions at the 16-week test period. These results indicate that the patient moved her head less distance (overall) and less frequently during gait activities in which the speed of gait was controlled.

Discussion

Both patients demonstrated improvements in postural stability and reported improvements in the perception of disequilibrium and handicap following 8-week individually designed programs of vestibular physical therapy. The patient with BVH also reported a decrease in the perception of dizziness. For the patient with BVH, improvements in performance noted after an initial 8-week period of treatment continued to occur during the second 8-week period when the patient continued exercises at home with telephone supervision.

Although there were some similarities in the patients' response to treatment, there were important differences between these two patients. The patient with UVD was 6 months postonset of her vestibular damage and reported persistent and stable symptoms for 3 months prior to beginning vestibular physical therapy. Although most of the spontaneous resolution of symptoms associated with UVD occur within 3 to 6 months,[7,14] recovery can also be delayed or incomplete.[7,26] That this patient demonstrated documented improvements in SVAR testing from pretreatment to posttreatment

In the next paragraphs, the authors describe differences between the two patients and explore alternative hypotheses to explain the outcomes. Notice that they do not attempt to establish a cause-and-effect relationship between the intervention and the outcomes. They even acknowledge that spontaneous recovery is a possibility.

Table 6. *Percentage of Improvement From Pretreatment in Kinematic Indicators of Stability[a] During Activities of Daily Living and Locomotor Performance for Patient With Bilateral Vestibular Hypofunction*

	Improvement (%)[b]	
	Change From 0 to 8 Weeks	Overall Change From 0 to 16 Weeks
Feet together, eyes open		
AP COG excursion[c]	60	66
ML COG excursion[c]	27	48
Feet together, eyes closed		
AP COG excursion[c]	87	76
ML COG excursion[c]	45	91
Free gait		
Average velocity	13	36
ML COG excursion[c]	59	44
Head flex/ext acceleration[c]	12	60
Head lateral flex acceleration[c]	−8[d]	20
Paced gait		
Average velocity	11	19
ML COG excursion[c]	46	57
Double support time	20	8
Stance duration time	17	3
Head flex/ext displacement[c]	−46[d]	31
Head lateral flex displacement[c]	328	146
Head rotation displacement[c]	−58[d]	−3[d]
Head flex/ext acceleration[c]	7	52
Head lateral flex acceleration[c]	20	50
Head rotation acceleration[c]	7	50
Paced chair rise		
COG-COG maximum moment arm[e]	14	9

[a] AP=anterior-posterior; ML=medial-lateral; COG=center of gravity; COP=center of pressure, flex=flexion; ext=extension.

[b] Improvement corresponds to a decrease in the values for all kinematic indicators of stability except velocity and COG-COP maximum moment arm; for these items, improvement reflects an increase in these values.

[c] Measurements are relative to the room.

[d] These values represent a decline in kinematic indicators of stability.

[e] COG-COP maximum movement arm is the difference between the body's COP and COG.

suggests that central adaptation to her right-sided vestibular damage occurred during the course of treatment. At least two possibilities exist to explain this finding: (1) that spontaneous recovery, perhaps delayed in this patient, occurred and could have occurred regardless of her participation in treatment and (2) that the vestibular adaptation program was effective in promoting compensation in this patient with an incomplete vestibular deficit.[7] In contrast, the patient with BVH experienced no change in baseline vestibular function (as tested by SVAR) during the course of the 16-week treatment period. This patient had some remaining vestibular function as evidenced by SVAR testing at higher frequencies of rotation (0.2, 0.5, and 1.0 Hz). For this reason, a treatment program that focused on both the adaptative capability of the central nervous system and the substitution of alternative sensory information for postural control and gait was used. This patient demonstrated the ability to progress from less difficult (phase 1) to more difficult (phase 3) exercises during the course of treatment and also demonstrated improvements in performance—both factors that support the use of this treatment approach as a logical one.

If the treatment program for the patient with UVD were related to the improvements that were made, why might they have occurred? One possibility is that the patient was able to "train" her central nervous system, through the repetition of the various activities performed, to reinterpret the available vestibular information so that it more accurately represented what was truly occurring (ie, the interpretation of the vestibular input was more in agreement with that of the somatosensory and visual inputs in situations in which sensory conflict was absent).[7,10] Another possibility is that the patient's increased range of cervical mobility, combined with the experience of performing activities and movements that she had been avoiding since her initial onset, allowed her central nervous system to "realize" that she indeed had some postural control that was present and available for use on a daily basis.[10] A third possibility is that the patient, through the repetition of the various activities performed, was trained to more efficiently use any available sensory input (visual, somatosensory, or vestibular) for postural control and to choose among the various sensory information available as a situation required.[7] Finally, a combination of these factors may be operative.

If the improvements demonstrated by the patient with BVH were related to the treatment intervention, why might these have occurred? Clearly an improvement (or recovery) of vestibular function did not occur. One possibility is that the patient was trained to better use somatosensory and visual inputs for postural control in situations in which this sensory information was available (eg, the ADL tasks).[7] Another possibility is that the patient

13. Summary. In the summary, the authors succinctly summarize the report. They also suggest topics for research with a larger number of participants. A thoughtful discussion of specific variables to be tested, based on their experiences with the two patients, would have been more useful.

Summary

After participation in individually designed programs of vestibular physical therapy, two patients with distinctly different vestibular pathology demonstrated improvements in postural stability, as noted by self-report, posturography testing, and three-dimensional movement analysis of ADL tests. One patient demonstrated changes in baseline vestibular function during the course of treatment, whereas the other patient showed no change, suggesting the possibility that different explanations need to be considered to understand why these changes might have occurred. Improvements in performance noted cannot be attributed to practice of the tasks, as the three-dimensional movement analysis of the ADL tasks included activities not performed as part of the treatment program. There were similarities in the two patients' responses to treatment, even though the treatment programs differed. Further research is necessary with a similar, but larger, patient population to continue to investigate the effectiveness of this treatment approach for patients with peripheral vestibular dysfunction.

References

1 Igarashi M. Vestibular compensation: an overview. *Acta Otolaryngol Suppl (Stockh)*. 1984;406:78–82.

2 Baloh RW. *Dizziness, Hearing Loss and Tinnitus: The Essentials of Neuro-otology*. Philadelphia, Pa: FA Davis Co; 1984:182–185.

3 Herdman SJ. Exercise strategies in vestibular disorders. *Ear Nose Throat J*. 1989;68:961–964.

4 Tangemann PT, Wheeler J. Inner ear concussive syndrome: vestibular implications and physical therapy treatment. *Topics in Acute Rehabilitation*. 1986;1:72–83.

5 Parker SW. Modern approaches to dizziness and vertigo. *Drug Therapy*. 1980;10:109–120.

6 Fisch U. Surgical treatment of vertigo. *J Laryngol Otol*. 1976;90:75–82.

7 Herdman SJ. Assessment and treatment of balance disorders in the vestibular deficient patient. In: Duncan P, ed. *Balance: Proceedings of the APTA Forum*. Alexandria, Va: American Physical Therapy Association; 1980:87–94.

8 Shumway-Cook A, Horak FB. Vestibular rehabilitation: an exercise approach to managing symptoms of vestibular dysfunction. *Sem Hear*. 1984;10:194–204.

9 Smith-Wheelock M, Shepard NT, Telian SA. Physical therapy program for vestibular rehabilitation. *Am J Otol*. 1991;12:218–225.

10 Shumway-Cook A, Horak FB. Rehabilitation strategies for patients with vestibular deficits. *Neurol Clin*. 1990;8:441–457.

11 Cawthorne T. Vestibular injuries. *Proc Roy Soc Med*. 1946;39:270–273.

12 Gauthier GM, Robinson DA. Adaption of the human vestibular ocular reflex to magnifying lenses. *Brain Res*. 1975;92:331–335.

13 Shepard NT, Telian SA, Smith-Wheelock M. Habituation and balance retraining: a retrospective review. In: Arenberg I, Smith D, eds. Diagnostic neurology. *Neurol Clin*. 1990;8:459–475.

14 Horak FB, Jones-Rycewicz C, Black FO, Shumway-Cook A. Effects of vestibular rehabilitation on dizziness and imbalance. *Otolaryngol Head Neck Surg*. 1992;106:175–180.

15 Black FO, Nashner LM. Postural control in four classes of vestibular abnormalities. In: Igarashi M, Black FO, eds. *Vestibular and Visual Control on Posture and Locomotor Equilibrium*. Basel, Switzerland: S Karger AG, Scientific Publishers; 1985:271–281.

16 Parker SW, Krebs DE, Gill KM, Riley PO. Varying sway-referencing gain to quantify measurement of standing balance in patients with bilateral vestibular hypofunction. In: Woolacott M, Horak FB, eds. *Posture and Gait: Control Mechanisms*. Eugene, Ore: University of Oregon Books; 1992;1:315–318.

17 Krebs DE, Lockert J. Vestibulopathy and gait. In: Spivack BS, ed. *Neurologic Diseases and Therapy: Mobility and Gait*. New York, NY: Marcel Dekker Inc. In press.

18 Riley PO, Hodge WA, Mann RW. Modelling the biomechanics of posture and balance. *J Biomech*. 1990;23:503–505.

19 Krebs DE, Wong DK, Jevsevar DS, et al. Trunk kinematics during locomotor activities. *Phys Ther*. 1992;72:505–514.

20 Winter DA. *Biomechanics and Motor Control of Human Movement*. 2nd ed. New York, NY: John Wiley & Sons Inc; 1990.

21 Baloh RW, Honrubia V, Yee K. Changes in the human vestibular-ocular reflex after loss of peripheral sensitivity. *Ann Neurol*. 1984;16:222–228.

22 Hirsch BE. Computed sinusoidal harmonic acceleration. *Ear Hear*. 1986;7:198–203.

23 Jacobson GP, Newman CW. The development of the dizziness handicap inventory. *Arch Otolaryngol Head Neck Surg*. 1990;116:424–427.

24 Honrubia V, Marco J, Andrews J, et al. Vestibular-ocular reflexes in peripheral labyrinthine lesions, III: bilateral dysfunction. *Am J Otolaryngol*. 1985;6:342–352.

25 Hamid MA, Hughes GB, Kinney SE. Criteria for diagnosing bilateral vestibular dysfunction. In: Graham MD, Kemink JL, eds. *The Vestibular System: Neurophysiologic and Clinical Research*. New York, NY: Raven Press Inc; 1987:115–118.

26 Herdman SJ. Patients with vestibular disorders: physical therapy assessment and treatment. In: *Post-graduate Advances in Physical Therapy*. Alexandria, Va: American Physical Therapy Association; 1987.

Appendix 6

Review of a "Submitted" Case Report

To point out problems that are common to many of the case reports that are submitted for review by *Physical Therapy*, we've modified a case report that the Journal actually published (Brach JS, VanSwearingen JM. Physical therapy for facial paralysis: a tailored treatment approach. *Phys Ther*. 1999;79:379-404). We've altered this case report with the permission of the authors; the problems you'll see are ones that we—not the authors—created.

Review the manuscript, and try to find the problems. (We've added line numbering to make it easier for you to discuss the article with your colleagues.) Then read the sample review.

Did you catch the same problems that our hypothetical reviewer did? Refer to the real case report to see how the authors avoided them.

1   **Bell's Palsy Rehabilitation: A Case Study**

2

3   **Background and Purpose.** Bell's palsy is an acute facial paralysis. Although recovery from Bell's

4   palsy is expected without intervention, recovery is often incomplete. This case study describes a

5   classification system used to guide treatment, which improved the recovery of an individual with facial

6   paralysis. **Case Description.** The patient was a 71-year-old woman with complete left facial paralysis

7   secondary to Bell's palsy. Signs and symptoms were assessed using a standardized measure of facial

8   impairment and questions regarding functional limitations. A treatment-based category was assigned

9   based on signs and symptoms. **Outcomes.** Physical therapy resulted in improved facial impairments and

10   no reported functional limitations. **Discussion.** Recovery from Bell's palsy can be a complicated and

11   lengthy process. The use of a classification system helps to simplify the rehabilitation process.

12   **Key Words:** *Bell's palsy, Classification system, Facial neuromuscular re-education, Facial*

13   *paralysis.*

1   Bell's palsy is an acute facial paralysis. Bell's palsy most commonly occurs between the

2   ages of 15 and 60 years, with 15- to 44-year-olds experiencing the highest incidence.[1] In 1982,

3   Peitersen[1] outlined the natural history of Bell's palsy after studying 1,011 patients for 1 year

4   following their development of facial paralysis. Thirty-one percent of the patients had

5   incomplete paralysis, and 69% of the patients had complete paralysis of the facial muscles.

6   Normal facial function returned in 71% of the patients.[1] Peitersen[1] reported that age has a strong

7   influence on the recovery process. Ninety percent of the patients aged 0 to 14 years recovered

8   completely, whereas only 37% of the patients over 60 years of age recovered completely. It was

9   concluded that the sooner some facial function returned, the more favorable the overall outcome.

10   Individuals with Bell's palsy seldom receive physical therapy. Typically, the patients are

11   told to do nothing and that facial movement will return without intervention.[2-4] Patients referred

12   to physical therapy are often treated with electrical stimulation of the facial muscles and facial

13   movement exercises to be completed with maximal effort. The outcomes of such interventions

14   were less than optimal, with the patients often developing mass action or synkinesis.[5] Several

15   studies indicate that the use of electrical stimulation is disruptive to reinnervation[6-8] and thus may

16   be contraindicated for individuals with facial nerve disorders.[5]

17   Facial neuromuscular re-education is a conservative approach to facial rehabilitation.

18   Demonstrated outcomes of facial neuromuscular re-education include improvements in

19   impairments associated with facial paralysis.[9-12] Subgroups of patients with facial nerve disorder

20   have characteristic signs and symptoms that can be recognized prior to treatment. Based on these

21   signs and symptoms, clinicians can identify the impairment that respond to a certain intervention.

22   Therefore, we developed a classification scheme based on the intervention tailored to the signs

23   and symptoms that could also be used to guide treatment [13] After the treatment-based category is

2

1   identified, a physical therapy program consisting of neuromuscular re-education matched to the

2   assigned category is then initiated.

3   Surface electromyography (sEMG) biofeedback or a mirror may be used as an adjunct to the

4   retraining exercises in each of the treatment-based categories. The sEMG biofeedback is not the

5   treatment; exercises are the treatment. The facial muscles have few, if any, muscle

6   spindles.[12,14,15] Thus, little information about muscle length and action is available to the

7   individual. Learning facial movements is difficult without the feedback. We have found that the

8   use of sEMG or a hand mirror is a means of providing a visual or auditory representation of

9   facial muscle activity (sEMG) or movement (mirror). Patients are also instructed in a home facial

10   movement exercise program, which is based on the treatment-based category and the patients'

11   performance during the rehabilitation session. The purpose of this case study is to describe how

12   the facial rehabilitation process using facial neuromuscular re-education and a treatment-based

13   classification system resulted in improved facial functioning of an individual with Bell's palsy.

14

15   **Case Description**

16   The patient ("MC") was a 71-year-old woman who was diagnosed with Bell's palsy of

17   the left facial nerve and complete left facial paralysis. At the time of the initial evaluation, the

18   patient had no other active medical problems. The patient reported that her facial paralysis came

19   on suddenly and was accompanied by pain in her left ear and a funny feeling in her tongue. The

20   paralysis was associated with no pain or sensory deficits in the left side of the face. The patient

21   reported no hearing loss, but she reported hearing swishing sounds in her left ear. She had a

22   magnetic resonance imaging scan of her head, and no abnormalities were found. Electro-

23   diagnostic testing was not performed. One week after the onset of her symptoms, she started a 7-

24   day tapered dosage of steroid therapy.

3

1   The physical therapy evaluation consisted of grading resting posture, voluntary

2   movement, and the presence of synkinesis or abnormal movement, using the Facial Grading

3   System (FGS) developed by Ross and colleagues.[16] The FGS is an observer-based rating scale

4   that is responsive to change.[16] Ross et al indicated that the changes in scores on the resting

5   symmetry component of the scale occur more slowly with rehabilitation than scores on the

6   movement or synkinesis components of the scale. The scores of the FGS range from 0 (complete

7   paralysis) to 100 (normal facial function). The 3 sections to the FGS--resting posture (FGS rest),

8   voluntary movement (FGS movement), and synkinesis (FGS synkinesis)--are scored

9   individually, and the scores are combined for a total or composite score. The FGS rest section

10   consists of rating 3 facial areas for symmetry: (1) palpebral fissure (normal [0], narrow [1], wide

11   [1], or eyelid surgery [1]), (2) nasolabial fold (normal [0], absent [2], less pronounced [1], or

12   more pronounced [1]), and (3) corner of the mouth (normal [0], drooped [1], or pulled up and out

13   [1]).

14   The FGS rest section scores range from 0 to 4 and are weighted by a multiplier of 5 for a

15   total FGS rest score of 0 to 20. The symmetry of 5 voluntary facial movements (brow raise, eye

16   closure, snarl, smile, and pucker) are rated on a 5-point scale to determine the FGS movement

17   score. The FGS movement scores range from 5 to 25 and are weighted by a multiplier of 4 for a

18   total FGS movement score of 20 to 100. The degree of synkinesis associated with each of the

19   voluntary movements is graded on a 4-point scale from 0 (no synkinesis, or no abnormal or pass

20   movement patterns) to 3 (severe synkinesis, or disfiguring abnormal movement or gross mass

21   movement of several muscles). The FGS synkinesis scores range from 0 to 15. For both the FGS

22   rest and FGS synkinesis sections, a higher score relates to greater impairments. For the FGS

23   movement section, a lower score relates to greater impairment. The FGS score is calculated as

24   follows: FGS=FGS movement-FGS rest-FGS synkinesis. Ross et al[16] demonstrated that the FGS

4

1. is sensitive to change by comparing prerehabilitation and postrehabilitation scores for 19 patients

2. with facial nerve disorders.

3.   We used the FGS to monitor progress and to describe the patient at different stages of

4. recovery. The FGS scores were not used to determine the treatment-based category.

5.   The patient's functional limitations were determined through an interview process

6. consisting of a set of questions asked at each subsequent visit. The patient was asked questions

7. regarding her eye and mouth function and how this function may have interfered with her daily

8. activities.

9.   During the initial evaluation, the patient had severe asymmetry in resting facial posture.

10. Voluntary movement, as compared with movement of the uninvolved side, was trace to minimal.

11. She initiated slight movement with severe asymmetry throughout all regions of the face. As is

12. typical in this stage of recovery when movement is minimal, the patient had no signs of

13. synkinesis or abnormal movement patterns.

14.   MC was retired and lived alone. She reported little difficulty in eating, drinking,

15. speaking, and closing her eye; however, she relied on compensatory techniques such as drinking

16. from the uninvolved side of her mouth, lifting her cheek with her hand while speaking, and

17. manually closing her eye.

18.

19. **Intervention**

20. *Overview of Intervention*

21.   The patient was treated with facial neuromuscular retraining (NMR) techniques, using a

22. handheld mirror or sEMG biofeedback.[5,11-13] Treatment planning was based on the evaluation

23. findings and on treatment-based categories. Treatment sessions were one on one with a physical

24. therapist for approximately 1 hour. A typical physical therapy session consisted of a brief re-

5

1   evaluation, training with sEMG or a mirror, and instruction in an exercise program to be

2   completed at home.

3   Surface EMG biofeedback was used initially to measure muscle activity associated with

4   voluntary facial movements. As she was able to move more, she used the surface EMG

5   biofeedback less and a mirror more.

6

7   *Initiation*

8   Based on the initial signs and symptoms (severe resting asymmetry, minimal voluntary

9   movement, absent synkinesis, and impaired function), MC was considered to be in an initiation

10   treatment category. Exercises typical for the initiation category include active assisted range of

11   motion exercises. Often, patients find that it is easier to hold a position with a muscle than it is to

12   move to the desired position. MC used these techniques, as part of her home exercise program,

13   for the following facial expressions: smile, pucker, brow raise, and frown.

14   Because MC could not voluntarily close her eye and had signs and symptoms of corneal

15   irritation typical of patients in the initiation category, exercises focused on closing the eye.

16   Squinting or raising the lower eyelid was also included in the home facial exercise program. An

17   exercise that appears to allow the patient control over Bell's reflex[18] (eye rolling backward) is

18   helpful to achieve a more complete eye closure. The patient is instructed to focus both eyes on an

19   object positioned 30.5 cm (12 in) down and in front of the patient and then to attempt to close

20   both eyes. The eyes are to remain focused on this point until they are closed. Focusing the eyes

21   downward helps to initiate the lowering of the upper eyelid. Maintaining the focused position

22   until the eyes are closed prevents Bell's reflex, which can trick the patient into thinking that the

23   eye is closed.

24

1 *Facilitation*

2   A re-evaluation done 6 weeks and 3 physical therapy sessions later revealed that the

3 patient's resting posture was unchanged. Her face was less drooped but still not symmetrical.

4 Voluntary movement had increased to minimal to moderate movement. She initiated movement

5 with mid-excursion and moderate asymmetry for all facial movements, and there was no

6 evidence of synkinesis. MC reported less difficulty with eating and drinking than at the initiation

7 of treatment, but she had continued difficulty protecting the cornea of her eye. She was able to

8 close her eye completely, but only with conscious effort.

9   At this point in her recovery, the patient was considered to be in the facilitation category

10 of treatment. The patient was instructed in active and resisted facial movement exercises. She

11 was instructed to do symmetrical active facial movements without allowing the voluntary

12 movement of the uninvolved side of the face to distort the movement of the involved side of the

13 face. Maintaining symmetry is an important part of facial movement exercises. When the

14 uninvolved facial muscles overpower the involved facial muscles, the facial posture tends to shift

15 to the uninvolved side.

16   When some active movements are difficult to perform, such as lowering the bottom lip,

17 functional activities, such as saying specific sounds, are used for exercise. The activity of

18 lowering the bottom lip is an important component of saying words that begin with the letter "F."

19 MC reported practicing a word list to be easier than doing lip movement exercises, presumably

20 because of her greater familiarity with the word task than with isolated oral movements.

21   Resistive facial exercises may be appropriate if the patient has no signs of synkinesis.

22 Care must be taken not to overstrengthen the uninvolved facial muscles, which would cause an

23 even greater imbalance.

24

7

Movement Control

Seven months after the initiation of therapy and 11 physical therapy sessions, MC's resting posture had changed from a drooping brow, lower eyelid, cheek, and mouth corner to a raised lower eyelid and a retracted cheek and mouth corner. Voluntary movement had improved throughout the left side of the patient's face and was almost symmetrical with that of the uninvolved side. At this point, MC had started to develop mild abnormal movement patterns or synkinesis with brow raise and snarl motions. When she would raise her eyebrows or snarl, her left eye would close slightly.

Physical therapy had led to improvements in the patient's facial functioning. She had no problems with eating or performing oral hygiene (brushing her teeth). She reported only slight difficulty drinking from a glass without compensation techniques and only occasional problems with eye closure and protection.

The patient was now considered to be in the movement control category of treatment, with the facilitation category a secondary classification. Exercises focused on controlling the abnormal or synkinetic movement, such as raising the brow while keeping the eye open and controlling the ocular synkinesis. Movement control facial exercises emphasize moving only as much as the patient can without triggering the abnormal facial movement. The range of the movement is increased as long as the abnormal movement is controlled. The patient is told to concentrate on the quality of the exercise and not the quantity of the exercises completed. It is better for a patient to do 5 repetitions of an exercise correctly than it is to do 20 repetitions incorrectly.

Because facial muscle tightness often accompanies synkinesis, it is important to teach the patient facial muscle stretching exercises. Strengthening exercises for specific movements were continued as long as they did not cause synkinesis.

8

The patient's last physical therapy visit was 13 months after the initiation of therapy. She continued to demonstrate asymmetry in resting posture, which consisted of a narrow eye and a tight cheek. Voluntary movement had improved slightly to almost complete to complete movement between the sides, and the abnormal movement or synkinesis had increased slightly to minimal with all movements. The biggest change appeared to be in function. The patient reported no difficulties with eating, drinking, speaking, or protecting the cornea of her eye.

Based on these signs and symptoms, we still considered the patient to be in the movement control treatment category, with relaxation the secondary treatment category. Because minimal changes were noticed in voluntary movement in the previous 7 months, strengthening was no longer, in our opinion, a reasonable goal. We instructed the patient in a final program to help maintain her facial function and to prevent any inappropriate muscle activity or synkinesis. The program consisted of isolated facial movements, stretching, facial massage, and relaxation exercises[19] typical for patients in the movement control and relaxation treatment categories. Jacobsen's relaxation exercises[19] and the same technique of progressively contracting and relaxing of muscles was applied to specific facial muscles.

Outcomes

Service Delivery

The patient was treated over a 13-month period and seen for only 14 physical therapy sessions. Initially, the treatment sessions were more frequent (2-4 times per month) because of the need for instruction and for the patient to become familiar with the exercise process. As the patient became more aware of her facial movements, she was treated less frequently (once every 3 months).

9

1   **Impairment and Functional Limitation**

2   The patient demonstrated improvements as facial impairments and functional limitations

3   became less severe. In our opinion, moderate improvements were made in symmetry of the face

4   at rest, even though these improvements were not evident in the FGS rest scores. The FGS

5   grades resting posture as being either symmetrical or asymmetrical and does not account for

6   levels of severity. The most noticeable changes were the improvement of her voluntary

7   movement (FGS movement), which occurred in the first 7 months of treatment, and the

8   development of synkinesis (FGS synkinesis) in the seventh month.

9   The patient's functional activities improved so that after 13 months she had no difficulty

10   eating, drinking, speaking, or protecting the cornea of her eye. She no longer had to rely on

11   compensatory techniques to complete her activities of daily living.

12

13   **Discussion**

14   Individuals with Bell's palsy are seldom referred for physical therapy at the onset of the

15   disorder. Often, they are told to wait and that this condition will get better on its own. Complete

16   recovery does not always occur, especially in high-risk populations such as people who are

17   elderly or who have delayed recovery.[1]

18   Physical therapists rarely continue to treat patients for 13 months. We believed, however,

19   that this treatment duration was necessary to achieve the outcomes for this patient. For the first 7

20   months, the patient had facial weakness and was treated with strengthening exercises. At the 7-

21   month visit, she had facial muscle overactivity and synkinesis. At this point, the treatment plan

22   was adjusted to fit the changes in her facial impairments. If the physical therapy had been

23   terminated prior to this 7-month mark, her problems of facial muscle tightness and synkinesis

24   would not have been addressed. Instructing the patient in a maintenance program at the last

10

physical therapy session may help to prevent an increase in facial muscle tightness and synkinesis over time. Although 13 months may seem like a long time to treat a patient, the total number of physical therapy visits was only 14 visits.

Physical therapy for patients with facial paralysis traditionally has consisted of generic facial exercises or electrical stimulation.[4] Facial neuromuscular re-education techniques (ie, the use of facial exercises to address a patient's impairments and functional limitations) are different from the traditional intervention for facial paralysis. In our approach, the exercise program changes over time as the patient's impairments change with recovery. The facial neuromuscular re-education exercise program emphasizes accuracy of facial movement patterns and isolated muscle control, and it excludes exercises that promote mass contraction of muscles related to more than one facial expression. In our approach, the number of exercise repetitions and the frequency of the exercise program depend on the treatment-based categories, which are based on the patient's impairments.

References

1 Peitersen E. Natural history of Bell's palsy. In: Graham MD, House WF, eds. *Disorders of the Facial Nerve.* New York, NY: Raven Press; 1982:307-312.

2 Ohye RG, Altenberger EA. Bell's palsy. *Am Fam Physician.* 1989;40:159-166.

3 Bateman DE. Facial palsy. *Br J Hosp Med.* 1992;47:430-431.

4 Waxman B. Electrotherapy for treatment of facial nerve paralysis (Bell's palsy). In: *Anonymous Health Technology Assessment Reports.* 3rd ed. Rockville, Md: National Center for Health Services Research; 1984:27.

5 Diels JH. New concepts in nonsurgical facial nerve rehabilitation. *Advances in Otolaryngology-Head and Neck Surgery.* 1995;9:289-315.

6 Cohan CS, Kater SB. Suppression of neurite elongation and growth cone motility by electrical activity. *Science.* 1986;232:1638-1640.

7 Brown MC, Holland RL. A central role for denervated tissues in causing nerve sprouting. *Nature.* 1979;282:724-726.

8 Girlanda P, Dattola R, Vita G, et al. Effect of electrotherapy on denervated muscles in rabbits: an electrophysiological and morphological study. *Exp Neurol.* 1982;77:483-491.

9 Ross B, Nedzelski JM, McLean JA. Efficacy of feedback training in long-standing facial nerve paresis. *Laryngoscope.* 1991;101:744-750.

10 Brudny J, Hammerschlag PE, Cohen NL, Ransehoff J. Electromyographic rehabilitation of facial function and introduction of a facial paralysis grading scale for hypoglossal-facial nerve anastomosis. *Laryngoscope.* 1988;98:405-410.

11 Brach JS, VanSwearingen JM, Lennert J, Johnson PC. Facial neuromuscular retraining for oral synkinesis. *Plast Reconstr Surg.* 1997;99:1922-1931.

12 Brudny J. Biofeedback in facial paralysis: electromyographic rehabilitation. In: Rubin L, eds. *The Paralyzed Face.* St Louis, Mo: Mosby-Year Book; 1991:247-264.

13 VanSwearingen JM, Brach JS. Validation of a treatment-based classification system for individuals with facial neuromotor disorders. *Phys Ther.* 1998;78:678-689.

14 Baumel JJ. Trigeminal-facial nerve communications: their function in facial muscle innervation and reinnervation. *Arch Otolaryngol.* 1974;99:34-44.

15 Burgess PR, Wei JY, Clark FJ, Simon J. Signaling of kinesthetic information by peripheral sensory receptors. *Annu Rev Neurosci.* 1982;5:171-187.

16 Ross BG, Fradet G, Nedzelski JM. Development of a sensitive clinical facial grading system. *Otolaryngol Head Neck Surg.* 1996;114:380-386.

1 **17** Brach JS, VanSwearingen JM, Delitto A, Johnson PC. Impairment and disability in patients

2 with facial neuromuscular dysfunction. *Otolaryngol Head Neck Surg.* 1997;117:315-321.

3 **18** Jelks GW, Smith B, Bosniak S. The evaluation and management of the eye in facial palsy.

4 *Clin Plast Surg.* 1979;6:397-419.

5 **19** Jacobson E. *Progressive Relaxation.* 2nd ed. Chicago, Ill: University of Chicago Press; 1938.

13

R-1
Reviewer's Comments
Physical Therapy Manuscript Review

Author Copy

MS # ███████
Reviewer # 1
Date: ████████
Masked? Yes
Title: *Bell's Palsy Rehabilitation: A Case Study*

Category CR

The reviewer has provided general comments in the spaces below. Specific comments are provided on the attached sheets. On these attached sheets, comments are keyed to the corresponding page and paragraph number in the manuscript.

1. Credibility of material in the manuscript (eg, comprehensive and critical discussion of recent literature; scholarly basis for arguments and suppositions; appropriate design and analysis [issues relating to internal and external validity]; if appropriate, discussion of clinical implications):

The literature review is generally appropriate and credible, but has a few holes that need to be filled. For example, the authors did not cover the cause of Bell palsy and the usual recovery time, which are important for putting this patient's experience in context. They also made several statements that need literature support or, if literature support is not available, they need to acknowledge that the statements are based on their own experience and/or opinion. Some terms also need to be defined, such as "synkinesis" and "facial neuromuscular re-education." The literature review seems somewhat dated (8 of the 19 references were published in the 1990s), but it may be the most recent or the most credible literature available. Suggest that the authors check to see if it is.

The case description section also omitted important information. The examination and intervention, for example, need to be described so clearly that another clinician could replicate them with a similar patient. The reliability and validity of the Facial Grading System (FGS) and the reliability of the measurements need to be addressed. The treatment categories, the timeline of the intervention, the FGS data, and the patient's goals also need to be reported.

The discussion section is generally appropriate and credible. Suggestions for future research need to be added. Please see my specific comments for details of these and other recommendations to strengthen the credibility of the material in the manuscript.

2. Organization and writing (eg, coherence, tone for audience, correct and contemporary use of terms, sections properly organized, material in appropriate sections):

The manuscript is well organized and written. As mentioned above and in my specific comments, a few terms need to be defined.

3. Appropriateness of the manuscript for the Journal (eg, relevance of content, significance of contribution to the field, relationship of manuscript to existing knowledge):

The author's approach is an interesting one that could make a nice contribution to the case report literature on management of patients with Bell palsy. As indicated above and in the specific comments, the manuscript needs revision to strengthen its contribution.

4. Summary (general observations about the manuscript):

This manuscript reports an approach to intervention with patients with Bell palsy that would be of interest to readers of the Journal. The introduction, case description, and discussion sections, in particular, need additional information to strengthen the contribution that the manuscript can make. Please see my specific comments for details.

MS # ▮▮▮▮▮▮▮
Reviewer # 1

Page Number	Paragraph Number	Specific Comments
Title		Here and throughout the manuscript, please change "Bell'" to "Bell." The *American Medical Association Manual of Style* (9th ed) generally recommends the nonpossessive form for eponymous terms.
		Please use the term "case report," not case "study." As the Journal uses the term, a case study is a type of research.
		"Rehabilitation" is broad. Can you modify the title to make it describe your approach more specifically?
Abstract	Background and Purpose	Case reports cannot establish cause and effect relationships between interventions and outcomes, so avoid suggesting that physical therapy caused the outcomes, as in "improved the outcome."
	Case Description	What "standardized measure of facial impairment" did you use?
		Briefly explain what the intervention was and explain how much intervention the patient received and over what period of time.
	Outcomes	Again, in a case report it's not appropriate to say that physical therapy resulted improved function.
	Discussion	A classification system <u>might</u> help simplify the rehabilitation process. We need research to determine if it does.
2	1	What causes Bell palsy?
		How long does recovery usually take?
		In the last sentence of this paragraph, who concluded? Peitersen? Use of passive voice construction ("it was concluded") hides who did.

3

2	2	Please provide a reference for the statement that individuals with Bell palsy seldom receive physical therapy.
		Patients are referred for physical therapy, not "to" physical therapy. Physical therapy is a service, not a place.
		The statement that patients are treated with electrical stimulation and exercises to be completed with maximal effort needs to be supported with a reference.
		Please define "mass action or synkinesis."
		I believe the studies cited (6-8) that found electrical simulation is disruptive to reinnervation used animal models -- if so, this needs to be acknowledged.
2	3	Please explain what you mean by "facial neuromuscular re-education."
		Either provide a reference to support your statement about sub-groups having certain signs and symptoms or explain that the classification system is based on your own experience, if it is.
		Please clearly explain your classification scheme and treatment-based categories.
3	2	Again, this is a case report, which can only describe practice. It cannot determine if an intervention causes an outcome.
3	3	How long after the onset of Bell palsy was the "initial physical therapy evaluation"?
		Please use terminology consistent with the Guide to Physical Therapist Practice, such as "examination" instead of "evaluation" and "intervention" instead of "treatment," when appropriate.
5	1	Please provide information about the reliability and validity of the Facial Grading System (FGS).
		What were the patient's goals?
5	2	How did you measure the patient's facial posture and movements? What was the reliability of your measurements?
5	4	How many treatment sessions did the patient have, over what period of time, and with what frequency?

4

6	1	What was the purpose of measuring muscle activity associated with voluntary facial movements? Please give an example of how the patient used the biofeedback. Where did you place the electrodes?
6	2	What is the "initiation" treatment category?
		Please describe the active assisted range of motion clearly, so another clinician could replicate what you did.
		Please explain how many of each exercise the patient did, how many times a day she did them, and your rationale for this intensity. Can you provide any information to support whether she did the home program?
7	1	Please define the "facilitation" treatment category.
		How were the 3 physical therapy sessions distributed over the 6-week period?
		Please provide the FGS data (if this is what you used) to support your statements about the patient's facial functioning.
7	2	On what did you base your statement that the patient now was in the "facilitation category of treatment"? Please explain in such a way that other clinicians could replicate your decision-making process.
		Please explain why a facial posture shift to the uninvolved side is a problem.
7	4	Please explain how the patient did resistive exercises and give an example. Also explain how many of each exercise she did how many times a day and provide your rationale for this intensity
8	1	The "movement control" category needs to be defined.
		How did you measure the patient's facial functioning? Did you use the FGS? If so, what were the data?
8	2	Again, case reports cannot establish cause and effect relationships. Saying that physical therapy led to the improvements is inappropriate.

5

| 8 | 3 | On what did you base your decision that the patient was now in the "movement control" category, with the facilitation category secondary?

How many repetitions did you ask the patient to do? How many times a day? |
8	4	Please explain how the patient did the stretching exercises. Include repetitions for each one, times per day, and your rationale for both stretching and strengthening exercises.
9	1	Do you have FGS scores or other data to support these statements about the patient's facial functioning?
9	2	Please give an example of relaxation exercises and specify which exercises and how many of them she did and how often she did them.
9	3	Please provide details of the frequency of physical therapy sessions over the 13 months of intervention.
10	1	The changes in the patient's function would be easier for readers to grasp if you provided a table with FGS scores and function over time.
10	2	Please report the outcomes from the patient's point of view. Did she accomplish her goal(s)? Did she think she had improved?
10	3	A reference is needed for the statement that patients seldom are referred for physical therapy or, if it is based on your experience or opinion, simply say so.
10	4	How do the number of repetitions and frequency of exercise relate to the treatment-based categories?
11		Based on your experience with this patient, what suggestions do you have for future research? Please avoid simply recommending replication with a larger number of subjects.

6

MS # ▮▮▮▮▮▮   **Category** CR
Reviewer # 1
Date: ▮▮▮▮▮▮
Masked? Yes
Title: *Bell's Palsy Rehabilitation: A Case Study*

Recommendation of Reviewer (Circle one)

Accept   No changes needed from author(s). Staff will edit.

(**Revise**)   Minor to moderate changes needed from author(s) before manuscript can be accepted.

No Decision   Revisions are needed before a decision can be made. This category should be used only when a small number of specific questions bring into doubt the credibility of the paper. If there are major questions or a large number of questions, the paper should be rejected, with suggestions for revision supplied.

Reject (Check one)

_____ Suggest that author(s) revise manuscript and resubmit.

_____ Suggest that author(s) resubmit as a different type of paper.

Suggestion: _____

_____ Rewrite not encouraged.

Please summarize why you have made your recommendation. These comments are for the Editorial Board member and the Editor only; any comments for the author should be made on form R-1 or on the running narrative that accompanies form R-1.

Rationale: This manuscript has the potential to be a good case report. Its major problem is the lack of necessary information. Because so much information was omitted, I was tempted to recommend rejection with the suggestion for revision and resubmission. The missing information should not be difficult for the authors to provide, however. IF they make a good effort to address these concerns, they should be able to make the necessary modifications with one revision.

7